Diagnosis and Management of Heart Failure

Diagnosis and Management of Heart Failure

Editors

Inna P. Gladysheva
Ryan D. Sullivan

MDPI • Basel • Beijing • Wuhan • Barcelona • Belgrade • Manchester • Tokyo • Cluj • Tianjin

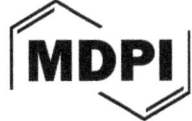

Editors
Inna P. Gladysheva
Medicine
University of Arizona
College of Medicine –Phoenix
Phoenix
United States

Ryan D. Sullivan
Medicine
University of Arizona
College of Medicine –Phoenix
Phoenix
United States

Editorial Office
MDPI
St. Alban-Anlage 66
4052 Basel, Switzerland

This is a reprint of articles from the Special Issue published online in the open access journal *Diagnostics* (ISSN 2075-4418) (available at: www.mdpi.com/journal/diagnostics/special_issues/Heart_Failure_Diagnosis).

For citation purposes, cite each article independently as indicated on the article page online and as indicated below:

LastName, A.A.; LastName, B.B.; LastName, C.C. Article Title. *Journal Name* **Year**, *Volume Number*, Page Range.

ISBN 978-3-0365-4154-9 (Hbk)
ISBN 978-3-0365-4153-2 (PDF)

© 2022 by the authors. Articles in this book are Open Access and distributed under the Creative Commons Attribution (CC BY) license, which allows users to download, copy and build upon published articles, as long as the author and publisher are properly credited, which ensures maximum dissemination and a wider impact of our publications.

The book as a whole is distributed by MDPI under the terms and conditions of the Creative Commons license CC BY-NC-ND.

Contents

Ryan D. Sullivan and Inna P. Gladysheva
Advances and Challenges in Diagnosis and Management of Heart Failure
Reprinted from: 2022, *12*, 1103, doi:10.3390/diagnostics12051103 1

Silvius-Alexandru Pescariu, Raluca Șoșdean, Cristina Tudoran, Adina Ionac, Gheorghe Nicusor Pop and Romulus Zorin Timar et al.
Echocardiographic Parameters as Predictors for the Efficiency of Resynchronization Therapy in Patients with Dilated Cardiomyopathy and HFrEF
Reprinted from: 2021, *12*, 35, doi:10.3390/diagnostics12010035 5

Marilena-Brîndușa Zamfirescu, Liviu Nicolae Ghilencea, Mihaela-Roxana Popescu, Gabriel Cristian Bejan, Ileana Maria Ghiordanescu and Andreea-Catarina Popescu et al.
A Practical Risk Score for Prediction of Early Readmission after a First Episode of Acute Heart Failure with Preserved Ejection Fraction
Reprinted from: 2021, *11*, 198, doi:10.3390/diagnostics11020198 15

Daniele Masarone, Michelle Kittleson, Rita Gravino, Fabio Valente, Andrea Petraio and Giuseppe Pacileo
The Role of Echocardiography in the Management of Heart Transplant Recipients
Reprinted from: 2021, *11*, 2338, doi:10.3390/diagnostics11122338 33

Raluca D. Ianoș, Călin Pop, Mihaela Iancu, Rodica Rahaian, Angela Cozma and Lucia M. Procopciuc
Diagnostic Performance of Serum Biomarkers Fibroblast Growth Factor 21, Galectin-3 and Copeptin for Heart Failure with Preserved Ejection Fraction in a Sample of Patients with Type 2 Diabetes Mellitus
Reprinted from: 2021, *11*, 1577, doi:10.3390/diagnostics11091577 45

Ioan Tilea, Andreea Varga and Razvan Constantin Serban
Past, Present, and Future of Blood Biomarkers for the Diagnosis of Acute Myocardial Infarction—Promises and Challenges
Reprinted from: 2021, *11*, 881, doi:10.3390/diagnostics11050881 59

Tamara Pecherina, Anton Kutikhin, Vasily Kashtalap, Victoria Karetnikova, Olga Gruzdeva and Oksana Hryachkova et al.
Serum and Echocardiographic Markers May Synergistically Predict Adverse Cardiac Remodeling after ST-Segment Elevation Myocardial Infarction in Patients with Preserved Ejection Fraction
Reprinted from: 2020, *10*, 301, doi:10.3390/diagnostics10050301 79

Valentin Oleynikov, Lyudmila Salyamova, Olga Kvasova and Nadezhda Burko
Prediction of Adverse Post-Infarction Left Ventricular Remodeling Using a Multivariate Regression Model
Reprinted from: 2022, *12*, 770, doi:10.3390/diagnostics12030770 93

Yau-Huei Lai, Cheng-Huang Su, Ta-Chuan Hung, Chun-Ho Yun, Cheng-Ting Tsai and Hung-I Yeh et al.
Association of Non-Alcoholic Fatty Liver Disease and Hepatic Fibrosis with Epicardial Adipose Tissue Volume and Atrial Deformation Mechanics in a Large Asian Population Free from Clinical Heart Failure
Reprinted from: 2022, *12*, 916, doi:10.3390/diagnostics12040916 105

Anna Adamska-Wełnicka, Marcin Wełnicki, Artur Mamcarz and Ryszard Gellert
Chronic Kidney Disease and Heart Failure–Everyday Diagnostic Challenges
Reprinted from: 2021, *11*, 2164, doi:10.3390/diagnostics11112164 117

Shyh-Ming Chen, Lin-Yi Wang, Po-Jui Wu, Mei-Yun Liaw, Yung-Lung Chen and An-Ni Chen et al.
The Interrelationship between Ventilatory Inefficiency and Left Ventricular Ejection Fraction in Terms of Cardiovascular Outcomes in Heart Failure Outpatients
Reprinted from: 2020, *10*, 469, doi:10.3390/diagnostics10070469 131

Filippo Pirrotta, Benedetto Mazza, Luigi Gennari and Alberto Palazzuoli
Pulmonary Congestion Assessment in Heart Failure: Traditional and New Tools
Reprinted from: 2021, *11*, 1306, doi:10.3390/diagnostics11081306 143

Michelle Hernandez, Ryan D. Sullivan, Mariana E. McCune, Guy L. Reed and Inna P. Gladysheva
Sodium-Glucose Cotransporter-2 Inhibitors Improve Heart Failure with Reduced Ejection Fraction Outcomes by Reducing Edema and Congestion
Reprinted from: 2022, *12*, 989, doi:10.3390/diagnostics12040989 157

Valentin Elievich Oleynikov, Elena Vladimirovna Averyanova, Anastasia Aleksandrovna Oreshkina, Nadezhda Valerievna Burko, Yulia Andreevna Barmenkova and Alena Vladimirovna Golubeva et al.
A Multivariate Model to Predict Chronic Heart Failure after Acute ST-Segment Elevation Myocardial Infarction: Preliminary Study
Reprinted from: 2021, *11*, 1925, doi:10.3390/diagnostics11101925 175

Gregor Poglajen, Ajda Anžič-Drofenik, Gregor Zemljič, Sabina Frljak, Andraž Cerar and Renata Okrajšek et al.
Long-Term Effects of Angiotensin Receptor–Neprilysin Inhibitors on Myocardial Function in Chronic Heart Failure Patients with Reduced Ejection Fraction
Reprinted from: 2020, *10*, 522, doi:10.3390/diagnostics10080522 183

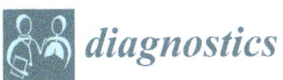

Editorial

Advances and Challenges in Diagnosis and Management of Heart Failure

Ryan D. Sullivan * and Inna P. Gladysheva *

Department of Medicine, University of Arizona College of Medicine—Phoenix, Phoenix, AZ 85004, USA
* Correspondence: ryansullivan@arizona.edu (R.D.S.); innagladysheva@arizona.edu (I.P.G.);
Tel.: +1-(602)-827-2850 (R.D.S.); +1-(602)-827-2919 (I.P.G.)

Citation: Sullivan, R.D.; Gladysheva, I.P. Advances and Challenges in Diagnosis and Management of Heart Failure. *Diagnostics* **2022**, *12*, 1103. https://doi.org/10.3390/diagnostics12051103

Received: 21 April 2022
Accepted: 24 April 2022
Published: 28 April 2022

Publisher's Note: MDPI stays neutral with regard to jurisdictional claims in published maps and institutional affiliations.

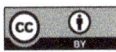

Copyright: © 2022 by the authors. Licensee MDPI, Basel, Switzerland. This article is an open access article distributed under the terms and conditions of the Creative Commons Attribution (CC BY) license (https://creativecommons.org/licenses/by/4.0/).

The prevalence of heart failure (HF) with reduced (r) and preserved (p) ejection fraction (EF) continues to rise globally despite current advances in diagnostics and improvements to medical management. Regardless of the underlying etiology, HF remains a progressive disease, which is largely irreversible and may ultimately require cardiac transplantation. This Special Issue focuses on the challenges and recent advances of diagnosis, treatment, and prevention of HF with or without associated comorbidities.

Existing clinical imaging modalities and methods continue to be optimized for HF. These advances allow for earlier initial diagnosis, improved prognostic timelines, and can even be used to provide personalized medical management. Echocardiography remains a clinical mainstay for point-of-care evaluation, identifying disease etiology, and longitudinal monitoring. From our issue, Pescariu, et al. utilized cardiac strain and left ventricular function to accurately predict resynchronization success in HFrEF patients [1]. Left ventricular end-diastolic diameter, mitral valve E/e' ratio, and left ventricular outflow tract velocity time integral were reported by Zamfirescu, et al. to predict HF readmission following initial acute HFpEF [2]. Masarone et al. reviewed how echocardiography is utilized to monitor graft function, pathology development and rejection following heart transplantation [3]. The ability to measure standardized views, while simultaneously having the versatility to explore new correlates has clearly earned cardiac ultrasound a top spot in HF patient evaluation and management.

Blood biomarkers are another well-established component for helping in the diagnosis of HF. While the natriuretic peptides (BNP/NT-proBNP and ANP/NT-proANP) are the most commonly used clinical biomarkers to confirm or exclude a HF diagnosis, other biomarkers are under investigation, Though there were no correlations with serum galectin-3 or copeptin, Ianos, et al. found fibroblast growth factor 21 (FGF21) to be a reliable biomarker for HFpEF with type-2 diabetes mellitus [4]. Considering acute myocardial infarction (AMI) as a risk for developing HF, Tilea et al. reviewed biomarkers in the pathophysiology that are altered earlier than myocyte necrosis needed to release cardiac troponins [5] which are commonly assessed during emergency workups. By combining modalities, echocardiography and blood biomarkers, clinicians can more confidently diagnose HF and likely stage the disease severity. Pecherina et al. found using both modalities (diastolic dysfunction + NT-proBNP, sST2, galectin-3, and MMP-3) can predict risk for adverse cardiac remodeling in patients with HFpEF following ST-segment elevation myocardial infarction (STEMI) [6]. Similarly in both HFrEF and HFpEF STEMI patients, Oleynikov et al. used acute left ventricular remodeling (ALVR vs. non-ALVR) status to predict and stratify outcome risks with statistical significance [7].

Even with proper imaging and great blood biomarkers, common comorbidities (diabetes mellitus, COPD, chronic kidney disease, etc.) can complicate accurate and timely diagnosis of HF. Lai et al. found that non-alcoholic fatty liver disease without HF is associated with left ventricular diastolic dysfunction and subclinical changes in left atrial contractility [8]. Adamska-Welnicka et al. reviewed the difficulty associated with proper

HF diagnosis when comorbidities of chronic kidney disease or pulmonary hypertension are present [9].

Part of the confusion from the comorbidities is the non-cardiac-systemic involvement; notably, the lungs. Ventilatory inefficiency, measured during cardiopulmonary exercise test, was used to stratify left ventricular ejection fraction in HFrEF outpatients for prognostic predictability of HF outcomes [10]. Chen et al. reiterated that ventilatory inefficiency (due to tachypnea) can in part be due to receptors responding to pulmonary congestion [10]. Early detection of pulmonary edema and congestion responsible for HF decompensation is lacking clinically, Pirrotta et al. reviewed traditional methods and chest radiography vs. lung ultrasonography (LUS) [11] as an alternative method to access decompensation. The standardization of LUS in HF evaluations would improve outcomes by diagnosing the initiation of lung fluid rather than relying on peripheral edema (advanced) or other HF symptoms to begin diuretic treatment. Edema, regardless of anatomical location, is synonymous with clinical symptoms and late stage HF. Thankfully a new drug class reviewed by Hernandez et al., sodium-glucose cotransporter-2 inhibitors (SGLT-2i), are helping to delay HFrEF progression, rehospitalization and improve quality of life by reducing HF associated edema [12].

HF medical management effectiveness can be longitudinally evaluated using all the above methods. This improvement in patient monitoring allows for a personized medicine approach–run the diagnostics and alter therapy according to the patient's own data. As an example, Oleynikov, et al. were able to generate patient risk stratification using a developed model (formula) to predict chronic HF progression within 48 weeks after STEMI [13]. Though not as effective in cardiomyopathy of ischemic origin, Poglajen et al. found that the addition of angiotensin receptor blocker–neprilysin inhibitor (ARNI) therapy improved left and right ventricular function beyond that of control patients on optimal medical treatment after one year [14].

We thank the authors, reviewers, Ms Lassie Shu and the rest of the editorial staff that contributed to this Special Issue. We hope that readers will appreciate the wide breadth of topics and clinical utility of the articles and reviews published within "Diagnosis and Management of Heart Failure".

Funding: Supported by research funds from the University of Arizona, College of Medicine-Phoenix.

Conflicts of Interest: The authors declare no conflict of interest.

References

1. Pescariu, S.-A.; Şoşdean, R.; Tudoran, C.; Ionac, A.; Pop, G.N.; Timar, R.Z.; Pescariu, S.; Tudoran, M. Echocardiographic Parameters as Predictors for the Efficiency of Resynchronization Therapy in Patients with Dilated Cardiomyopathy and HFrEF. *Diagnostics* **2021**, *12*, 35. [CrossRef] [PubMed]
2. Zamfirescu, M.-B.; Ghilencea, L.; Popescu, M.-R.; Bejan, G.; Ghiordanescu, I.; Popescu, A.-C.; Dorobanțu, S. A Practical Risk Score for Prediction of Early Readmission after a First Episode of Acute Heart Failure with Preserved Ejection Fraction. *Diagnostics* **2021**, *11*, 198. [CrossRef] [PubMed]
3. Masarone, D.; Kittleson, M.; Gravino, R.; Valente, F.; Petraio, A.; Pacileo, G. The Role of Echocardiography in the Management of Heart Transplant Recipients. *Diagnostics* **2021**, *11*, 2338. [CrossRef] [PubMed]
4. Ianoş, R.D.; Pop, C.; Iancu, M.; Rahaian, R.; Cozma, A.; Procopciuc, L.M. Diagnostic Performance of Serum Biomarkers Fibroblast Growth Factor 21, Galectin-3 and Copeptin for Heart Failure with Preserved Ejection Fraction in a Sample of Patients with Type 2 Diabetes Mellitus. *Diagnostics* **2021**, *11*, 1577. [CrossRef] [PubMed]
5. Tilea, I.; Varga, A.; Serban, R. Past, Present, and Future of Blood Biomarkers for the Diagnosis of Acute Myocardial Infarction—Promises and Challenges. *Diagnostics* **2021**, *11*, 881. [CrossRef] [PubMed]
6. Pecherina, T.; Kutikhin, A.; Kashtalap, V.; Karetnikova, V.; Gruzdeva, O.; Hryachkova, O.; Barbarash, O. Serum and Echocardiographic Markers May Synergistically Predict Adverse Cardiac Remodeling after ST-Segment Elevation Myocardial Infarction in Patients with Preserved Ejection Fraction. *Diagnostics* **2020**, *10*, 301. [CrossRef] [PubMed]
7. Oleynikov, V.; Salyamova, L.; Kvasova, O.; Burko, N. Prediction of Adverse Post-Infarction Left Ventricular Remodeling Using a Multivariate Regression Model. *Diagnostics* **2022**, *12*, 770. [CrossRef] [PubMed]
8. Lai, Y.-H.; Su, C.-H.; Hung, T.-C.; Yun, C.-H.; Tsai, C.-T.; Yeh, H.-I.; Hung, C.-L. Association of Non-Alcoholic Fatty Liver Disease and Hepatic Fibrosis with Epicardial Adipose Tissue Volume and Atrial Deformation Mechanics in a Large Asian Population Free from Clinical Heart Failure. *Diagnostics* **2022**, *12*, 916. [CrossRef] [PubMed]

9. Adamska-Wełnicka, A.; Wełnicki, M.; Mamcarz, A.; Gellert, R. Chronic Kidney Disease and Heart Failure–Everyday Diagnostic Challenges. *Diagnostics* **2021**, *11*, 2164. [CrossRef] [PubMed]
10. Chen, S.-M.; Wang, L.-Y.; Wu, P.-J.; Liaw, M.-Y.; Chen, Y.-L.; Chen, A.-N.; Tsai, T.-H.; Hang, C.-L.; Lin, M.-C. The Interrelationship between Ventilatory Inefficiency and Left Ventricular Ejection Fraction in Terms of Cardiovascular Outcomes in Heart Failure Outpatients. *Diagnostics* **2020**, *10*, 469. [CrossRef]
11. Pirrotta, F.; Mazza, B.; Gennari, L.; Palazzuoli, A. Pulmonary Congestion Assessment in Heart Failure: Traditional and New Tools. *Diagnostics* **2021**, *11*, 1306. [CrossRef] [PubMed]
12. Hernandez, M.; Sullivan, R.D.; McCune, M.E.; Reed, G.L.; Gladysheva, I.P. Sodium-Glucose Cotransporter-2 Inhibitors Improve Heart Failure with Reduced Ejection Fraction Outcomes by Reducing Edema and Congestion. *Diagnostics* **2022**, *12*, 989. [CrossRef] [PubMed]
13. Oleynikov, V.E.; Averyanova, E.V.; Oreshkina, A.A.; Burko, N.V.; Barmenkova, Y.A.; Golubeva, A.V.; Galimskaya, V.A. A Multivariate Model to Predict Chronic Heart Failure after Acute ST-Segment Elevation Myocardial Infarction: Preliminary Study. *Diagnostics* **2021**, *11*, 1925. [CrossRef] [PubMed]
14. Poglajen, G.; Anžič-Drofenik, A.; Zemljič, G.; Frljak, S.; Cerar, A.; Okrajšek, R.; Šebeštjen, M.; Vrtovec, B. Long-Term Effects of Angiotensin Receptor–Neprilysin Inhibitors on Myocardial Function in Chronic Heart Failure Patients with Reduced Ejection Fraction. *Diagnostics* **2020**, *10*, 522. [CrossRef]

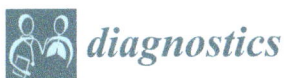

Article

Echocardiographic Parameters as Predictors for the Efficiency of Resynchronization Therapy in Patients with Dilated Cardiomyopathy and HFrEF

Silvius-Alexandru Pescariu [1,2,3,4], Raluca Șoșdean [1,2,3,*], Cristina Tudoran [5,6,7,*], Adina Ionac [1,2,3], Gheorghe Nicusor Pop [1], Romulus Zorin Timar [5,6,7], Sorin Pescariu [1,2,3] and Mariana Tudoran [5,6,7]

1. Department VI, Discipline of Cardiology, University of Medicine and Pharmacy "Victor Babes" Timisoara, E. Murgu Square, Nr. 2, 300041 Timisoara, Romania; pescariu.alexandru@umft.ro (S.-A.P.); ionac.adina@umft.ro (A.I.); pop.nicusor@umft.ro (G.N.P.); pescariu.sorin@umft.ro (S.P.)
2. Cardiology Clinic, Institute of Cardiovascular Medicine Timişoara, 13A, Gheorghe Adam Street, 300310 Timisoara, Romania
3. Research Center for Cardiovascular Diseases, Institute of Cardiovascular Diseases, 300310 Timisoara, Romania
4. Doctoral School, "Victor Babes" University of Medicine and Pharmacy Timisoara, E. Murgu Square, Nr. 2, 300041 Timisoara, Romania
5. Department VII, Internal Medicine II, Discipline of Cardiology, University of Medicine and Pharmacy "Victor Babes" Timisoara, E. Murgu Square, Nr. 2, 300041 Timisoara, Romania; timar.romulu@umft.ro (R.Z.T.); tudoran.mariana@umft.ro (M.T.)
6. Center of Molecular Research in Nephrology and Vascular Disease, Faculty of Medicine, University of Medicine and Pharmacy "Victor Babes" Timisoara, E. Murgu Square, Nr. 2, 300041 Timisoara, Romania
7. County Emergency Hospital, L. Rebreanu Str., Nr. 156, 300723 Timisoara, Romania
* Correspondence: sosdean.raluca@umft.ro (R.Ș.); tudoran.cristina@umft.ro (C.T.); Tel.: +40-745538055 (R.Ș.); +40-722669086 (C.T.); Fax: +40-256207352 (R.Ș.)

Abstract: Cardiac resynchronization therapy (CRT) represents an increasingly recommended solution to alleviate symptomatology and improve the quality of life in individuals with dilated cardiomyopathy (DCM) and heart failure (HF) with reduced ejection fraction (HFrEF) who remain symptomatic despite optimal medical therapy (OMT). However, this therapy does have the desired results all cases, in that sometimes low sensing and high voltage stimulation are needed to obtain some degree of resynchronization, even in the case of perfectly placed cardiac pacing leads. Our study aims to identify whether there is a relationship between several transthoracic echocardiographic (TTE) parameters characterizing left ventricular (LV) performance, especially strain results, and sensing and pacing parameters. Between 2020–2021, CRT was performed to treat persistent symptoms in 48 patients with a mean age of 64 (53.25–70) years, who were diagnosed with DCM and HFrEF, and who were still symptomatic despite OMT. We documented statistically significant correlations between global longitudinal strain, posterolateral strain, and ejection fraction and LV sensing (r = 0.65, 0.469, and 0.534, respectively, $p < 0.001$) and LV pacing parameters (r = −0.567, −0.555, and −0.363, respectively, $p < 0.001$). Modern imaging techniques, such as TTE with cardiac strain, are contributing to the evaluation of patients with HFrEF, increasing the chances of CRT success, and allowing physicians to anticipate and plan for case management.

Keywords: transthoracic echocardiography; longitudinal strain; sensing parameters; pacing parameters

1. Introduction

Dilated cardiomyopathy (DCM) carries a significant burden for the patients and for the health care system and physicians as well. As the disease progresses, treatment options involving medication become limited as heart failure (HF) continues to worsen, severely limiting the patient's ability to perform even the smallest of daily tasks [1]. Fortunately, modern imaging techniques provide superior insight into the extent of the disease. Speckle tracking with cardiac strain is a modern imaging technique that analyses in detail the segmental shortening of the ventricular myocardium [2,3]. These ultrasonographic investigations are vital in assessing the severity of the disease as well as its progression. As the disease progresses, an increasing amount of left ventricular (LV) intramyocardial fibrosis is detected. This happens independent of the etiology of HF, although in ischemic patients the amount of fibrosis and scar burden is much more evident and detected earlier in the disease evolution [4]. This aspect may interfere with the pacing and sensing thresholds of a cardiac resynchronization therapy (CRT) system, by altering them. Currently, the best way to evaluate intramyocardial fibrosis is by use of cardiac magnetic resonance imaging (cMRI) with late gadolinium enhancement for scar evaluation and T1 mapping for diffuse fibrosis. This imaging modality is not always available and is time consuming; however, the evaluation of longitudinal strain by the echocardiographic speckle tracking technique has concordant results and is more widely available [4,5]. Longitudinal strain is more reproducible as compared to radial and circumferential strain, and it evaluates the contraction of the longitudinal fibers, which are the first to be affected [4,6,7]. In terms of current treatment options, currently, interventional cardiology comes to the aid of these patients employing CRT [8,9]. Patients with left bundle branch block (LBBB) and significant systolic dysfunction, expressed by HF with reduced ejection fraction (HFrEF), can benefit from this course of treatment according to current guidelines [1,10]. CRT has been proven to be superior to conventional medical treatment by decreasing mortality and morbidity among patients who suffer from DCM, be it of ischemic or idiopathic etiology [11,12]. However, CRT poses a set of particular challenges, being less successful in certain patients who have high pacing thresholds which need constant adjustment and intermediate sensing values, despite the optimal lead placement. High acute pacing thresholds are especially detrimental since a higher voltage for pacing translates into a higher rate of pulse generator battery discharge, leading to an important decrease in the battery's longevity, which consequently leads to the need for earlier generator replacement [13–15]. With pacing thresholds being known to vary, sometimes failure-to-capture can occur over time, requiring even further amplification of the stimulation voltage. Interventions for replacing the pulse generator carry some degree of risk for the patient as infections of the device pocket are extremely dangerous since they can lead to exteriorization, endocarditis, or even sepsis and are seldom curative without the extraction of the entire pacing system, a difficult maneuver with considerable risks [14,16,17]. Individuals implanted with CRT defibrillator (CRT-D) are especially vulnerable in the event of discharged generators, since they require the additional protection that the defibrillator offers. As a result of the thresholds increasing over time, a failure in the impulse capturing can result in pacing deficits and/or inefficient CRT therapy.

This study aims to investigate whether several TTE parameters characterizing cardiac performance, and especially the strain imaging techniques such as LV global longitudinal strain (LV-GLS) and LV postero-lateral strain (LV-PLS) could be considered as predictors for suboptimal CRT functional parameters, namely low sensing, and high pacing, in patients with DCM and HFrEF.

2. Materials and Methods

2.1. Study Population

A single cohort of 48 patients suffering from DCM and HFrEF, who were implanted during January 2020 and June 2021 with three-lead pacemaker CRT (CRT-P) and three-lead intracardiac defibrillator (CRT-D) devices at the Institute of Cardiovascular Diseases from Timisoara, Romania, represent our study population. All patients were symptomatic despite optimal medical therapy (OMT), all had LBBB and were implanted with these devices according to current European Society of Cardiology (ESC) guidelines [1,10]. Patients with permanent atrial fibrillation who received biventricular pacemakers (CRT-P) were also included in the study as the main goal was to evaluate the impact of global and focal longitudinal strain on pacing parameters. All patients were evaluated by TTE before the implantation procedure.

All patients signed the standardized informed consent form required by the Health Authority of Romania at hospital admission, and their data were anonymized before data collection. The Ethics Committee of the Institute of Cardiovascular Diseases, Timisoara approved this study, Nr. 4052/19.06.2020.

2.2. Echocardiography

A complete bidimensional TTE evaluation was performed by a single blinded cardiologist, with advanced training in echocardiography, in all patients approximately 1 day before CRT intervention, using the General Electric VIVID E95 ultrasound system (GEMS Ultrasound, Horten, Norway). Several parameters reflecting LV (end-diastolic volume, ejection fraction, global and segmental longitudinal strain, volume) and right ventricular (RV, including longitudinal contraction, pulmonary artery systolic pressures) morphological and functional status, as well as atrial morphological status (left atrial volume), were selected to be analyzed for this study.

The left atrial volume (LAV) was measured by planimetry in a biplane manner, in 4 chambers and 2 chambers views, respectively, according to the European Association of Cardiovascular Imaging (EACVI) recommendations [18].

The LV volumes (end-diastolic volume—EDV and end-systolic volume—ESV) were measured by planimetry (tracing the interface between the myocardium and the cavity), also in a biplane manner, in 4 chambers and 2 chambers views, respectively. The LV ejection fraction (LVEF) was measured by using the biplane modified Simpson's method [3,19].

The longitudinal strain was evaluated by using the speckle tracking technique, in 4, 2, and 3 chamber views. The region of interest (ROI) was automatically rendered, with subsequent manual adjustments to obtain the best delineation of the myocardium to be analyzed. Care was taken not to include the pericardium in the ROI, and thus obtain falsely decreased absolute strain values. The LV was divided into 6 segments to be analyzed-basal, mid-ventricular, and apical, in each view. Three cardiac cycles were recorded for offline analysis in each view, at a frame rate between 40 and 90 frames/s, depending on the heart rate (higher frame rate for higher heart rates). The global longitudinal strain was calculated on the resultant bull's eye model [2,19–21].

The longitudinal contraction of the RV was evaluated by measuring the tricuspid annular plane systolic excursion (TAPSE). This parameter was measured according to the EACVI chamber quantification recommendations, by M-mode, between end-diastole and peak-systole [3,19].

The systolic pulmonary artery pressure (sPAP) was evaluated by measuring the tricuspid regurgitation flow maximal pressure. The estimated right atrial pressure (RAP) was added to this value (5 mmHg if the diameter of the inferior vena cava (IVC) was <2.1 cm with >50% inspiratory collapse, 10 mmHg if the diameter of the IVC was >2.1 cm with >50% inspiratory collapse or the diameter of the IVC was <2.1 cm with <50% inspiratory collapse and 15 mmHg if the diameter of the IVC was >2.1 cm with <50% inspiratory collapse).

2.3. Resynchronization Therapy (CRT)

In most patients, the implantation technique consisted of inserting a defibrillator/RV pacing lead into the RV cavity via the cephalic vein which was isolated in the deltopectoral groove. If the vein permitted, the atrial lead was inserted using the same route, if not, the atrial lead was inserted via the subclavian vein after positioning the coronary-sinus (CS) lead. Using the cephalic vein for the insertion of the RV lead allowed us to avoid difficulties in positioning because of lead interactions via the route of the subclavian vein, thus facilitating our control in cannulating the CS and maneuvering the CS lead into the optimal position. Arguably the most difficult step of the procedure is positioning the LV lead. This is mainly due to two anatomical variabilities (1) CS ostium and (2) cardiac veins themselves. Once the CS has been cannulated using the purpose built catheters, contrast is injected to visualize the particular anatomy of the cardiac veins, which presents significant interindividual variety [22]. A guidewire is advanced in order to offer support as well as a pathway for advancing the actual LV lead. The guidewire is then manipulated in such a way that it enters one of the posterolateral branches. These branches allow for stable placement of the LV lead. Despite satisfactory radiological positioning of the lead, sensing and pacing parameters can be substandard, possibly due to an area rich in fibrous tissue. In order to electrically assess the positioning of the leads, sensing and pacing thresholds are evaluated to discern whether it is necessary to adjust the position or possibly relocate the lead to another branch of the CS due to low sensing or high pacing thresholds. After positioning the lead optimally in the CS, by using the cephalic vein for the other two leads, the risk of dislodgement was decreased, as this is an extremely unwanted event that threatens the success of the overall resynchronization therapy. By inserting the defibrillator lead first into the RV cavity, we secured the means of delivering an internal shock if malignant ventricular tachycardia arises during the procedure. This measure is especially important in patients with previously diagnosed ventricular tachycardia who benefited from implantable cardiac defibrillator therapy for secondary prevention.

We consider ideal functioning parameters for pacing around 1 ± 0.5 V for the RV and right atrium leads and around 2 ± 0.5 V for the CS lead with ideal sensing parameters exceeding 10 mV in the case of the CS and RV lead and over 3 mV for the right atrium lead.

2.4. Statistical Methods

We employed the Shapiro–Wilk test to evaluate the distribution of numeric variables. Numeric variables were presented as the median and interquartile range (IQR), and categorical variables were presented as frequency and percentages. We employed Wilcoxon test to compare the QRS duration before and after CRT implantation. To evaluate the association between LV sensing/pacing and different echocardiographic parameters we used the Spearman correlation test. To assess the independent factors that influenced the LV sensing/pacing we built several multivariate linear regression models. In the final regression equations, the predictors were accepted according to a repeated backward-stepwise algorithm (inclusion criteria $p < 0.05$, exclusion criteria $p > 0.10$) so as to obtain the most appropriate theoretical model that fit the collected data. The quality of the model was described using the accuracy of prediction and R squared. Data analysis was performed using the Statistical Package for the Social Sciences v.26 (SPSS, Chicago, IL, USA). A p-value < 0.05 was considered statistically significant.

3. Results

This study included 48 patients with DCM, aged between 39 and 73 years, with a median of 64 (53.25–70) years. Thirty-seven of them were men (77%) and 11 women (23%). Referring to the etiology, 37 had idiopathic DCM (64.6%) and 17 ischemic forms (35.4%). According to their symptomatology, most patients were in class NYHA III (47.9%), followed by class II (41.6%) and class IV (10.4%). The characteristics of the study population, as well as their therapy, are presented in Table 1 and their initial electrocardiographic and TTE parameters in Table 2.

All patients were treated according to the ESC guidelines [1] with OMT according to indications, associated diseases, and side effects, with doses adjusted according to the individual tolerance, Table 1. All of them underwent a detailed TTE examination before the CRT implantation, and their echocardiographic, but also the electrocardiographic parameters before and after the implantation are presented in Table 2.

We observed a statistically significant shorter QRS duration after the CRT implantation ($p < 0.001$, Wilcoxon test). The median values of sensing and pacing parameters of CRT' devices are presented in Table 3.

Table 1. Patients' characteristics before CRT implantation.

Parameter	ValueTitle
Age (years)	64 (53–70)
Sex: male	37 (77%)
female	11 (23%)
Etiology of DCM: ischemic	17 (35.4%)
idiopathic	31 (64.6%)
NYHA class: II	20 (41.6%)
III	23 (47.9%)
IV	5 (10.4%)
Associated diabetes mellitus	20 (41.66%)
Nondiabetics	28 (58.33%)
Therapy: Beta-blockers	43 (89.58%)
ACE/ARB	22 (45.83%)
Sacubitril/valsartan	20 (41.66%)
Spironolactone	38 (79.16%)
Digoxin	10 (20.83%)
Furosemide	47 (97.91%)

Legend: CRT—cardiac resynchronization therapy; DCM—dilated cardiomyopathy; NYHA—New York Heart Association; ACE—angiotensin-converting enzyme inhibitors; ARB—angiotensin receptor blockers.

Table 2. Echocardiographic parameters before CRT implantation.

Electrocardiography	
QRS (ms): initial	160 (160–200)
post CRT implantation	130 (120–140)
Episodes of ventricular tachycardia	13 patients (27.08%)
Atrial fibrillation	9 patients (18.75%)
Echocardiographic Parameters	**Mean (min–max)**
LAV (mL)	101.5 (83.25–142)
LVEDV (mL)	236.5 (200–296.25)
LVEF (%—Simpson)	26 (20.25–30)
LV-GLS (%)	5.85 (3.82–7.2)
LV-PLS (%)	5 (2.125–8)
TAPSE cm	1.7 (1.5–1.97)
sPAP (mmHg)	35 (27–46.75)

Legend: CRT—cardiac resynchronization therapy; LAV—left atrial volume; LVEDD—left ventricular end-diastolic volume; LVEF—left ventricular ejection fraction; LV-GLS—left ventricular global longitudinal strain; LV-PLD—left ventricular postero-lateral strain; TAPSE—tricuspid annular plane systolic excursion; sPAP—systolic pulmonary artery pressure.

Table 3. Sensing and pacing parameters after CRT implantation.

CRT Parameter	Value
LV sensing (mV)	12 (9.5–17.5)
Pacing threshold LV (V)	3.5 (2.5–4)
Acute pacing threshold RV (V)	1 (0.625–1.5)
Acute sensing threshold RV (mV)	11 (8–12)
RA sensing (mV)	3.45 (2.5–3.8)

Legend: CRT—cardiac resynchronization therapy; LV—left ventricle; V—volt; RV—right ventricle.

By analyzing the existence of statistically significant correlations between several echocardiographic results and LV sensing and pacing, we identified that the most significant ones were evidenced between the strain parameters, followed by the LVEF and LAV both for LV sensing, but especially for LV pacing, Table 4. We also observed a weak, but still statistically significant correlation between sPAP and RV pacing (r = 0.286, p = 0.049).

Table 4. Correlations between the TTE parameters and LV sensing and pacing.

Parameter	LV Sensing			LV Pacing		
	r	95% CI	p	r	95% CI	p
LVEF (Simpson)	0.534	0.301; 0.716	<0.001	−0.363	−0.608; −0.113	0.011
LV-GLS	0.650	0.407; 0.816	<0.001	−0.567	−0.765; −0.317	<0.001
LV-PLS	0.469	0.159; 0.726	0.001	−0.555	−0.793; −0.271	<0.001
LAV (mL)	−0.574	−0.750; −0.333	<0.001	0.385	0.122; 0.599	0.007
TAPSE (cm)	0.417	0.179; 0.616	0.003	−0.373	−0.597; −0.078	0.009
sPAP (mmHg)	−0.270	−0.497; −0.002	0.064	0.124	−0.169; 0.401	0.402

Legend: LV—left ventricle; LVEF—left ventricular ejection fraction; LV-GLS—left ventricular global longitudinal strain; LV-PLD—left ventricular postero-lateral strain; r—correlation coefficient; CI—confidence interval; p—statistical significance; Spearman correlation test. Statistically significant $p < 0.05$.

To determine which independent factors, namely the LV sensing and LV pacing thresholds, could be predicted in our study group we employed a multivariate linear regression model. We used the forward stepwise method, and the best models were selected based on Akaike information criteria (AIC). We included in our models parameters such as age, sex, echocardiographic parameters, and patients' comorbidities.

The regression equation for the LV sensing proved to be adequate for the model, explaining 72.1% of the LV sensing variance ($R^2 = 0.721$), the details being presented in Table 5. The LV sensing threshold increased directly proportional with the elevation of LV-GLS and LAV values. The presence of ventricular tachycardia or diabetes mellitus decrease the LV sensing threshold. Additionally, more advanced stages of HF (NYHA) decrease the LV sensing value.

Table 5. Multivariate linear regression of independent factors for LV sensing.

Variable	β	Standard Error	p	95% CI for β
LVEDD (mL)	−0.016	0.005	0.006	−0.027; −0.005
LV-GLS (%)	1.046	0.148	<0.001	0.747; 0.145
LAV (mL)	0.023	0.007	0.003	−0.037; −0.008
Ventricular tachycardia	−2.187	0.936	0.025	−4.079; −0.296
NYHA class	−1.626	0.562	0.006	−2.761; −0.491
Diabetes Mellitus	−1.491	0.743	0.052	−2.994; 0.012

Legend: LAV—left atrial volume; LV-GLS—left ventricular global longitudinal strain; LVEDD—left ventricular end-diastolic volume; NYHA—New York Heart Association; β—regression coefficient; SE—standard error; p—statistical significance; CI—confidence interval; statistical method: multivariate stepwise linear regression (Akaike information criteria). Statistically significant $p < 0.05$.

Referring to the LV pacing, the model presented in Table 6 explains 44.6% of its variance ($R^2 = 0.446$). Lower values of LV-GLS, RV-GLS, and TAPSE increase the LV pacing threshold, as well as the presence of diabetes mellitus.

Table 6. Multivariate linear regression of independent factors for LV pacing.

Variable	β	Standard Error	p	95% CI for β
LV-GLS	−0.116	0.057	0.049	−0.231; 0.000
LV-PLS	−0.095	0.038	0.015	−0.171; −0.019
TAPSE	−0.508	0.282	0.049	−1.078; 0.061
Diabetes Mellitus	0.504	0.210	0.021	0.080; 0.929

Legend: LV-GLS—left ventricular global longitudinal strain; LVEDD—left ventricular end-diastolic volume; LV-PLS—left ventricular postero-lateral strain; TAPSE—tricuspid annular plane systolic excursion; β—regression coefficient; SE—standard error; p—statistical significance; CI—confidence interval; statistical method: multivariate stepwise linear regression (Akaike information criteria). Statistically significant $p < 0.05$.

4. Discussion

According to the newest ESC guidelines, CRT represents a Class I, Level A recommendation for the treatment of HFrEF, with LVEF under 35%, regardless of the NYHA class, in patients who are still symptomatic, despite OMT, to reduce morbidity and mortality, and especially, to alleviate their complaints and to improve their quality of life [1,10,23]. There is research that predicates that the benefits of this therapy are still underutilized [9,24]. All patients included in this study had an indication of Class I for CRT implantation and were referred for this therapy [1,10].

As they were evaluated before the procedure, a comprehensive TTE exam, followed by strain imaging was performed to characterize LV performance, to observe the severity of kinesis abnormalities, and the existence of mechanical asynchronism [25,26]. The results illustrated that ultrasound strain parameters, global and focal as well, can indeed be linked with sensing and stimulation thresholds. As well as finding LV-GLS relevant, we also found focal, LV-PLS to be just as relevant as it evaluates the strain in the regions where the coronary sinus lead will be positioned, which is vital to a successful CRT. As all patients had undergone strain echocardiography before implantation, the results from this noninvasive investigation can help us to guide the interventional cardiologist in programming the device after the implantation has taken place. It is relevant as well as during the procedure when the interventionist is influenced by the acute sensing threshold. Acute sensing thresholds are important in regard to making intraoperative decisions towards positioning the leads, as interventionists seek the optimal position, which usually involves achieving the highest sensing value as this is a marker of how well the electrodes on the lead receive the electrical action potential generated by the myocardium. Pacing thresholds are an even more valuable parameter to predict [15,25,27], as the success of CRT depends on the ability to achieve successful LV and RV pacing. Without efficient impulse captures on either lead, the stimulation will mainly be achieved by just one of the ventricular leads, thus possibly decreasing the ejection fraction even further as well as further altering intra- and interventricular synchronism, consequently having possible effects on the LV-GLS [13,23,28]. Fortunately, the efficiency of CRT therapy can also be evaluated by the simpler means of the surface ECG, with the end optimal result being the reduction in the duration of the QRS complex. The modern CRT devices and leads we use in our patients, mainly manufactured by Biotronik (Berlin, Germany), offer an array of possible programming polarities. By modifying the combination of electrodes, the electrical impulse travels between, we achieve, in most patients, significant reductions in the QRS complex duration, especially in those with significantly prolonged QRS complexes before the procedure [25,29,30].

As debated in the medical literature [23,24,29,31], CRT is one of the most effective therapeutic possibilities for the treatment of patients with HFrEF, which still remains widely underutilized, with only approximately one-third of eligible patients receiving a timely referral for this procedure [9,10,24]. An optimized collaborative work between the cardiologists responsible for the clinical care and evaluation of those patients with the interventional cardiologist could improve the management of patients with HFrEF [1,10,24,30], even in cases where it seems more difficult to obtains the optimal results.

Our results are explained by the fact that GLS (local and global) reflects the fibrosis burden in the myocardium. It is demonstrated that scar tissue does not have any electrical activity therefore no pacing and/or sensing is possible [32,33]. It is recommended to avoid placing the CS lead on scar tissue and also in its immediate proximity, as the scar induces fragmentation of the electrical impulse. Abozguia et al., used a multipolar LV lead in order to counteract the deleterious scar effects, with good results [34]. Mele et al., evaluated the response of patients with CRT with the LV pacing lead placed on, adjacent to and/or remote from a scared segment, considered as therapy responders the patients with at least 10% decrease in LV end-systolic volume at 6 months. They demonstrated that the CRT response depended on the quality of the pacing site underlying tissue in addition to the global LV scar burden [35]. Mendonca Costa et al., also demonstrated that pacing in the proximity of a scar may induce ventricular arrhythmias. Using images from a number of 24 patients with ischemic DCM, they created computational models (patient specific, LV anatomic, scar morphology included) through which they demonstrated an increased repolarization dispersion inducing an arrhythmogenic substrate [36].

In the same manner, even if there is no consistent scar on the LV lead targeted wall, a high amount of diffuse/interstitial or replacement fibrosis explain the altered of the pacing and sensing thresholds. The low response to CRT in these patients is induced, as demonstrated previously by several authors [32–35], using the fragmentation of the impulse conduction, with a significant increase in conduction delay and prolongation of the QRS length, but also by a possible intermittent loss of LV capture, which is sometimes hard to diagnose just by interrogating the device.

It is true that longitudinal strain evaluates the longitudinal fibers contraction, fibers that are best represented (but not exclusively) in the subendocardial layer [18], and the LV lead is placed in one of the CS branches, most of the time a postero-lateral branch to serve the most delayed contracting wall, which is on the epicardial side of the LV. However, the impulse must travel from the epicardial side to the endocardial side and meet the impulse induced by the RV lead, which travels from the endocardium to the epicardium, in order to obtain a homogenous and faster depolarization and synchronize the contraction. If the impulse is delivered in or in the proximity of a high fibrosis area, its quality will be compromised, as this type of tissue has altered fiber orientation and a reduced electrical conductivity [37].

The main limitation of our study is represented by the small number of patients treated with CRT. The low case numbers were due to the COVID-19 pandemic with admission of non-COVID patients and reduced access to the interventional laboratory. As a consequence of the small patient population, we could not further analyze the impact of other factors, especially of associated diseases, on our results.

5. Conclusions

Modern imagistic techniques, such as cardiac strain, are contributing to the evaluation of patients with heart failure with HFrEF who are referred for CRT implantation, also suggesting a course of treatment. Cardiac strain imaging results might be able to predict the chances of CRT being successful or not, allowing the interventional cardiologist to anticipate and plan for improved patient outcomes.

Author Contributions: Conceptualization, S.-A.P., R.Ş., C.T., A.I., G.N.P., R.Z.T., S.P. and M.T.; methodology, S.-A.P., R.Ş., C.T. and M.T.; software, C.T. and G.N.P.; validation, S.-A.P., R.Ş., C.T., A.I., G.N.P., R.Z.T., S.P. and M.T.; formal analysis, S.-A.P., R.Ş., C.T. and M.T.; investigation, S.-A.P., R.Ş., C.T. and M.T.; resources, S.-A.P., R.Ş., C.T. and M.T.; data curation, S.-A.P., R.Ş., C.T. and M.T.; writing—original draft preparation, S.-A.P., R.Ş., C.T., A.I., G.N.P., R.Z.T., S.P. and M.T.; writing—review and editing, S.-A.P., R.Ş., C.T. and M.T.; visualization, S.-A.P., R.Ş., C.T., A.I., G.N.P., R.Z.T., S.P. and M.T.; supervision, S.-A.P., R.Ş., C.T. and M.T.; project administration, S.-A.P., R.Ş., C.T. and M.T.;. All authors have read and agreed to the published version of the manuscript.

Funding: This research received no external funding.

Institutional Review Board Statement: The study was conducted according to the guidelines of the Declaration of Helsinki and approved by Ethics Committee of the Institute for Cardio-vascular Diseases from Timisoara, Romania, Nr. 4052/19.06.2020.

Informed Consent Statement: Written informed consent was obtained from all subjects involved in the study.

Data Availability Statement: Our data are available at https://doi.org/10.17632/w4536c7gpd.1.

Conflicts of Interest: The authors declare no conflict of interest.

References

1. McDonagh, T.A.; Metra, M.; Adamo, M.; Gardner, R.S.; Baumbach, A.; Böhm, M.; Burri, H.; Butler, J.; Čelutkienė, J.; Chioncel, O.; et al. 2021 ESC Guidelines for the Diagnosis and Treatment of Acute and Chronic Heart Failure. *Eur. Heart J.* 2021, 42, 3599–3726. [CrossRef] [PubMed]
2. Trivedi, S.J.; Altman, M.; Stanton, T.; Thomas, L. Echocardiographic Strain in Clinical Practice. *Heart Lung Circ.* 2019, 28, 1320–1330. [CrossRef]
3. Badano, L.P.; Kolias, T.J.; Muraru, D.; Abraham, T.P.; Aurigemma, G.; Edvardsen, T.; D'Hooge, J.; Donal, E.; Fraser, A.G.; Marwick, T.; et al. Standardization of Left Atrial, Right Ventricular, and Right Atrial Deformation Imaging Using Two-Dimensional Speckle Tracking Echocardiography: A Consensus Document of the EACVI/ASE/Industry Task Force to Standardize Deformation Imaging. *Eur. Heart J. Cardiovasc. Imaging* 2018, 19, 591–600. [CrossRef] [PubMed]
4. Jung, I.H.; Park, J.H.; Lee, J.-A.; Kim, G.S.; Lee, H.Y.; Byun, Y.S.; Kim, B.O. Left Ventricular Global Longitudinal Strain as a Predictor for Left Ventricular Reverse Remodeling in Dilated Cardiomyopathy. *J. Cardiovasc. Imaging* 2020, 28, 137. [CrossRef]
5. Hoffmann, R.; Altiok, E.; Friedman, Z.; Becker, M.; Frick, M. Myocardial Deformation Imaging by Two-Dimensional Speckle-Tracking Echocardiography in Comparison to Late Gadolinium Enhancement Cardiac Magnetic Resonance for Analysis of Myocardial Fibrosis in Severe Aortic Stenosis. *Am. J. Cardiol.* 2014, 114, 1083–1088. [CrossRef]
6. Mirea, O.; Pagourelias, E.D.; Duchenne, J.; Bogaert, J.; Thomas, J.D.; Badano, L.P.; Voigt, J.-U.; Badano, L.P.; Thomas, J.D.; Hamilton, J.; et al. Intervendor Differences in the Accuracy of Detecting Regional Functional Abnormalities. *JACC Cardiovasc. Imaging* 2018, 11, 25–34. [CrossRef]
7. Sugimoto, T.; Dulgheru, R.; Bernard, A.; Ilardi, F.; Contu, L.; Addetia, K.; Caballero, L.; Akhaladze, N.; Athanassopoulos, G.D.; Barone, D.; et al. Echocardiographic Reference Ranges for Normal Left Ventricular 2D Strain: Results from the EACVI NORRE Study. *Eur. Heart J. Cardiovasc. Imaging* 2017, 18, 833–840. [CrossRef] [PubMed]
8. Boriani, G.; Berti, E.; Belotti, L.M.B.; Biffi, M.; Carboni, A.; Bandini, A.; Casali, E.; Tomasi, C.; Toselli, T.; Baraldi, P.; et al. Cardiac Resynchronization Therapy: Implant Rates, Temporal Trends and Relationships with Heart Failure Epidemiology. *J. Cardiovasc. Med.* 2014, 15, 147–154. [CrossRef] [PubMed]
9. Lawin, D.; Stellbrink, C. Change in Indication for Cardiac Resynchronization Therapy? *Eur. J. Cardio-Thorac. Surg.* 2019, 55, i11–i16. [CrossRef]
10. 2021 ESC Guidelines on Cardiac Pacing and Cardiac Resynchronization Therapy. *Eur. Heart J.* 2021, 42, 3427–3520. Available online: https://academic.oup.com/eurheartj/article/42/35/3427/6358547 (accessed on 10 November 2021). [CrossRef]
11. Epstein, A.E.; DiMarco, J.P.; Ellenbogen, K.A.; Estes, N.A.M.; Freedman, R.A.; Gettes, L.S.; Gillinov, A.M.; Gregoratos, G.; Hammill, S.C.; Hayes, D.L.; et al. ACC/AHA/HRS 2008 Guidelines for Device-Based Therapy of Cardiac Rhythm Abnormalities. *J. Am. Coll. Cardiol.* 2008, 51, e1–e62. [CrossRef] [PubMed]
12. Authors/Task Force Members; Brignole, M.; Auricchio, A.; Baron-Esquivias, G.; Bordachar, P.; Boriani, G.; Breithardt, O.-A.; Cleland, J.; Deharo, J.-C.; Delgado, V.; et al. 2013 ESC Guidelines on Cardiac Pacing and Cardiac Resynchronization Therapy: The Task Force on Cardiac Pacing and Resynchronization Therapy of the European Society of Cardiology (ESC). Developed in Collaboration with the European Heart Rhythm Association (EHRA). *Europace* 2013, 15, 1070–1118. [CrossRef]
13. Chugh, S.S. Clinical Cardiac Pacing, Defibrillation, and Resynchronization Therapy, 5th Edition. By Kenneth A. Ellenbogen, Bruce L. Wilkoff, G. Neal Kay, Chu-Pak Lau, and Angelo Auricchio. Philadelphia, PA: Elsevier, Inc., 1232 Pages, ISBN: 978-0-323-37804-8.: BOOK REVIEW. *Pacing Clin. Electrophysiol.* 2017, 40, 221. [CrossRef]
14. Udo, E.O.; Zuithoff, N.P.A.; van Hemel, N.M.; de Cock, C.C.; Hendriks, T.; Doevendans, P.A.; Moons, K.G.M. Incidence and Predictors of Short- and Long-Term Complications in Pacemaker Therapy: The FOLLOWPACE Study. *Heart Rhythm* 2012, 9, 728–735. [CrossRef] [PubMed]
15. Huang, C.-C.; Tuan, T.-C.; Fong, M.-C.; Lee, W.-S.; Kong, C.-W. Predictors of Inappropriate Atrial Sensing in Long-Term VDD-Pacing Systems. *Europace* 2010, 12, 1251–1255. [CrossRef] [PubMed]
16. Poole, J.E.; Gleva, M.J.; Mela, T.; Chung, M.K.; Uslan, D.Z.; Borge, R.; Gottipaty, V.; Shinn, T.; Dan, D.; Feldman, L.A.; et al. Complication Rates Associated with Pacemaker or Implantable Cardioverter-Defibrillator Generator Replacements and Upgrade Procedures: Results From the REPLACE Registry. *Circulation* 2010, 122, 1553–1561. [CrossRef]
17. Sohail, M.R.; Uslan, D.Z.; Khan, A.H.; Friedman, P.A.; Hayes, D.L.; Wilson, W.R.; Steckelberg, J.M.; Stoner, S.; Baddour, L.M. Management and Outcome of Permanent Pacemaker and Implantable Cardioverter-Defibrillator Infections. *J. Am. Coll. Cardiol.* 2007, 49, 1851–1859. [CrossRef]
18. Lang, R.M.; Bierig, M.; Devereux, R.B.; Flachskampf, F.A.; Foster, E.; Pellikka, P.A.; Picard, M.H.; Roman, M.J.; Seward, J.; Shanewise, J.S.; et al. Recommendations for Chamber Quantification: A Report from the American Society of Echocardiography's Guidelines and Standards Committee and the Chamber Quantification Writing Group, Developed in Conjunction with the European Association of Echocardiography, a Branch of the European Society of Cardiology. *J. Am. Soc. Echocardiogr.* 2005, 18, 1440–1463. [CrossRef]
19. Lang, R.M.; Badano, L.P.; Mor-Avi, V.; Afilalo, J.; Armstrong, A.; Ernande, L.; Flachskampf, F.A.; Foster, E.; Goldstein, S.A.; Kuznetsova, T.; et al. Recommendations for Cardiac Chamber Quantification by Echocardiography in Adults: An Update from the American Society of Echocardiography and the European Association of Cardiovascular Imaging. *J. Am. Soc. Echocardiogr.* 2015, 28, 1–39.e14. [CrossRef]
20. Normal Ranges of Left Ventricular Strain: A Meta-Analysis. *J. Am. Soc. Echocardiogr.* 2013, 26, 185–191. [CrossRef]

21. Croft, L.B.; Krishnamoorthy, P.; Ro, R.; Anastasius, M.; Zhao, W.; Buckley, S.; Goldman, M.; Argulian, E.; Sharma, S.K.; Kini, A.; et al. Abnormal Left Ventricular Global Longitudinal Strain by Speckle Tracking Echocardiography in COVID-19 Patients. *Future Cardiol.* 2020, *17*, 655–661. [CrossRef] [PubMed]
22. Saremi, F.; Muresian, H.; Sánchez-Quintana, D. Coronary Veins: Comprehensive CT-Anatomic Classification and Review of Variants and Clinical Implications. *Radiographics* 2012, *32*, E1–E32. [CrossRef]
23. Khazanie, P.; Hammill, B.G.; Qualls, L.G.; Fonarow, G.C.; Hammill, S.C.; Heidenreich, P.A.; Al-Khatib, S.M.; Piccini, J.P.; Masoudi, F.A.; Peterson, P.N.; et al. Clinical Effectiveness of Cardiac Resynchronization Therapy Versus Medical Therapy Alone Among Patients with Heart Failure: Analysis of the ICD Registry and ADHERE. *Circ. Heart Fail.* 2014, *7*, 926–934. [CrossRef]
24. Mullens, W.; Auricchio, A.; Martens, P.; Witte, K.; Cowie, M.R.; Delgado, V.; Dickstein, K.; Linde, C.; Vernooy, K.; Leyva, F.; et al. Optimized Implementation of Cardiac Resynchronization Therapy: A Call for Action for Referral and Optimization of Care: A Joint Position Statement from the Heart Failure Association (HFA), European Heart Rhythm Association (EHRA), and European Association of Cardiovascular Imaging (EACVI) of the European Society of Cardiology. *Eur. J. Heart Fail.* 2020, *22*, 2349–2369. [CrossRef]
25. Gage, R.M.; Burns, K.V.; Bank, A.J. Echocardiographic and Clinical Response to Cardiac Resynchronization Therapy in Heart Failure Patients with and without Previous Right Ventricular Pacing. *Eur. J. Heart Fail.* 2014, *16*, 1199–1205. [CrossRef]
26. Beela, A.S.; Ünlü, S.; Duchenne, J.; Ciarka, A.; Daraban, A.M.; Kotrc, M.; Aarones, M.; Szulik, M.; Winter, S.; Penicka, M.; et al. Assessment of Mechanical Dyssynchrony Can Improve the Prognostic Value of Guideline-Based Patient Selection for Cardiac Resynchronization Therapy. *Eur. Heart J. Cardiovasc. Imaging* 2019, *20*, 66–74. [CrossRef] [PubMed]
27. Freemantle, N.; Tharmanathan, P.; Calvert, M.J.; Abraham, W.T.; Ghosh, J.; Cleland, J.G.F. Cardiac Resynchronisation for Patients with Heart Failure Due to Left Ventricular Systolic Dysfunction—A Systematic Review and Meta-Analysis. *Eur. J. Heart Fail.* 2006, *8*, 433–440. [CrossRef]
28. Hayes, D.L.; Boehmer, J.P.; Day, J.D.; Gilliam, F.R.; Heidenreich, P.A.; Seth, M.; Jones, P.W.; Saxon, L.A. Cardiac Resynchronization Therapy and the Relationship of Percent Biventricular Pacing to Symptoms and Survival. *Heart Rhythm* 2011, *8*, 1469–1475. [CrossRef]
29. Normand, C.; Linde, C.; Singh, J.; Dickstein, K. Indications for Cardiac Resynchronization Therapy. *JACC Heart Fail.* 2018, *6*, 308–316. [CrossRef]
30. Normand, C.; Linde, C.; Blomström-Lundqvist, C.; Stellbrink, C.; Gasparini, M.; Anker, S.D.; Plummer, C.; Sarigul, N.U.; Papiashvili, G.; Iovev, S.; et al. Adherence to ESC Cardiac Resynchronization Therapy Guidelines: Findings from the ESC CRT Survey II. *Europace* 2020, *22*, 932–938. [CrossRef] [PubMed]
31. Al-Majed, N.S.; McAlister, F.A.; Bakal, J.A.; Ezekowitz, J.A. Meta-Analysis: Cardiac Resynchronization Therapy for Patients with Less Symptomatic Heart Failure. *Ann. Intern. Med.* 2011, *154*, 401. [CrossRef] [PubMed]
32. Adelstein, E.C.; Tanaka, H.; Soman, P.; Miske, G.; Haberman, S.C.; Saba, S.F.; Gorcsan, J. Impact of Scar Burden by Single-Photon Emission Computed Tomography Myocardial Perfusion Imaging on Patient Outcomes Following Cardiac Resynchronization Therapy. *Eur. Heart. J.* 2011, *32*, 93–103. [CrossRef]
33. Chalil, S.; Foley, P.W.X.; Muyhaldeen, S.A.; Patel, K.C.R.; Yousef, Z.R.; Smith, R.E.A.; Frenneaux, M.P.; Leyva, F. Late Gadolinium Enhancement-Cardiovascular Magnetic Resonance as a Predictor of Response to Cardiac Resynchronization Therapy in Patients with Ischaemic Cardiomyopathy. *Europace* 2007, *9*, 1031–1037. [CrossRef] [PubMed]
34. Abozguia, K.; Leyva, F. Targeting Viable Myocardium in Cardiac Resynchronization Therapy Using a Multipolar Left Ventricular Lead. *Circulation* 2011, *123*, e617–e618. [CrossRef] [PubMed]
35. Mele, D.; Agricola, E.; Monte, A.D.; Galderisi, M.; D'Andrea, A.; Rigo, F.; Citro, R.; Chiodi, E.; Marchese, G.; Valentina, P.D.; et al. Pacing Transmural Scar Tissue Reduces Left Ventricle Reverse Remodeling after Cardiac Resynchronization Therapy. *Int. J. Cardiol.* 2013, *167*, 94–101. [CrossRef]
36. Mendonca Costa, C.; Neic, A.; Kerfoot, E.; Porter, B.; Sieniewicz, B.; Gould, J.; Sidhu, B.; Chen, Z.; Plank, G.; Rinaldi, C.A.; et al. Pacing in Proximity to Scar during Cardiac Resynchronization Therapy Increases Local Dispersion of Repolarization and Susceptibility to Ventricular Arrhythmogenesis. *Heart Rhythm* 2019, *16*, 1475–1483. [CrossRef] [PubMed]
37. Lee, A.W.C.; Costa, C.M.; Strocchi, M.; Rinaldi, C.A.; Niederer, S.A. Computational Modeling for Cardiac Resynchronization Therapy. *J. Cardiovasc. Transl. Res.* 2018, *11*, 92–108. [CrossRef] [PubMed]

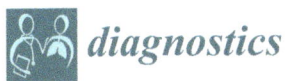

Article

A Practical Risk Score for Prediction of Early Readmission after a First Episode of Acute Heart Failure with Preserved Ejection Fraction

Marilena-Brîndușa Zamfirescu [1,2,†], Liviu Nicolae Ghilencea [1,2,*,†], Mihaela-Roxana Popescu [1,2,*,†], Gabriel Cristian Bejan [1,†], Ileana Maria Ghiordanescu [1,3], Andreea-Catarina Popescu [1,2], Saul G. Myerson [4,5] and Maria Dorobanțu [1,6]

1. Cardiothoracic Pathology Department, Carol Davila University of Medicine and Pharmacy, 020021 Bucharest, Romania; brindusa.zamfirescu@gmail.com (M.-B.Z.); crrsty1@yahoo.com (G.C.B.); ileana.ghiordanescu@gmail.com (I.M.G.); andreea.popescu@umfcd.ro (A.-C.P.); maria.dorobantu@gmail.com (M.D.)
2. Department of Cardiology, Elias Emergency University Hospital, "Carol Davila" University of Medicine and Pharmacy, 011227 Bucharest, Romania
3. Department of Allergology, Elias Emergency University Hospital, 011416 Bucharest, Romania
4. Oxford Heart Centre, John Radcliffe Hospital, Oxford OX4 2PG, UK; saul.myerson@cardiov.ox.ac.uk
5. Radcliffe Department of Medicine, University of Oxford, Oxford OX1 2JD, UK
6. Department of Cardiology, Clinic Emergency Hospital, 011227 Bucharest, Romania
* Correspondence: liviu.ghilencea@yahoo.com (L.N.G.); roxana.popescu@umfcd.ro (M.-R.P.); Tel.: +44-753-504-3647 (L.N.G.)
† M.-B.Z., L.N.G., M.-R.P. and G.C.B. equally contributed to the research and manuscript development.

Abstract: Background: The first admission for acute heart failure with preserved ejection fraction (HFpEF) drastically influences the short-term prognosis. Baseline characteristics may predict repeat hospitalization or death in these patients. Methods: A 103 patient-cohort, admitted for the first acute HFpEF episode, was monitored for six months. Baseline characteristics were recorded and their relation to the primary outcome of heart failure readmission (HFR) and secondary outcome of all-cause mortality was assessed. Results: We identified six independent determinants for HFR: estimated glomerular filtration rate (eGFR) ($p = 0.07$), hemoglobin ($p = 0.04$), left ventricle end-diastolic diameter (LVEDD) ($p = 0.07$), E/e' ratio ($p = 0.004$), left ventricle outflow tract velocity-time integral (LVOT VTI) ($p = 0.045$), and diabetes mellitus ($p = 0.06$). Three of the variables were used to generate a risk score for HFR: LVEDD, E/e', LVOT VTI -DEI Score = − 28.763 + 4.558 × log (LVEDD (mm)) + 1.961 × log (E/e' ratio) + 1.759 × log (LVOT VTI (cm)). Our model predicts a relative amount of 20.50% of HFR during the first 6 months after the first acute hospitalization within the general population with HFpEF with a DEI Score over −0.747. Conclusions: We have identified three echocardiographic parameters (LVEDD, E/e', and LVOT VTI) that predict HFR following an initial acute HFpEF hospitalization. The prognostic DEI score demonstrated good accuracy.

Keywords: risk stratification; left ventricle end-diastolic diameter; E/e' ratio; left ventricle outflow tract velocity-time integral; hospitalization predictor; short-term prognosis; heart failure readmission

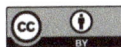

1. Introduction

As the population ages, the number of heart failure (HF) patients appears to be increasing [1–3]. Heart failure with preserved ejection fraction (HFpEF) is becoming a common occurrence in daily practice. From the total number of HF patients, around half have HFpEF [4,5], accounting for a considerable burden on the healthcare system, both as in- and outpatients [3]. Over 90% of the patients with HFpEF are ≥60 years old [6] at the time of diagnosis, and as life expectancy increases the public-health impact of HFpEF is likely to follow the same escalating trend.

HFpEF patients do not respond well to the standard treatment used for patients with heart failure with reduced ejection fraction (HFrEF) and have similar mortality rates [7–9]. Readmission rates increase in parallel with the average number of days spent in the hospital during the initial hospitalization for acute HFpEF [10]. The complex pathophysiology of HFpEF, the heterogeneity of the patient population, and a large number of comorbidities at the age of onset could explain the limited number of therapeutic options and the poor response to treatment. Both US and European HF guidelines have highlighted the importance of recognizing and managing multiple comorbidities, adjusting treatment to the patient phenotype [4,11]. Furthermore, there is an urgent need to identify predictors and trends of HFpEF readmission, as an initial step towards the personalized management of this specific group of patients.

Echocardiography is invaluable in the risk stratification of patients with HFpEF. It is, however, unclear how clinical and echocardiographic data should integrate into the monitoring and prognostic assessment of HFpEF. This study aimed to identify clinical and echocardiographic predictors of disease progression in HFpEF, focusing on the risk of rehospitalization or death after an index hospital admission. As the first hospital admission for HFpEF has a significant impact on short-term prognosis [12,13], we focused our research on patients in this particular group.

2. Materials and Methods

2.1. Study Design

This prospective observational study was performed between April 2017 and March 2020 at Elias Emergency University Hospital (EEUH). A total of 103 consecutive patients during their first hospitalization for acute HFpEF and their characteristics have been analyzed. The study protocol complied with the Declaration of Helsinki and was approved by the Ethics Committee of EEUH. All patients provided written informed consent.

The documented data included: cardiovascular risk factors, associated conditions, medication upon discharge, hemoglobin level, estimated glomerular filtration rate (eGFR), blood sodium, and n-terminal pro-B type natriuretic peptide (NT proBNP) levels. The echocardiography parameters were assessed within the first 24 h according to the ESC guidelines [14–16] using a Vivid T8 Pro (GE Healthcare). Follow-up data were collected at six months.

Patients inclusion criteria were: (1) first hospitalization for acute HF (with clinical signs and symptoms of HF, according to the Framingham criteria) [17], (2) left ventricular ejection fraction (LVEF) $\geq 50\%$ (assessed by echocardiography with the modified Simpson's rule) [4], (3) NT-proBNP >220 pg/mL (in sinus rhythm) and >660 pg/mL (in atrial fibrillation) [18–20], and at least one additional criterion: (A) left ventricle mass index (LVMI) ≥ 115 g/m^2 for males and ≥ 95 g/m^2 for females, or (B) diastolic dysfunction (defined as at least 3 of the following: average E/e'>14, septal e' velocity <7 cm/s or lateral e' velocity <10 cm/s, tricuspid regurgitation velocity >2.8 m/s, left atrial volume index (LAVI) >34 mL/m^2).

Patients exclusion criteria were: (1) significant left heart valve disease (mitral or aortic regurgitation above moderate, mitral or aortic stenosis above mild), (2) severe mitral annulus calcification, (3) acute coronary syndrome, (4) acute pulmonary embolism, (5) pericardial constriction, (6) severe kidney failure (clearance <15 mL/min/1.73 m^2 or dialysis).

Patient follow-up was performed prospectively at six months after admission. Vital status was assessed through scheduled outpatient department appointments, by phone call, or alternatively during readmissions to our hospital.

2.2. End-Points and Study Aim

The primary end-point was the number of heart failure readmissions (HFR). The secondary endpoint was all-cause mortality.

We aimed to identify clinical, biological, and echocardiographic predictors for HFR, and design a prediction score for HFR and all-cause mortality at six months after discharge of patients with first acute event attributable to HFpEF.

2.3. Statistical Analysis

Data for continuous variables are presented as mean ± SD (standard deviation) (%) for uniform distribution or as medians (interquartile range (IQR)) for non-uniform distribution. A t-test or Mann-Whitney U rank-sum/ Wilcoxon rank-difference test was used to compare numerical variables between groups.

Categorical data are reported as numbers (percentages %), and group comparisons have been performed with Pearson's chi-square test and Fischer's exact test.

The variables that were statistically different between patients with HFR and patients without HFR in the cohort were modeled in a univariate fashion using binary logistic regression in order to identify univariable independent predictors among variables, each at a time, with a p-value < 0.05. For each variable we used AUROC (area under the ROC curve) >0.60 and a Hosmer-Lemeshow goodness-of-fit test, p-value > 0.05 as criteria to identify independent variables for the model. The validated independent variables were initially transformed using natural logarithm (ln), and were afterward assembled in multivariate models, which were compared for both discrimination and calibration [21]. The estimation of the multivariate model consisted of a backward stepwise approach (p < 0.10 to enter, p > 0.15 to be removed). The calibration of the predicted models used Akaike's Information Criterion (AIC) and Bayesian Information Criterion (BIC) as tests for Goodness-of-Fit at the lowest values [21]. The probability of HFR at six months according to the modeled score was computed as a function with the remaining variables included. The validation of the results was performed after a random selection of an internal validation contingent of 46 patients from the studied cohort [21].

An optimal threshold was identified in the training cohort (with a maximum Youden index), and the sensitivity and specificity identified were reported. The difference between the two AUROC curves of the training (study) cohort and the validation contingent was calculated using the Hanley & McNeal test.

The odds ratio (OR) was generated for each of the variables identified.

The Kaplan-Meier method was applied to create survival estimates. A Chi-square test was also used to compare the rates of HFR and death between the two groups. All p-values were two-sided and a p-value < 0.05 was considered statistically significant. The statistical analysis was performed with SPSS version 26 (Statistical Package for Social Science, IBM, Armonk, NY, USA: IBM Corp.).

3. Results

3.1. Study Cohort

The study population included 103 hospitalized patients in EEUH between April 2017 and October 2019. Within six months twelve patients were lost to follow-up and eight patients died. Thirty patients were readmitted due to acute decompensation of HFpEF (See Figure 1).

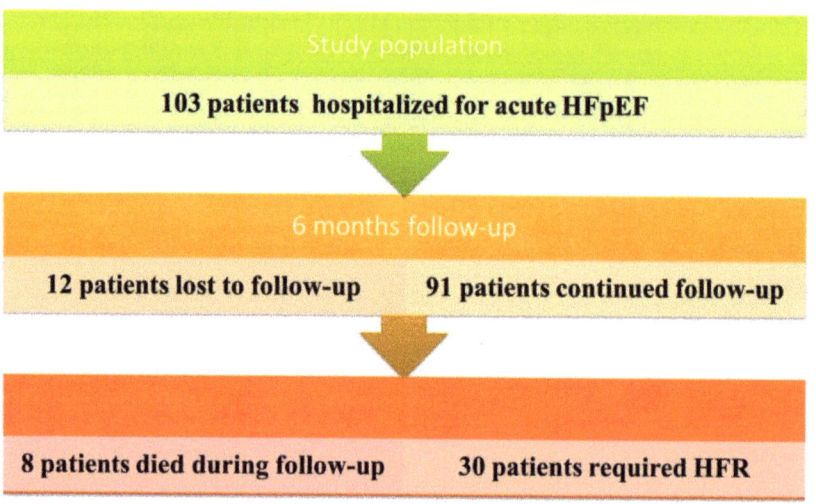

Figure 1. Patient flow-chart at six months. HFR: heart failure readmission, HFpEF: Heart failure with preserved ejection fraction.

3.2. Baseline Characteristics

Overall, 62 women (68%), and 29 men with a mean age of 73.0 years (±10 years) have been included in the study. Demographic, clinical, and laboratory key baseline characteristics of the patients with and without HFR are summarized in Table 1.

Table 1. Complete baseline characteristics of the patients with acute HfpEF according to HFR status ($n = 91$).

Characteristics	No HFR	HFR	p-Value
Number (%)	61 (67.03)	30 (32.96)	
Age at diagnosis, yo, mean ± SD (95% CI)	73.57 ± 10.85 (70.80–75.00)	71.97 ± 10.21 (68.16–75.78)	0.50 *
Female gender, n (%)	39 (63.90%)	23 (76.70%)	
Male gender, n (%)	22 (36.10%)	7 (23.30%)	
Cardiovascular risk factors			
High blood pressure, n (%)	61 (100%)	30 (100%)	1
Diabetes mellitus, n (%)	30 (49.2%)	21 (70%)	0.06 **
Tobacco smoking (current or former), n (%)	17 (27.90%)	8 (26.70%)	0.90 **
Hypercholesterolemia, n (%)	48 (78.70%)	27 (90%)	0.183 **
BMI, median (IQR)	31 (9)	31.50 (7)	0.351 *
Previous medical history			
Medical history of CAD, n (%)	14 (23%)	7 (23.30%)	0.968 **
Medical history of MI, n (%)	9 (14.80%)	4 (13.30%)	0.856 **
Medical history of stroke, n (%)	10 (16.40%)	8 (26.70%)	0.247 **
History of Atrial fibrillation, n (%)	44 (72.10%)	19 (63.30%)	0.393 **
Medical history of lung disease, n (%)	27 (44.30%)	17 (56.70%)	0.266 **
Medical history of sleep apnea, n (%)	6 (9.80%)	6 (20%)	0.178 **

Table 1. Cont.

Characteristics	No HFR	HFR	p-Value
Assessment on admission			
Non-Invasive ventilation on admission, n (%)	12 (19.70%)	8 (26.70%)	0.449 **
Mechanical ventilation on admission, n (%)	5 (8.20%)	1 (3.30%)	0.379 **
Peripheral edema on admission, n (%)	32 (52.50%)	21 (70%)	0.111 **
SaO$_2$ on admission, median (IQR)	90 (7)	88.50 (5)	0.378 ***
HR on admission, median (IQR)	96 (53)	101 (51)	0.609 ***
SBP, mm Hg, mean ± SD (95% CI)	185.25 ± 33.83 (176.58–193.91)	185.83 ± 37.18 (171.95–199.72)	0.94 *
DBP, mm Hg, mean ± SD (95% CI)	98.10 ± 17.18 (93.70–102.50)	101.50 ± 19.83 (94.09–108.91)	0.40 *
Serum natremia, mmol/L, median (IQR)	140 (6)	139 (3)	0.141 ***
eGFR, mL/min/1.73 sqm, mean ± SD (95% CI)	70.29 ± 28.64 (62.95–77.62)	58.86 ± 27.92 (48.43–69.29)	0.075 *
Hb, g/dl, mean±SD (95% CI)	12.27 ± 2.12 (11.73–12.91)	11.36 ± 1.70 (10.72–11.99)	0.043 *
NTproBNP, ng/L, median (IQR)	3563 (6907)	2928 (4256)	0.886 ***
Length of in-hospital stay, days, median (IQR)	7 (5)	8.50 (4)	0.135
Mortality of any cause at six months, n (%)	5 (8.20%)	3 (10%)	0.775

Data are presented as mean ± SD (%), medians, and as numbers (percentages). 95% CI = 95% confidence interval of the difference; IQR: interquartile range. * The p-value was calculated with t-test; ** The p-value was assessed using Pearson Chi Square test for non-parametric variables such as percentages of occurrence of an ordinal or nominal variable, *** The p-value was assessed using Mann-Whitney U test for the continuous variables with abnormal distribution, where skewness and kurtosis were outside the range (−1, +1) and (−2, +2), respectively; ACEI: angiotensin-converting enzyme inhibitors, ARB: angiotensin receptor blockers, BMI: body mass index, CAD: Coronary Artery Disease; DBP: diastolic blood pressure, eGFR: estimated glomerular filtration rate, Hb: Hemoglobin, HR: heart rate, IQR: interquartile range, MI: Myocardial Infarction, SaO2: arterial oxygen saturation, SBP: systolic blood pressure.

A significant proportion of the study population had comorbidities including known cardiovascular risk factors such as: obesity (63%), arterial hypertension (100%), coronary artery disease (23%), hypercholesterolemia (82%), diabetes mellitus (56%), paroxysmal or persistent atrial fibrillation (69%), and chronic kidney disease (43%). Besides the cardiovascular conditions, the patients' medical records included other comorbidities, such as chronic obstructive pulmonary disease (13%), asthma (8%), sleep apnoea syndrome (13%), and cerebrovascular disease (19%). Thirty-nine patients (42%) had impaired lung function tests.

The mean/median values for echocardiographic parameters were calculated, see Table 2.

Table 2. Transthoracic echocardiography features in patients with HFpEF, with and without HFR.

Characteristics	No HFR	HFR	p-Value
Left ventricle			
LV end-diastolic diameter, mm, mean ± SD (95% CI)	46.92 ± 5.97 (45.39–48.45)	49.10 ± 4.02 (47.60–50.60)	0.074 *
LVEF on admission, vol%, mean ± SD (95% CI)	55.62 ± 5.43 (54.23–57.01)	56.27 ± 6.95 (53.67–58.86)	0.63 *
Septal s velocity, cm/s, mean ± SD (95% CI)	6.31 ± 1.23 (5.99–6.62)	6.03 ± 1.11 (5.61–6.45)	0.224 ***
Lateral s velocity, cm/s, mean ± SD (95% CI)	7.37 ± 1.28 (7.04–7.70)	7.28 ± 1.35 (6.77–7.78)	0.918 ***
Left ventricle mass, g/m^2, median (IQR)	120 (36)	127 (37.25)	0.422 ***
LVOT VTI, cm, mean ± SD (95% CI)	18.60 ± 1.74 (17.29–19.91)	21.19 ± 6.41 (18.80–23.59)	0.04
LA index volume, mL, mean ± SD (95% CI)	50.83 ± 11.86 (47.79–53.87)	53.36 ± 12.61 (48.65–58.06)	0.353 *
E/e' ratio, median (IQR)	12.8 (5.25)	15.75 (4.50)	0.001 ***
E/e' > 9, n (%)	52 (85.20%)	30 (100%)	0.027 **
E/e' > 14, n (%)	25 (41%)	22 (73.30%)	0.004 **
Septal e' velocity < 7 cm/s, n (%)	42 (68.90%)	23 (76.70%)	0.438 **
Lateral e' velocity < 10 cm/s, n (%)	39 (69.60%)	25 (83.30%)	0.168 *
Right ventricle, IVC, and right atrium			
Free wall RV S < 9.5, n (%)	8 (13.10%)	4 (13.30%)	0.977 **
TAPSE < 17 mm, n (%)	16 (26.20%)	7 (23.30%)	0.765 **
RA area over 18 cm^2, n (%)	44 (72.10%)	19 (63.30%)	0.393 **
IVC over 21 mm, n (%)	28 (45.90%)	12 (40%)	0.594 **
IVC collapse < 50%, n (%)	25 (41%)	10 (33.30%)	0.481 **
PAPS, mm Hg, mean ± SD (95% CI)	41.22 ± 13.67 (37.72–44.73)	39.90 ± 17.42 (33.39–46.40)	0.692 *
PAPS > 35 mm Hg, n (%)	43 (70.50%)	16 (53.30%)	0.107 **

Data are presented as mean ± SD (%), medians, and as numbers (percentages). 95% CI = 95% confidence interval of the difference. IQR: interquartile range. * The p-value was calculated with t-test; ** The p-value was assessed using Pearson Chi-Square test for non-parametric variables such as percentages of occurrence of an ordinal or nominal variable, *** The p-value was assessed using Mann-Whitney U test for the continuous variables with abnormal distribution, where skewness and kurtosis were outside the range (−1, +1) and (−2, +2), respectively. HF: heart failure, Hb: Hemoglobin, HR: heart rate, IQR: interquartile range, IVC: inferior vena cava, MI: Myocardial Infarction, PAPS: systolic pulmonary artery pressure, SaO2: arterial oxygen saturation, SBP: systolic blood pressure, TAPSE: tricuspid annular plane systolic excursion, LA: left atrium, LV: left ventricle; LVEF: Left ventricle ejection fraction, LVOT VTI: left ventricular outflow tract velocity time integral; RA: right atrium, RV: right ventricle.

3.3. Clinical Features and Outcomes

The clinical presentation of acute HFpEF syndrome was mainly as acute left heart failure (75%) while 25% of the patients presented with predominantly right heart failure. 23% of these patients required respiratory support either as invasive ventilation (6.6%) or non-invasive positive pressure ventilation (22%). The median duration of the index hospitalization was 7.5 (IQR = 5) days.

After six months of follow-up, 30 patients (33%) required HFR, and eight patients (9%) died. Of the 30 patients needing heart failure readmission, two also suffered a stroke. Mortality was classified as: cardiovascular (63%), non-cardiovascular (25%) and of unknown cause (12%).

3.4. Independent Predictors for Short Term HFR

We identified six independent determinants for HFR at six months with a difference ($p < 0.10$) between the two groups of the cohort (with and without HFR at six months). The determinants are: E/e' ratio, level of hemoglobin, left ventricular outflow tract velocity time integral (LVOT VTI), LV end-diastolic diameter (LVEDD), eGFR, and presence of DM. These variables had the highest value at Hosmer and Lemeshow test and an AUC over 0.600 (see Table 3, Table A1). However, these predictors for HFR at six months did not seem to have an influence on all-cause mortality (See Table 1).

Table 3. Selection of the independent variables by bivariate linear regression/univariate analysis.

Variables	Nagelkerke R Square	Hosmer and Lemeshow Test	p-Value Regression Coefficient	AUC	p-Value AUC
E/e' ratio	0.136	0.148	0.004	0.710	0.001
Hb	0.062	0.305	0.047	0.665	0.011
LVOT VTI	0.063	0.888	0.045	0.611	0.085
LVEDD	0.049	0.379	0.079	0.630	0.045
eGFR	0.050	0.584	0.078	0.623	0.056
Diabetes mellitus	0.054	N/A	0.063	0.604	0.108
Serum sodium	0.018	0.124	0.284	0.595	0.143
Lateral s velocity	0.002	0.207	0.745	0.507	0.919
Septal s velocity	0.017	0.343	0.296	0.576	0.239
Medium s velocity	0.009	0.652	0.444	0.523	0.717
BMI	0.013	0.806	0.349	0.545	0.483
LV mass	0.006	0.364	0.524	0.552	0.423
NTproBNP	0.006	0.031	0.550	0.695	0.101

AUC: area under the curve; BMI: body mass index; eGFR: estimated glomerular filtration rate; Hb: hemoglobin; LV: left ventricle; LVOT VTI: left ventricular outflow tract velocity time integral; MI: Myocardial infarction; N/A: not applicable.

Next, the odds ratio (OR) of the six selected clinical and echocardiographic characteristics for HFR at six months were calculated with univariate analysis and are detailed in Table A3, Figure A1.

3.5. Modeling the Score

The six aforementioned parameters, with statistically significant OR for causing an early HFR, were included and computed in a binary logistic regression, with a backward approach in order to identify the predictors to be included in a risk score for readmission at six months after the first hospitalization for acute HFpEF.

The power of prediction of each variable, considered for the role of predictor in the score, was assessed according to the coefficient of determination (Nagelkerke R-square value) between the outcome and each variable determinant.

The model was constructed with binary regression with a backward stepwise method, which started with a model that included all the six independent predictors. At each step a predictor was eliminated from the model, using the Nagelkerke R square and Hosmer & Lemeshow tests for the whole model [21].

In the first step, the initial model (model 1) incorporated all the six variables considered to be predictors: E/e' ratio, level of hemoglobin, LVOT VTI, LVEDD, eGFR, and presence of DM. In the second step, eGFR was eliminated; the second model loses a statistically insignificant ($p = 0.907$) power of prediction (-0.014) compared to model 1 (with all six predictors). In the third step, DM was rejected, as model three has lost -0.707 of its prediction power, with no statistical significance ($p = 0.401$). In step four, Hb was removed from the general model, with a loss of -1.220 of the power of prediction ($p = 0.269$). The general observation was that three variables were cast away from the general model with no significant loss of prediction power, which proves that eGFR, DM, and Hb are not predictors of the model. The other three variables that remained (LVEDD, E/e' ratio, LVOT

VTI) were taken into consideration for the final model of predicting the HFR at six months (see Table A2).

All the three mentioned predictors have an AUC over 0.600 (0.630; 0.710; 0.611), with good statistical significance ($p = 0.059; 0.056; 0.063$) for LVEDD, E/e' ratio, and LVOT VTI respectively (see Figure 2).

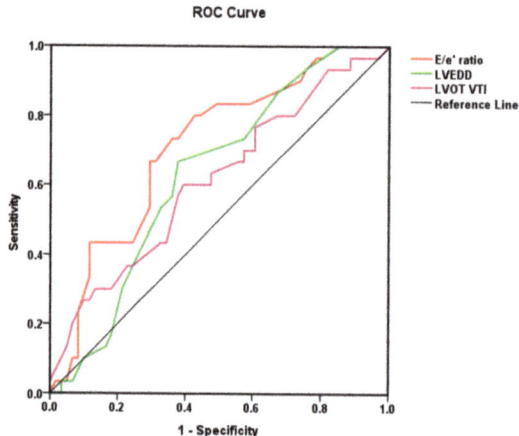

Figure 2. The ROC curve for each of the three independent determinants (LVEDD—green, E/e' ratio—red, LVOT VTI—purple) for HFR at 6 months. AUC are as follows: E/E' ratio = 0.710 ($p = 0.001$), LVEDD = 0.630 ($p = 0.045$), LVOTVTI = 0.611 ($p = 0.085$).

The validation of each predictor variable was assessed by computing the normalized residuals for each of them (see Figure 3). There is no relationship between each of the variables assumed to be predictors of our model and the residuals of the final model, which means each variable forecasts correctly the HFR at six months.

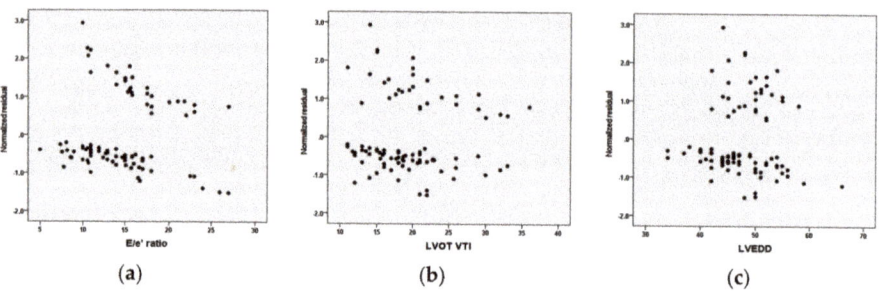

Figure 3. The normalized residuals for the model's predictors: (**a**) E/e' ratio, (**b**) LVOT VTI—left ventricular outflow tract velocity time integral, (**c**) LVEDD- left ventricle end-diastolic diameter.

The next step in modeling the score was to assess the out-of-the-sample prediction error and thereby the relative quality of statistical models for our set of data using the AIC (Aikake's Information Criterion) and BIC (Bayesian Information Criterion) (see Table A4). We have selected model 4 with three predicting variables: E/e' ratio, EDDLV, and LVOT VTI, of all the four prediction models presented in Table A4, according to the lowest AIC and BIC values for the model compared with the three previous models.

3.6. The DEI Score Model

The acronym for the modeled score is DEI, and was constructed based on the components of the scoring system: D (left ventricle end-**D**iastolic diameter), E (**E**/e'ratio), I (left ventricle outflow tract velocity-time **I**ntegral).

The variables used to build the model must fulfill strict criteria at univariate regression such as AUROC > 0.60 and a Hosmer–Lemeshow *p*-Value > 0.05. Non-parametric variables were transformed into parametric variables using natural logarithmic functions. Overall the model proved to be much more balanced and with a better predictive power than each other of the univariate models (see Tables 4 and A4).

Table 4. Multivariate Model Information- statistical characteristics of model 4.

Multivariate Model	Variable 1 $\log_e$ (E/e' Ratio)	Variable 2 $\log_e$ (LVEDD)	Variable 3 $\log_e$ (LVOT VTI)
VIF	1.147	1.113	1.139
Coefficient	1.961	4.558	1.759
Coefficient-Standard Error	0.860	2.488	1.002
Coefficient- Significance	$p = 0.023$	$p = 0.067$	$p = 0.079$
Intercept		−28,763	
Intercept-Standard Error		10.951	
Intercept- Significance		$p = 0.009$	
AUROC		0.746 (0.640—0.853)	
Nagelkerke Pseudo-R^2		0.228	
Hosmer-Lemeshow *p*-value		0.760	
Akaike's Information Criterion (AIC)		107.106	
Bayesian Information Criterion (BIC)		117.150	

The regression equation for our model (LVEDD, E/e' ratio, LVOT VTI) is: Log ODDS RATIO (for HFR at 6 months) = −8.394 + 0.114 × E/e' + 0.088 × LVEDD + 0.087 × VTI LVOT.

The computation of the DEI score is made according to the following formula:

$$\text{DEI Score} = -28.763 + 4.558 \times \log(\text{LVEDD (mm)}) + 1.961 \times \log(\text{E/e' ratio}) + 1.759 \times \log(\text{LVOT VTI (cm)})$$

The cut-off of the DEI score for HFR at six months is over −0.747 (Sensitivity = 73.33%, 95% CI = 54.10–87.70, Specificity = 72.13%, 95% CI = 59.20–82.90) with a positive LR = 2.63 and a negative LR of 0.37 (35).

The Kaplan-Meier curve for HFR according to the DEI score showed that patients with a score over −0.747 presented a statistically significantly higher number of HFR at six months compared to those with a score below −0.747 (Log Rank test $p = 0.001$) (see Figure 4).

A relative amount of 20.50% of HFR during the first six months of follow-up is predicted by our model within the general population with acute HFpEF and a DEI score over −0.747.

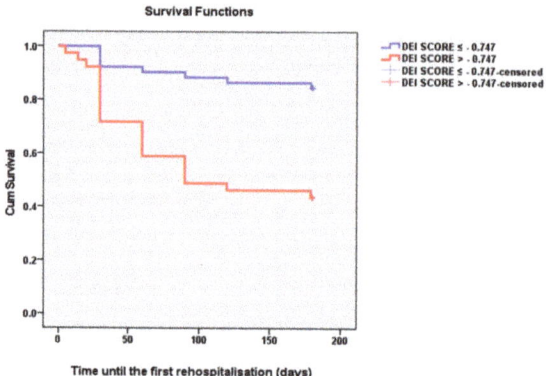

Figure 4. Kaplan-Meier curves according to DEI score for HFR (time in days to readmission) at six months in patients with acute hospitalized HFpEF. The two Kaplan-Meier curves are significantly apart ($p = 0.001$). Low DEI score (≤ -0.747) in blue, high DEI score (> -0.747) in red.

3.7. Validation of the DEI Score

We applied the DEI Score to the validation contingent initially randomized (www.random.com) (See Figure 5). The validation cohort comprised 46 patients, with a ratio of HFR and non-HFR similar to that of the training cohort (1:2).

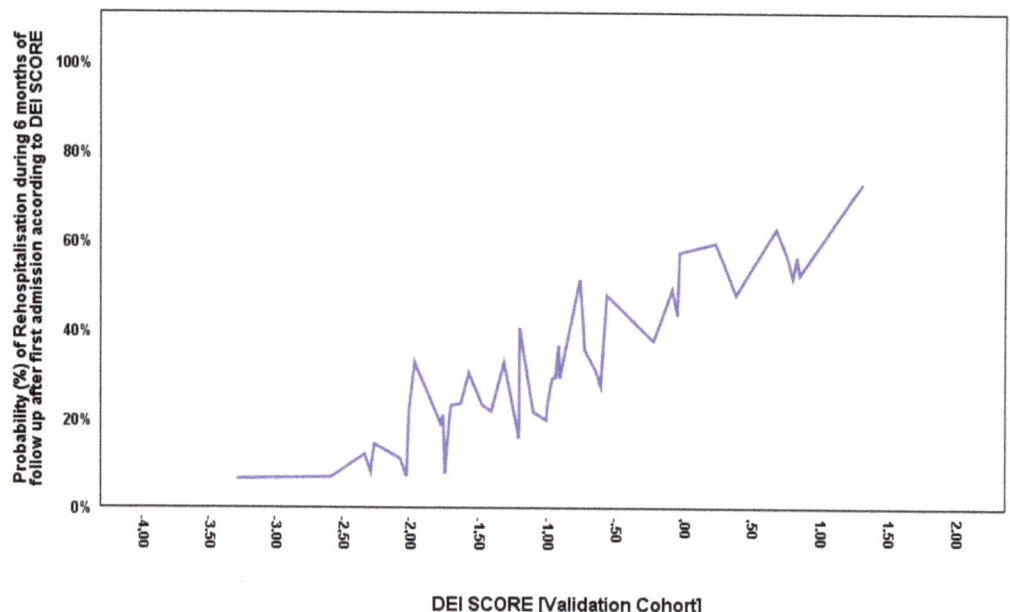

Figure 5. Probability plot of the rehospitalization during six months of follow-up after the first admission according to DEI score, according to the validation cohort.

The validation of the model was assessed further by using ROC curves of the training cohort (AUROC = 0.746, 95% CI = 0.640–0.853, $p = 0.0001$) (see Figures A2 and A3) and validation group (AUROC = 0.690 (95% CI = 0.520–0.861, $p = 0.038$). We computed the possibility of predicting the HFR at six months by comparing AUROC of the training cohort and validation cohort (see Figure 6). The Hanley Mc Neil test has a p-value = 0.47, which means that there is no statistical difference between the two ROC curves of the DEI score (the training cohort of 91 patients and the 46 patients validation contingent) in regard to the HFR at six months after a first acute event of HFpEF.

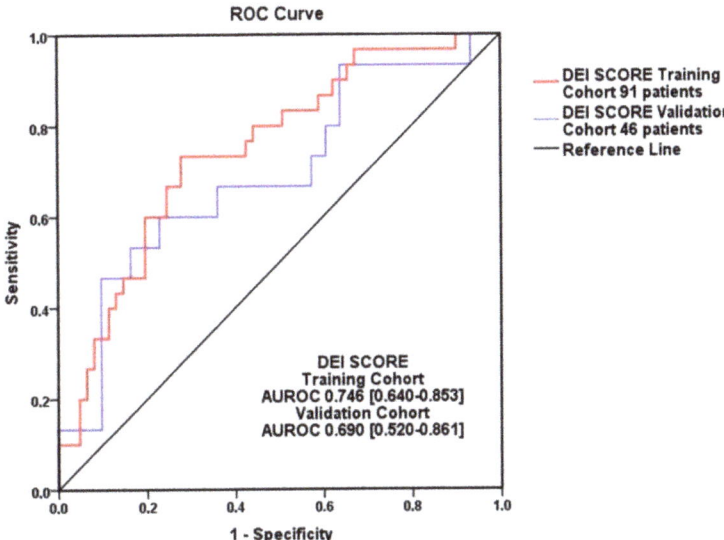

Figure 6. ROC curves of the training cohort (91 patients-red) and validation cohort (46 patients-blue). The two AUROC show close values and no significant differences (Hanley & McNeil test, $p = 0.47$).

We performed an analysis of the DEI Score in the training cohort based on its cut-off values in terms of maximizing sensitivity, specificity, or according to the Youden's Index criteria, and the result is reported in Table A5: (A) a DEI Score ≤ -2.605 showed a 100% sensitivity, 9.84% specificity, 5.5% PPV, 100% NVP, 1.11 +LR; (B) a DEI Score ≥ -0.747 showed a 73.33% sensitivity, 72.13% specificity, 12.2% PPV, 98.1% NVP, 2.63 +LR, 0.37 −LR; (C) a DEI Score ≥ 0.812 showed a 10% sensitivity, 100% specificity, 100% PPV, 95.6% NVP, 0.90 −LR.

We applied this pattern of validation according to cut-off values in the analysis of DEI Score to the validation cohort and noticed a comparable performance.

4. Discussion

Rationale for the study. As the world's population continues to age, a thorough understanding of the characteristics and outcomes of patients with acute HFpEF becomes crucial in reducing the burden of morbidity and mortality caused by this affliction. Therefore the development of risk prediction tools can prove effective in guiding the medical decision for these patients. Consequently, patients estimated to be at higher risk for rehospitalization or death may be treated in a personalized manner.

Added value to current literature. To date, there is a limited number of studies that specifically address heart failure with preserved ejection fraction, especially since the current registries report on heart failure, in general, as one entity [22,23]. The current literature also largely fails to concentrate on the subject of HFpEF with acute presentations.

To the best of our knowledge, the current study is the first to include only patients hospitalized for the first time with acute HFpEF. The study looks for prognostic and prediction tools to be used in this group of patients, considering that the specific moment of the first hospital admission is a turning point in the evolution of heart failure.

The DEI risk score, based on echocardiographic predictors, could prove to be a convenient instrument to evaluate the patient's prognosis and, at the same time, prescribe recommendations for follow-up as early as the initial presentation in the emergency department. These features render it a useful tool, with good accuracy for the management of patients suffering from acute heart failure with preserved ejection fraction.

In the era of COVID-19, when emergency rooms and intensive care facilities are facing high pressure, we propose assessment of patients with acute HFpEF by means of the DEI risk score in order to estimate their short-term prognosis and those in need of closer monitoring.

Comparison to similar studies. The study population and several characteristics were found to be relatively similar to other studies. For instance, lower hemoglobin levels seemed to enhance the need for rehospitalization in our study group, as previously demonstrated [24]. Moreover, lower hemoglobin levels have been associated with a longer hospital stay. Studies using machine learning have managed to identify prediction models for chronic HFpEF [25] that included the hemoglobin level and the glomerular filtration rate, two parameters we have also found to be of importance in our population.

Our study identified some interesting correlations between echo-graphic findings and the likelihood of rehospitalization at six months for patients with acute HFpEF. Our finding that LVOT VTI is a determinant of HFR, with higher values predicting HFR, is in contrast with a recent study of Omote et al. which associated a lower value with a worse outcome [26]. However, Omote et.al used a composite index (all-cause mortality and HFR) and followed the patients in the long-term. The present study focused on the first six months, and the outcome was HFR alone, not a composite index. Our data show that early on in the evolution of HFpEF, a slightly higher LVOT VTI is associated with more hospitalizations. This might indicate that, in the course of the disease, LVOT VTI does not show a linear decline. After an initial adaptative rise, linked to an increased left ventricular mass and increased filling pressures associated with more hospitalizations, the LVOT VTI starts to decline and the prognosis is worse in the long term. The higher ventricular mass is explained in part by the fact that 100% of our study population was hypertensive, thus explaining a worse relaxation profile.

Currently, risk assessment is based on a combination of clinical biomarkers and several generally recognized echocardiographic parameters [27]. Still, risk prediction can be improved by including left ventricle echocardiographic parameters such as LVEDD, LVOT VTI, and the E/e' ratio in the diagnostic algorithm. The applicability of non-sophisticated, accessible parameters such as these is what renders the DEI score a useful clinical instrument.

Ultimately, in our study, the predictors for HFR did not correlate with all-cause mortality which was not an unexpected finding since other studies have demonstrated that the predictors for rehospitalization and mortality are not the same [28]. On the other hand, a six months follow-up may not be enough to allow mortality predictors identification.

Study limitations. The calculations were made on a limited number of patients from a single-center. The relatively small number of patients was due to the strict inclusion criteria. Moreover, we included only patients hospitalized for the first episode of acute HFpEF. The follow-up period is short because the focus of our study was early heart failure readmissions. However, the monitoring will continue for another 18 months. A potential limit of the present study is the lack of evaluation of pulmonary congestion using lung ultrasound (LUS) that was shown to be of prognostic value in recent studies [29,30].

Future directions. The population characteristics, their correlations, and the risk score identified in this study need to be further addressed in larger randomized studies of acute HFpEF. Furthermore, a comparison between outpatients with HFpEF and patients presenting to the hospital with acute HFpEF would bring additional important information. We also plan to instate an online calculator for the DEI score.

5. Conclusions

Early rehospitalization of patients with a first acute HFpEF event is predicted by several echocardiographic parameters included in the DEI score ((left ventricle end-**D**iastolic diameter), (**E**/e'ratio), (left ventricle outflow tract velocity-time **I**ntegral).). However, all-cause mortality does not seem to be influenced by these heart failure readmission predictors in the short-term.

Author Contributions: Conceptualization, M.-B.Z., L.N.G. and M.-R.P.; data curation, M.-B.Z. and G.C.B.; formal analysis, L.N.G., M.-R.P. and G.C.B.; investigation, M.-B.Z., L.N.G. and M.-R.P.; Methodology, M.-B.Z.; project administration, M.-B.Z., S.G.M. and M.D.; software, L.N.G., M.-R.P. and G.C.B.; supervision, A.-C.P., S.G.M. and M.D.; validation, A.-C.P.; visualization, L.N.G. and M.-R.P.; writing original draft, M.-B.Z., L.N.G. and M.-R.P.; writing, review & editing, L.N.G., M.-R.P., I.M.G. and S.G.M. All authors have read and agreed to the published version of the manuscript.

Funding: This research received no external funding.

Institutional Review Board Statement: The study was conducted according to the guidelines of the Declaration of Helsinki, and approved by Ethics Committee of EEUH/April 2017 (protocol code 9433 and 20.10.2016 of approval).

Informed Consent Statement: Informed consent was obtained from all subjects involved in the study.

Data Availability Statement: All data is on hospital records, all data is available on request.

Acknowledgments: The authors of this paper would like to express gratitude to Kostantinos Dimopoulos from Royal Brompton Hospital, London, UK for the valuable suggestions and amendments, and to offer thanks to their colleagues from the Coronary Care Unit of EEUH for their dedication, support, and contribution.

Conflicts of Interest: The authors declare no conflict of interest.

Appendix A

Table A1. Univariate analysis. Intracohort statistically significant variables were studied univariately.

Univariate Analysis	E/e' Ratio	Hb	LVOT VTI	LVEDD	eGRF	DM
Intercept ($\beta 0$)	−3.015	2.012	−2.310	−4.345	0.249	−1.237
Intercept ($\beta 0$)-Standard Error	0.852	1.378	0.840	2.079	0.573	0.379
Intercept ($\beta 0$)-Significance (p-value)	<0.001	0.144	0.006	0.038	0.664	0.210
Coefficient ($\beta 1$)	0.154	−0.230	0.081	0.076	−0.015	0.880
Coefficient ($\beta 1$)- Standard Error	0.054	0.116	0.04	0.043	0.008	0.474
Coefficient ($\beta 1$)- Significance (p-value)	0.004	0.047	0.045	0.079	0.078	0.063
AUROC	0.710 (0.600–0.821)	0.665 (0.550–0.780)	0.611 (0.487–0.736)	0.630 (0.514–0.745)	0.623 (0.497–0.750)	0.604 (0.482–0.726)
Nagelkerke Pseudo-R^2	0.136	0.062	0.063	0.049	0.050	0.054
Hosmer-Lemeshow p-value	0.148	0.305	0.888	0.379	0.584	
AIC	70.532	91.807	68.154	51.665	110.504	12.162
BIC	75.554	96.828	73.176	56.687	115.525	17.184

Hb: hemoglobin; LVOT VTI: left ventricular outflow tract velocity time integral; LVEDD: left ventricular end-diastolic diameter; eGRF: estimated glomerular filtration rate; DM: diabetes mellitus.

Table A2. Variables in the Equation of the model, backward approach.

		B	S.E.	Wald	df	Sig.	Exp(B)	95% C.I. for EXP(B)	
								Lower	Upper
Step 1 [a]	E/e'	0.093	0.058	2.572	1	0.109	1.098	0.980	1.230
	VSTD	0.098	0.053	3.427	1	0.064	1.103	0.994	1.223
	VTI_LVOT	0.058	0.052	1.263	1	0.261	1.060	0.958	1.173
	Hb	−0.130	0.135	0.920	1	0.337	0.878	0.673	1.145
	eGFR	−0.001	0.010	0.014	1	0.907	0.999	0.979	1.019
	DM	−0.465	0.599	0.601	1	0.438	0.628	0.194	2.034
	Constant	−6.162	3.430	3.229	1	0.072	0.002		
Step 2 [a]	E/e'	0.093	0.058	2.603	1	0.107	1.098	0.980	1.230
	VSTD	0.099	0.052	3.607	1	0.058	1.104	0.997	1.222
	VTI_LVOT	0.059	0.051	1.304	1	0.253	1.060	0.959	1.173
	Hb	−0.135	0.129	1.099	1	0.295	0.874	0.679	1.125
	DM	−0.483	0.578	.699	1	0.403	0.617	0.199	1.915
	Constant	−6242	3.368	3.435	1	0.064	0.002		
Step 3 [a]	E/e'	0.107	0.056	3.624	1	0.057	1.112	0.997	1.241
	VSTD	0.091	0.050	3.282	1	0.070	1.095	0.993	1.208
	VTI_LVOT	0.070	0.049	1.974	1	0.160	1.072	0.973	1.181
	Hb	−0.141	0.129	1.194	1	0.275	0.869	0.675	1.118
	Constant	−6.390	3.345	3.649	1	0.056	0.002		
Step 4 [a]	E/e'	0.114	0.055	4.314	1	0.038	0.121	1.006	1.248
	VSTD	0.088	0.050	3.141	1	0.076	1.092	0.991	1.204
	VTI_LVOT	0.087	0.047	3.450	1	0.063	1.091	0.995	1.196
	Constant	−8.394	2.860	8.616	1	0.003	0.000		

[a] Variable(s) entered on step 1: E/E', VSTD, VTI_LVOT, Hb, eMDRD, DMtotal.

Table A3. Odds ratio (OR) for HFR at six months.

Characteristics	Odds Ratio	95% CI	p-Value *
DM present	2.411	0.953–6.101	0.06
Serum sodium	0.949	0.864–1.044	0.284
eGFR (mL/min/1.73 sqm)	0.985	0.969–1.002	0.078
Hb (g/dL)	0.794	0.633–0.997	0.047
LVEDD (mm)	1.079	0.991–1.174)	0.079
E/e' ratio	1.167	1.050–1.297	0.004
LVOT VTI (cm)	1.084	1.002–1.173	0.045

* p-value (Pearson chi-square); 95% CI: 95% confidence interval. CVR: cardiovascular readmission; DM: diabetes mellitus; eGFR: estimated glomerular filtration rate; Hb: hemoglobin; LVEDD: left ventricle end-diastolic diameter; LVOT VTI: left ventricle outflow tract velocity-time integral.

Table A4. Goodness of Fit assessment of the models. The AIC and BIC tests.

Nr.	MODEL	AIC	AICC	BIC	Nagelkerke R Square	Hosmer Lemeshow Test	p-Value Test OMNIBUS
1	E/e' Hb VSTD VTI LVOT DM eGFR	112.937	114.286	130.513	0.230	0.108	0.012
2	E/e' VSTD VTI LVOT Hb DM	110.951	111.951	126.016	0.230	0.033	0.006
3	E/e' VSTD VTI LVOT Hb	109.657	110.363	122.212	0.221	0.204	0.003
4	E/e' VSTD VTI LVOT	108.877	109.342	118.920	0.205	0.881	0.002

Table A5. Cut-off model. The criteria for choosing values of cut-off points in the training cohort were represented by maximizing either sensitivity or specificity or according to the Youden's Index criteria.

Cut-Off Value Selection	Maximize Sensitivity ≤ 2.605		Maximize Specificity > 0.812		Youden's Index = 0.454 Associated Criterion > 0.747	
	Training	Validation	Training	Validation	Training	Validation
Sensitivity (%)	100 (88.4–100)	100 (78.2–100)	10 (2.1–26.5)	13.33 (1.7–40.5)	73.33 (54.1–87.7)	60 (32.3–83.7)
Specificity (%)	9.84 (3.7–20.2)	6.45 (0.8–21.4)	100 (94.1–100)	100 (88.8–100)	72.13 (59.2–82.9)	77.42 (58.9–90.4)
PPV (%)	5.5 (5.1–6)	5.3 (4.9–5.8)%	100	100	12.2 (8.1–18)	12.3 (6.1–23.2)
NPV (%)	100	100	95.5 (94.9–96)	95.6 (94.7–96.4)	98.1 (96.5–99)	97.4 (95.1–98.6)
+LR	1.11 (1–1.1)	1.07 (1–1.2)	*	*	2.63 (1.7–4.2)	2.66 (1.2–5.7)
−LR	0	0	0.90 (0.8–1)	1 (1.0–1.0)	0.37 (0.2–0.7)	0.52 (0.3–1.0)

* very high value; PPV: positive predictive value; NPV: negative predictive value; +LR: positive likelihood ratio; −LR: negative likelihood ratio.

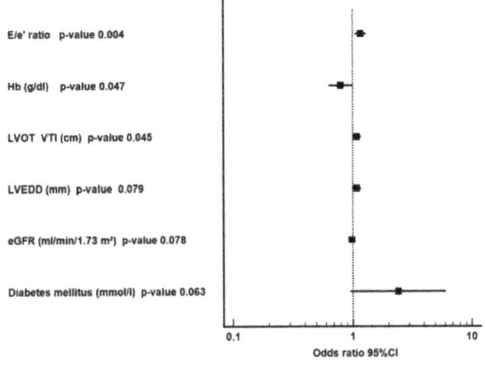

Figure A1. Forest plot for HFR predictors at 6 months. Point estimates represent the multivariable odds ratio for HFR after six months; whiskers indicate a 95% confidence interval (CI).

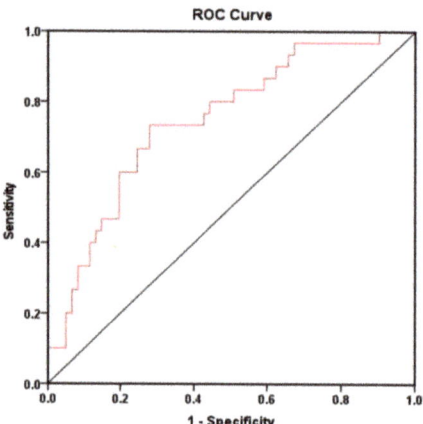

Figure A2. The ROC curve for the values of the DEI Score in the training cohort according to HFR during the 6 months from the first episode of HFpEF. AUROC = 0.746, 95% CI (0.640–0.853), $p = 0.0001$.

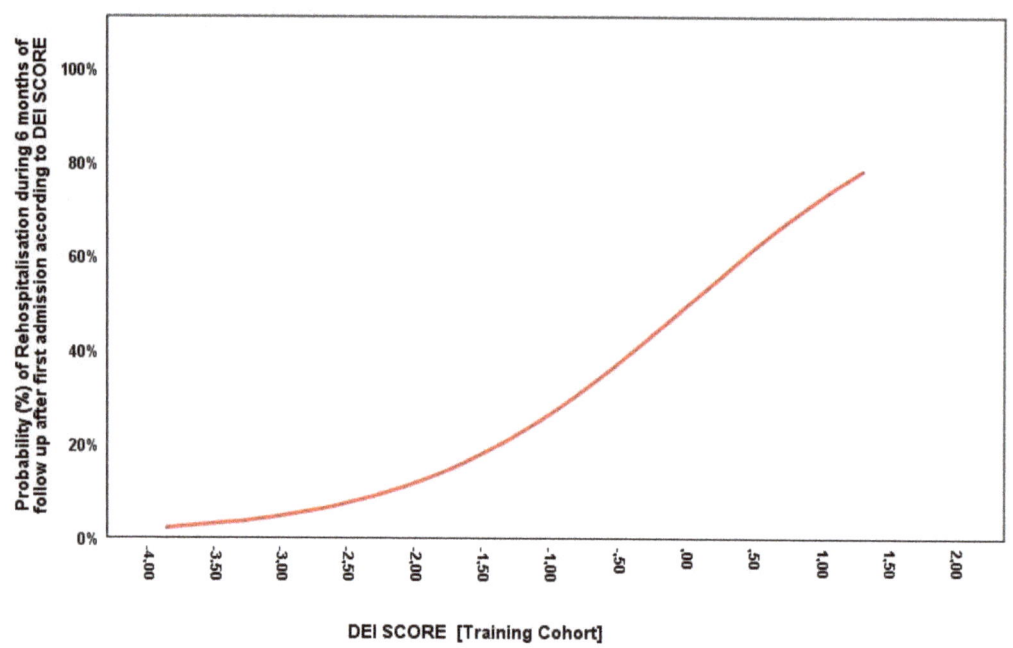

Figure A3. Probability plot of the HFR during 6 months of follow up after the first admission according to the DEI score.

References

1. Bleumink, G.S.; Knetsch, M.; Sturkenboom, M.C.J.M.; Straus, S.M.J.M.; Hofman, A.; Deckers, J.W.; Witteman, J.C.M.; Stricker, B.H.C. Quantifying the heart failure epidemic: Prevalence, incidence rate, lifetime risk and prognosis of heart failure—The Rotterdam Study. *Eur. Heart J.* **2004**, *25*, 1614–1619.
2. Owan, T.E.; Hodge, D.O.; Herges, R.M.; Jacobsen, S.J.; Roger, V.L.; Redfield, M.M. Trends in prevalence and outcome of heart failure with preserved ejection fraction. *N. Engl. J. Med.* **2006**, *355*, 251–259. Available online: https://pubmed.ncbi.nlm.nih.gov/16855265/ (accessed on 25 January 2021).

3. Hashemi, D.; Dettmann, L.; Trippel, T.D.; Holzendorf, V.; Petutschnigg, J.; Wachter, R.; Hasenfuß, G.; Pieske, B.; Zapf, A.; Edelmann, F. Economic impact of heart failure with preserved ejection fraction: Insights from the ALDO-DHF trial. *ESC Heart Fail.* **2020**, *7*, 786–793.
4. Ponikowski, P.; Voors, A.A.; Anker, S.D.; Bueno, H.; Cleland, J.G.F.; Coats, A.J.S.; Falk, V.; González-Juanatey, J.R.; Harjola, V.P.; Jankowska, E.A.; et al. 2016 ESC Guidelines for the diagnosis and treatment of acute and chronic heart failure. *Eur. Heart J.* **2016**, *37*, 2129–2200.
5. Arora, S.; Lahewala, S.; Hassan Virk, H.U.; Setareh-Shenas, S.; Patel, P.; Kumar, V.; Tripathi, B.; Shah, H.; Patel, V.; Gidwani, U.; et al. Etiologies, trends, and predictors of 30-day readmissions in patients with diastolic heart failure. *Am. J. Cardiol.* **2017**, *120*, 616–624. [CrossRef]
6. Borlaug, B.A. The pathophysiology of heart failure with preserved ejection fraction. *Nat. Rev. Cardiol.* **2014**, *11*, 507–515.
7. Metra, M.; Teerlink, J.R.; Cotter, G.; Davison, B.A.; Felker, G.M.; Filippatos, G.; Greenberg, B.H.; Pang, P.S.; Ponikowski, P.; Voors, A.A.; et al. Effects of serelaxin in patients with acute heart failure. *N. Engl. J. Med.* **2019**, *381*, 716–726. [CrossRef]
8. Tromp, J.; Bamadhaj, S.; Cleland, J.G.F.; Angermann, C.E.; Dahlstrom, U.; Ouwerkerk, W.; Tay, W.T.; Dickstein, K.; Ertl, G.; Hassanein, M.; et al. Post-discharge prognosis of patients admitted to hospital for heart failure by world region, and national level of income and income disparity (REPORT-HF): A cohort study. *Lancet Glob. Health* **2020**, *8*, e411–e422.
9. Shah, K.S.; Xu, H.; Matsouaka, R.A.; Bhatt, D.L.; Heidenreich, P.A.; Hernandez, A.F.; Devore, A.D.; Yancy, C.W.; Fonarow, G.C. Heart Failure With Preserved, Borderline, and Reduced Ejection Fraction 5-Year Outcomes. *J. Am. Coll. Cardiol.* **2017**, *70*, 2476–2486. [CrossRef]
10. Steinberg, B.A.; Zhao, X.; Heidenreich, P.A.; Peterson, E.D.; Bhatt, D.L.; Cannon, C.P.; Hernandez, A.F.; Fonarow, G.C. Trends in patients hospitalized with heart failure and preserved left ventricular ejection fraction: Prevalence, therapies, and outcomes. *Circulation* **2012**, *126*, 65–75.
11. Yancy, C.W.; Jessup, M.; Bozkurt, B.; Butler, J.; Casey, D.E.; Colvin, M.M.; Drazner, M.H.; Filippatos, G.S.; Fonarow, G.C.; Givertz, M.M.; et al. 2017 ACC/AHA/HFSA focused update of the 2013 ACCF/AHA guideline for the management of heart failure: A report of the american college of cardiology/American heart association task force on clinical practice guidelines and the heart failure society of amer. *Circulation* **2017**, *136*, e137–e161.
12. Gheorghiade, M.; De Luca, L.; Fonarow, G.C.; Filippatos, G.; Metra, M.; Francis, G.S. Pathophysiologic targets in the early phase of acute heart failure syndromes. *Am. J. Cardiol.* **2005**, *96*, 11–17.
13. Gheorghiade, M.; Zannad, F.; Sopko, G.; Klein, L.; Piña, I.L.; Konstam, M.A.; Massie, B.M.; Roland, E.; Targum, S.; Collins, S.P.; et al. Acute heart failure syndromes: Current state and framework for future research. *Circulation* **2005**, *112*, 3958–3968.
14. Lang, R.M.; Badano, L.P.; Victor, M.A.; Afilalo, J.; Armstrong, A.; Ernande, L.; Flachskampf, F.A.; Foster, E.; Goldstein, S.A.; Kuznetsova, T.; et al. Recommendations for cardiac chamber quantification by echocardiography in adults: An update from the American Society of Echocardiography and the European Association of Cardiovascular Imaging. *J. Am. Soc. Echocardiogr.* **2015**, *28*, 1–39.e14. [CrossRef]
15. Nagueh, S.F.; Smiseth, O.A.; Appleton, C.P.; Byrd, B.F.; Dokainish, H.; Edvardsen, T.; Flachskampf, F.A.; Gillebert, T.C.; Klein, A.L.; Lancellotti, P.; et al. Recommendations for the Evaluation of Left Ventricular Diastolic Function by Echocardiography: An Update from the American Society of Echocardiography and the European Association of Cardiovascular Imaging. *J. Am. Soc. Echocardiogr.* **2016**, *29*, 277–314. [CrossRef]
16. Chetrit, M.; Cremer, P.C.; Klein, A.L. Imaging of diastolic dysfunction in community-based epidemiological studies and randomized controlled trials of HFpEF. *JACC Cardiovasc. Imaging* **2020**, *13*, 310–326. [CrossRef]
17. Mckee, P.A.; Castelli, W.P.; Mcnamara, P.M.; Kannel, W.B. The natural history of congestive heart failure: The framingham study. *N. Engl. J. Med.* **1971**, *285*, 1441–1446. Available online: https://pubmed.ncbi.nlm.nih.gov/5122894/ (accessed on 25 January 2021).
18. Pieske, B.; Butler, J.; Filippatos, G.; Lam, C.; Maggioni, A.P.; Ponikowski, P.; Shah, S.; Solomon, S.; Kraigher-Krainer, E.; Samano, E.T.; et al. Rationale and design of the SOluble guanylate Cyclase stimulatoR in heArT failurE Studies (SOCRATES). *Eur. J. Heart Fail.* **2014**, *16*, 1026–1038.
19. Lam, C.S.P.; Rienstra, M.; Tay, W.T.; Liu, L.C.Y.; Hummel, Y.M.; Van der Meer, P.; De Boer, R.A.; Van Gelder, I.C.; Van Veldhuisen, D.J.; Voors, A.A.; et al. Atrial fibrillation in heart failure with preserved ejection fraction: Association with exercise capacity, left ventricular filling pressures, natriuretic peptides, and left atrial volume. *JACC Heart Fail.* **2017**, *5*, 92–98.
20. Pieske, B.; Tschö Pe, C.; De Boer, R.A.; Fraser, A.G.; Anker, S.D.; Donal, E.; Edelmann, F.; Fu, M.; Guazzi, M.; Lam, C.S.P.; et al. How to diagnose heart failure with preserved ejection fraction: The HFA-PEFF diagnostic algorithm: A consensus recommendation from the Heart Failure Association (HFA) of the European Society of Cardiology (ESC) Heart failure/cardiomyopathy. *Eur. Heart J.* **2019**, *40*, 3297–3317. Available online: https://academic.oup.com/eurheartj/article-abstract/40/40/3297/5557740 (accessed on 25 January 2021).
21. Sambataro, G.; Giuffrè, M.; Sambataro, D.; Palermo, A.; Vignigni, G.; Cesareo, R.; Crimi, N.; Torrisi, S.E.; Vancheri, C.; Malatino, L.; et al. The Model for Early COVID-19 Recognition (MECOR) score: A proof-of-concept for a simple and low-cost tool to recognize a possible viral etiology in community-acquired pneumonia patients during COVID-19 outbreak. *Diagnostics* **2020**, *10*, 619.

22. Chioncel, O.; Vinereanu, D.; Datcu, M.; Ionescu, D.D.; Capalneanu, R.; Brukner, I.; Dorobantu, M.; Ambrosy, A.; MacArie, C.; Gheorghiade, M. The Romanian Acute Heart Failure Syndromes (RO-AHFS) registry. *Am. Heart J.* **2011**, *162*, 142–153.e1. [CrossRef]
23. Chioncel, O.; Tatu-Chițoiu, G.; Christodorescu, R.; Coman, I.M.; Deleanu, D.; Vinereanu, D.; Macarie, C.; Crespo, M.; Laroche, C.; Fereirra, T.; et al. Characteristics of patients with heart failure from Romania enrolled in—ESC-HF Long-Term (ESC-HF-LT) Registry. *Rom. J. Cardiol.* **2015**, *25*, 413–420. Available online: https://www.romanianjournalcardiology.ro/arhiva/characteristics-of-patients-with-heart-failure-from-romania-enrolled-in-esc-hf-long-term-esc-hf-lt-registry/ (accessed on 25 January 2021).
24. Gupta, K.; Kalra, R.; Rajapreyar, I.; Joly, J.M.; Pate, M.; Cribbs, M.G.; Ather, S.; Prabhu, S.D.; Bajaj, N.S. Anemia, Mortality, and Hospitalizations in Heart Failure With a Preserved Ejection Fraction (from the TOPCAT Trial). *Am. J. Cardiol.* **2020**, *125*, 1347–1354.
25. Angraal, S.; Mortazavi, B.J.; Gupta, A.; Khera, R.; Ahmad, T.; Desai, N.R.; Jacoby, D.L.; Masoudi, F.A.; Spertus, J.A.; Krumholz, H.M. Machine Learning Prediction of Mortality and Hospitalization in Heart Failure With Preserved Ejection Fraction. *JACC Heart Fail.* **2020**, *8*, 12–21.
26. Omote, K.; Nagai, T.; Iwano, H.; Tsujinaga, S.; Kamiya, K.; Aikawa, T.; Konishi, T.; Sato, T.; Kato, Y.; Komoriyama, H.; et al. Left ventricular outflow tract velocity time integral in hospitalized heart failure with preserved ejection fraction. *ESC Heart Fail.* **2020**, *7*, 167–175.
27. Przewlocka-Kosmala, M.; Marwick, T.H.; Yang, H.; Wright, L.; Negishi, K.; Kosmala, W. Association of Reduced Apical Untwisting With Incident HF in Asymptomatic Patients With HF Risk Factors. *JACC Cardiovasc. Imaging* **2020**, *13*, 187–194.
28. Voors, A.A.; Ouwerkerk, W.; Zannad, F.; Van Veldhuisen, D.J.; Samani, N.J.; Ponikowski, P.; Ng, L.L.; Metra, M.; Ter Maaten, J.M.; Lang, C.C.; et al. Development and validation of multivariable models to predict mortality and hospitalization in patients with heart failure. *Eur. J. Heart Fail.* **2017**, *19*, 627–634.
29. Pugliese, N.R.; Biase, D.; Gargani, L.; Mazzola, M.; Conte, L.; Fabiani, I.; Natali, A.; Dini, F.L.; Frumento, P.; Rosada, J.; et al. Predicting the transition to and progression of heart failure with preserved ejection fraction: A weighted risk score using bio-humoural, cardiopulmonary, and echocardiographic stress testing. *Eur. J. Prev. Cardiol.* **2021**. [CrossRef]
30. Kobayashi, M.; Gargani, L.; Palazzuoli, A.; Ambrosio, G.; Bayés-Genis, A.; Lupon, J.; Pellicori, P.; Pugliese, N.R.; Reddy, Y.N.V.; Ruocco, G.; et al. Association between right-sided cardiac function and ultrasound-based pulmonary congestion on acutely decompensated heart failure: Findings from a pooled analysis of four cohort studies. *Clin. Res. Cardiol.* **2020**, 1–12. [CrossRef]

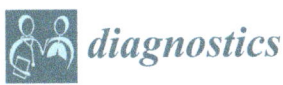

Review

The Role of Echocardiography in the Management of Heart Transplant Recipients

Daniele Masarone [1,*], Michelle Kittleson [2], Rita Gravino [1], Fabio Valente [1], Andrea Petraio [3] and Giuseppe Pacileo [1]

[1] Heart Failure Unit, Department of Cardiology, AORN dei Colli-Monaldi Hospital, 80131 Naples, Italy; rita.gravino@ospedalideicolli.it (R.G.); fabio.valente@ospedalideicolli.it (F.V.); giuseppe.pacileo@ospedalideicolli.it (G.P.)
[2] Department of Cardiology, Smidt Heart Institute, Cedars-Sinai, Los Angeles, CA 90048, USA; michelle.kittleson@cshs.org
[3] Heart Transplant Unit, Department of Cardiac Surgery and Transplantology, AORN dei Colli-Monaldi Hospital, 80131 Naples, Italy; andrea.petraio@ospedalideicolli.it
* Correspondence: daniele.masarone@ospedalideicolli.it

Abstract: Transthoracic echocardiography is the primary non-invasive modality for the investigation of heart transplant recipients. It is a versatile tool that provides comprehensive information on cardiac structure and function. Echocardiography is also helpful in diagnosing primary graft dysfunction and evaluating the effectiveness of therapeutic approaches for this condition. In acute rejection, echocardiography is useful with suspected cellular or antibody-mediated rejection, with findings confirmed and quantified by endomyocardial biopsy. For identifying chronic rejection, ultrasound has a more significant role and, in some specific patients (e.g., patients with renal failure), it may offer a role comparable to coronary angiography to identify cardiac allograft vasculopathy. This review highlights the usefulness of echocardiography in evaluating normal graft function and its role in the management of heart transplant recipients.

Keywords: echocardiography; heart transplant; cardiac allograft vasculopathy; heart transplant rejection

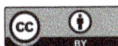

1. Introduction

Heart transplantation remains the gold-standard therapy for patients with advanced heart failure despite optimal medical treatment [1]. Over the past four decades, remarkable advances in diagnostic methods for early identification of acute and chronic rejection and in immunosuppressive therapy have resulted in a marked increase in long-term survival, with a current one-year survival rate after heart transplantation of 90% and a conditional half-life of over 13 years [2]. Echocardiography is a fundamental tool for adequately managing heart transplant recipients (HTRs), from monitoring the immediate post-operative period to surveillance of early and late post-transplant complications [3]. This review summarizes the basic principles for using echocardiography in cardiac transplant patients to allow even cardiologists not experienced in transplantation to apply this technology in the management of HTR correctly.

2. Normal Cardiac Allograft Structure and Function

Echocardiography is the first-line imaging modality for evaluating HTRs, providing accurate graft anatomy and function information, and should be part of all post-transplant follow-up visits. Current International Society for Heart and Lung Transplantation (ISHLT) guidelines for managing HTRs do not specify the timing of echocardiographic evaluations or recommend echocardiography as an alternative to endomyocardial biopsy in monitoring rejection [4]. However, echocardiography is routinely used when high clinical suspicion exists of acute graft rejection and for monitoring left ventricular function during episodes of acute graft rejection.

The echocardiographic evaluation of the graft is based on the assessment of the same morphological and functional parameters that are considered for the native heart. However, the results of this evaluation must be interpreted considering the pathophysiology of the transplanted heart; therefore, the main morphological and functional aspects to be considered normal in HTRs will be briefly described.

2.1. Left Ventricular Morphology and Function

In the first few months after heart transplantation, left ventricular mass and thickness increase due to graft edema and inflammatory cell infiltration (Figure 1) [5].

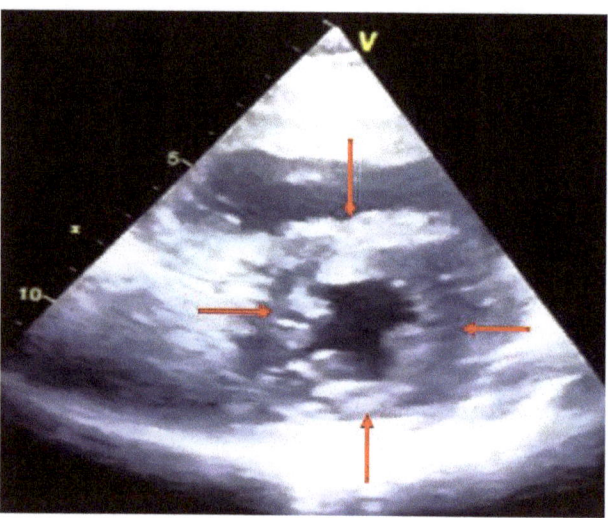

Figure 1. Short-axis view at trans thoracic echocardiography two months after heart transplantation. Note the concentric and symmetric hypertrophy of the left ventricle (red arrows).

Left ventricular mass and wall thicknesses generally normalize within three months, so the persistence of left ventricular hypertrophy after this period is typically due to arterial hypertension secondary to immunosuppressive treatment and/or repeated episodes of acute rejection. Typically, the left ventricular ejection fraction and regional wall motion (except for frequent and common septal dyskinesia) are preserved in most HTRs for 10 to 15 years, unless cardiac allograft vasculopathy (CAV) develops. In addition, a decrease in left ventricular systolic function during the first year is a predictor of allograft rejection or CAV. In contrast, a late (>5 years) reduction in ejection fraction after heart transplantation correlates with CAV progression [6].

In contrast to assessment of ejection fraction, the assessment of diastolic function in HTRs is complicated by several factors and no single parameter can identify diastolic dysfunction of the graft [7]. The elevated heart rate of the denervated heart results in E-wave and A-wave fusion [8]. Pulmonary vein flows are frequently from the contraction of the recipient's atrial tissue. Tissue Doppler imaging parameters are also altered in the graft; the e'- and a'-wave velocities are lower than those of the general population [9]. In addition, the diastolic function may be altered due to ischemia of the graft [10] or precapillary pulmonary hypertension of the recipient. Therefore, restrictive pathophysiology is common in the immediate post-transplant period and has no prognostic value. In contrast, the persistence of a significant alteration in diastolic function later after transplant [11] has a negative prognostic impact and is often related to inflammation, fibrosis, and allograft vasculopathy.

2.2. Right Ventricular Morphology and Function

In the early post-transplant stages, right ventricular volumes are increased due to the afterload mismatch with persistent high pulmonary pressures in the recipient. Within the first three months, a progressive reduction in right ventricular chamber size occurs, concomitant with a progressive decrease in pulmonary vascular resistance [12]. The right ventricular systolic functions of HTRs, measured by both classical echocardiographic methods (tricuspid annular plane systolic excursion (TAPSE)) and more sophisticated methods (S-wave at tissue Doppler imaging, fractional area change (FAC), and the global longitudinal strain of the right ventricular free wall) are all lower than those of healthy control participants [13]. These parameters do not tend to normalize during follow-up. However, after cardiac surgery, longitudinal parameters are known to be abnormal and not sensitive markers to assess global RV systolic function [14,15]. Despite abnormal right-sided function, in the absence of severe tricuspid regurgitation, clinical signs and symptoms of heart failure are usually not present in HTRs.

2.3. Atrial Morphology and Function

Atrial geometry and function are related to the surgical technique used for heart transplantation [16]. In patients who have undergone heart transplantation using the historical biatrial anastomosis, a unique morphological shape is visualized by echocardiography. This is best seen in the apical four-chamber view as an enlargement of the long-axis dimension of the atria with a ridge at the site of anastomosis (biatrial anastomosis involving the persistence of part of the recipient's atria; Figure 2).

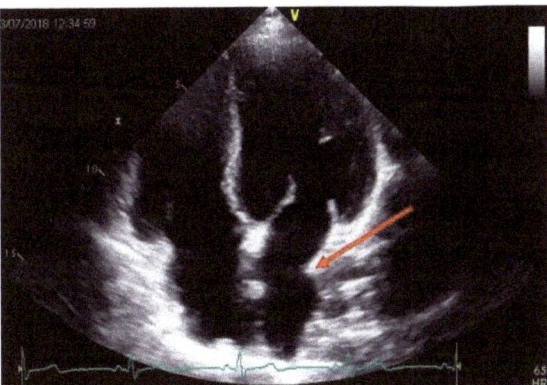

Figure 2. Apical four-chamber view, at trans thoracic echocardiography, after heart transplantation using a biatrial technique. Note the biatrial enlargement and the suture line in the left atrium that denotes the anastomosis between the donor and recipient atria (red arrow).

In contrast, in the now more standard bicaval approach, the geometry and function of the atria are comparable to those of healthy control participants. Few studies have evaluated atrial function using strain in patients with bicaval anastomosis [17]. In both atrial types of heart transplant technique, the left atrial contractile reserve is markedly reduced compared with healthy control participants [18].

2.4. Valve Morphology and Function

In general, the morphology of the valvular apparatus is normal in HTRs, and mild mitral and tricuspid regurgitation are common [19]. In the early post-transplantation phase, virtually all HTRs exhibit mitral valve regurgitation due to papillary muscle edema, but this is usually mild and tends to decrease over time [20]. After one year following transplantation, the most common valvular regurgitation is tricuspid, resulting from several mechanisms [21]. In the early post-transplant phases, tricuspid regurgitation is secondary to the high pulmonary pressures of the recipient; its magnitude decreases as the pulmonary vascular resistance decreases [22]. In the later stages, the leading causes of tricuspid regurgitation are the persistence of elevated pulmonary pressures, enlargement of the tricuspid annulus caused by right ventricular dilatation, and damage to the valvular and subvalvular apparatus due to frequent endomyocardial biopsies [23]. Finally, tricuspid regurgitation seems to be more prevalent with biatrial anastomosis because of altered right atrial morphology and annulus dilatation.

2.5. Pericardium

In HTRs, pericardial effusions are very common, particularly in the first year of follow-up [24]. After transplantation, small to moderate pericardial effusions are observed in around two-thirds of patients at three months and 25% of patients at six months [25] (Figure 3).

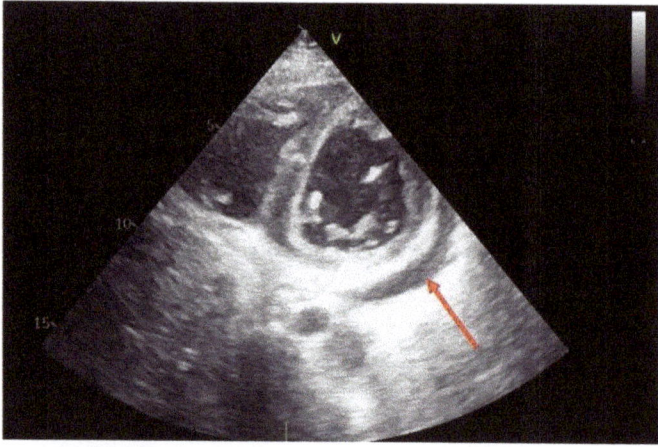

Figure 3. Short-axis view at trans thoracic echocardiography, one month after heart transplantation. Note the small pericardial effusion in the lateral position (red arrow).

Severe effusions causing cardiac tamponade are rarer and usually associated with undersized hearts for the recipient's body surface area [26]. The natural history of these effusions is variable and, in such patients, echocardiographic evaluation is required every 1–3 months to assess any changes in their extent, location, and hemodynamic impact. In cases of new-onset pericardial effusions, the main causes of effusion in HTRs should be excluded, such as right ventricle perforation due to endomyocardial biopsies, graft rejection, infection, or neoplasia.

3. Role of Echocardiography in the Evaluation of Primary Graft Dysfunction

Primary graft dysfunction (PGD) is the main cause of death in the first 30 days for HTRs [27]. PGD generally occurs within 24 h of transplantation, manifesting as cardiogenic shock, such as systolic blood pressure <90 mmHg for more than one hour and/or a cardiac index <2 L/min/m^2 despite adequate right ventricular filling pressures. A diagnosis of PGD requires that these hemodynamic conditions persist despite circulatory support based on at least two inotropes/vasopressors and/or short-term mechanical assistance devices [28,29]. Furthermore, other causes of early post-operative hemodynamic compromise must be excluded to make the diagnosis of PGD, including sepsis, cardiac tamponade, bleeding, immunological processes (hyperacute rejection), or persistent severe pulmonary hypertension not responsive to pharmacological treatment [30]. In this clinical context, echocardiography plays a key role by documenting the presence of systolic dysfunction (with a left ventricular ejection fraction <45%), loss of contractile reserve, and increased right ventricular volume with systolic dysfunction (TAPSE 15 mm or a right ventricular ejection fraction <45%). In addition, echocardiography is necessary to exclude other causes of early hemodynamic compromise such as cardiac tamponade, confirm the adequate filling status of the patient, and assess for improvement in hemodynamic conditions following the initiation of supportive therapy [31].

4. Role of Echocardiography in the Evaluation of Acute Graft Rejection

Acute graft rejection is the leading cause of mortality during the first year after heart transplant [32]. Although post-transplant mortality due to allograft rejection has decreased significantly with the introduction of appropriate anti-rejection protocols, acute allograft rejection still occurs in approximately 15% of HTRs during the first year [33].

Immunologically, acute rejection is due to the recognition of non-self-histocompatibility antigens, resulting in the elicitation of an immune response against cardiac muscle and/or graft endothelium [34]. This immune response may be either cellular (the most common) with lymphocyte infiltration of the myocyte, with or without necrosis [35], or antibody-mediated with deposition of immunoglobulins and complement in the microvasculature [36].

Acute rejection presents with extremely variable clinical patterns, ranging from asymptomatic systolic dysfunction (due to the appearance of mild and district changes in myocardial contractility) to cardiac shock (due to total and potentially irreversible graft dysfunction). Current ISHLT guidelines indicate endomyocardial biopsy as the current standard for diagnosing and grading rejection (Table 1) [37].

Table 1. International Society Heart and Lung Transplantation (ISHLT) grading of acute cellular rejection.

ISHLT Grading	Grading of Rejection	Histopathological Findings
Grade 0	No rejection	No rejection
Grade 1 R	Mild	Interstitial and/or perivascular infiltrate with up to one focus of myocyte damage
Grade 2 R	Moderate	Two or more foci of infiltrates with associated myocyte damage
Grade 3 R	Severe	Diffuse infiltrate with multifocal myocyte damage, with or without edema, hemorrhage, or vasculitis

However, in very few patients (0.5–1%), endomyocardial biopsy may cause complications (myocardial perforation, pericardial tamponade, tricuspid valve injury, thrombosis, or jugular vein infection) [38]. In addition, endomyocardial biopsy may be associated with sampling error and histological "false negatives", which occur in approximately 10–20% of HTRs [39]. Therefore, in many cardiac transplant management referral centers, echocardiography is considered a first-line complementary tool in addition to biopsy for monitoring acute graft rejection.

While reduced left ventricular systolic function early after transplantation warrants endomyocardial biopsy to exclude acute rejection, the degree of left ventricular systolic dysfunction may not correlate with the severity of rejection on biopsy [40]. Other echocardiographic indicators of acute rejection, including increased left ventricular mass and wall thickness [41], changed myocardial echogenicity, and the appearance of pericardial effusion [42], occur late in the rejection process and have low sensitivity and specificity. More recent studies have sought to identify early changes in myocardial function that can reliably identify the early phase of rejection.

Abnormalities in diastolic function are the first changes to occur in acute rejection. During episodes of acute rejection, myocardial edema, immune-mediated expansion of the extracellular compartment, and interstitial fibrosis stiffen the ventricles and impair relaxation [43]. Doppler changes include a decreased pressure interval, decreased isovolumetric relaxation time, and increased E velocity [44]. However, these parameters, although very specific, have poor sensitivity due to their dependence on preload, afterload, and heart rate.

Tissue Doppler assessment is less dependent on loading conditions and cardiac frequency. Studies with limited sample sizes have shown that reduced early and late diastolic peak mitral annulus (e′ and a′) and lower systolic velocities (s′) correlate with acute rejection episodes [45]. However, although tissue Doppler measurements are sensitive to rejection, their specificity is low, reflecting the abnormal diastolic function usually present in HTRs due to the physiology of the transplanted heart [46].

Considering that graft rejection is generally a focal process, myocardial deformation imaging could, in theory, more reliably identify the small changes in segmental myocardial function typical of acute rejection. Previous studies have found that the peak systolic global longitudinal strain and strain rate are reduced in patients with acute rejection confirmed at biopsy (Figure 4).

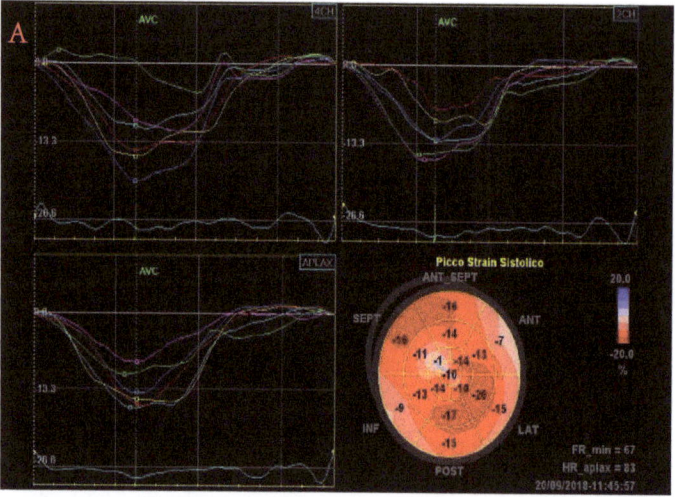

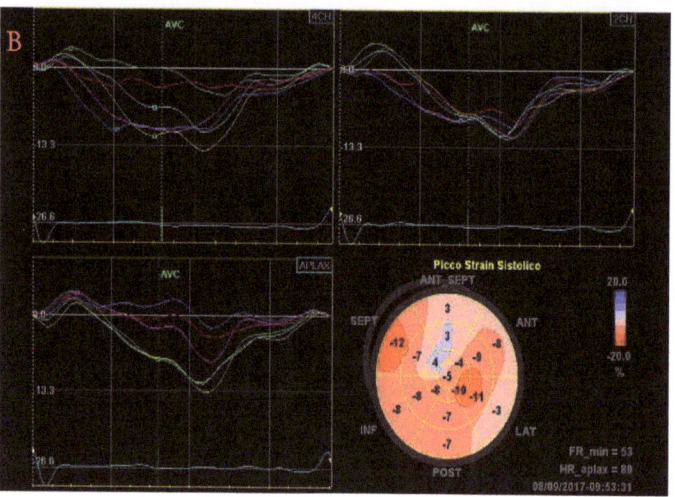

Figure 4. Evolution of global longitudinal strain in a patient with acute cellular rejection. Note the normal value at baseline (**A**) and the overall reduction during the rejection episode (**B**).

In a study enrolling 31 HTRs, Marciniak et al. found that during episodes of acute rejection, regional strain and strain rate were reduced in the left ventricular lateral wall but not in the septum [47]. This is the result of paradoxical septal motion that happens after cardiac surgery, including cardiac transplantation. Specifically, the lateral wall peak systolic longitudinal strain was $-21 \pm 6\%$ in patients with rejection grade $\leq$1B, compared with $-13 \pm 5\%$ in patients with rejection grade >1B ($p < 0.05$). In another study, a mean systolic strain cutoff value of -27.4% predicted grade 1B or higher acute rejection with a sensitivity of 82.2% and a specificity of 82.3% [48]. Tissue Doppler imaging findings should be interpreted cautiously because strain and strain rate parameters are dependent on the transducer angle, and images can be technically challenging to acquire, with poor reproducibility. Two-dimensional speckle tracking (2D STE) overcomes the limitation of angle dependence, and this technique has also been tested in identifying acute rejection [49].

Sato et al. used 2D STE to measure left ventricular torsion to detect acute rejection. This study showed that a reduction in torsion of more than 25% from baseline could predict the presence of acute rejection with a grade 2R or higher with high specificity (95.1%) and a high negative predictive value (92.9%) [50].

A prospective study of 34 HTRs identified an independent relationship between acute rejection of grade 2R or higher and two combined echocardiographic parameters, longitudinal right ventricular free wall deformation <17% and global left ventricular longitudinal deformation <15.5%, with a negative predictive value of 98.8% [51].

Although initial experience seems to indicate that echocardiography could be a reliable tool to diagnose acute rejection, notably, the studies cited were based on different echocardiographic methodologies, enrolled small samples, and were based on the experience of single centers. Therefore, before clear and evidence-based recommendations can be made, future studies are needed, aiming at standardizing the echocardiographic strategy for surveillance of acute rejection and the role of new echocardiographic techniques based on 2D STE, such as global longitudinal strain (GLS) and myocardial work.

5. Role of Echocardiography in the Evaluation of Cardiac Allograft Vasculopathy

Chronic graft rejection is manifested by CAV [52]. CAV is a diffuse process that involves not only the epicardial vessels but also the coronary microcirculation [53]. The etiology of CAV is multifactorial and based on the interaction of immunological and non-immunological factors (older donor age, cytomegalovirus infection, hyperlipidemia, and type II diabetes) [54]. Unlike what normally occurs in chronic coronary syndrome, CAV, due to cardiac denervation, may progress silently before manifesting clinically as myocardial ischemia, left ventricular dysfunction or heart failure, or ventricular arrhythmia or sudden cardiac death [55,56].

Resting echocardiography provides limited diagnostic accuracy to detect CAV [57,58]. Systolic function is generally preserved even in advanced forms of CAV, making left ventricular ejection fraction an unsuitable echocardiographic marker for early detection of coronary artery disease in the transplanted heart. Wall motion abnormalities should raise suspicion of the presence or progression of CAV [59]. However, these findings are not specific because wall motion abnormalities may also develop in the absence of CAV or be due to acute rejection.

Worsening diastolic function during follow-up may also indicate CAV (as well as acute rejection), necessitating an invasive diagnostic approach [60]. For example, patients with CAV have increased durations and reduced amplitudes of both systolic and diastolic waves on tissue Doppler imaging. For example, a Doppler-derived systolic radial velocity value of $\leq$10 m/s showed a sensitivity of approximately 90% for angiographically and/or intravenous ultrasound-detectable CAV, but this decreased to 51% when examining stenosed major epicardial vessels, even with a cutoff of 9 cm/s [61]. Resting tissue Doppler velocities also more frequently indicate advanced stages of CAV [62].

Reduced absolute GLS values are also associated with the presence of CAV and coronary microvascular dysfunction [63]. In a population of 128 HTRs, Clemmensen et al. found a significant correlation between the extent of GLS reduction and the presence and extent of CAV [64]. Another study noted an association of reduced left ventricular circumferential deformation with the presence of coronary artery stenosis (positive and negative predictive value $\geq$90%, considering proximal stenosis as $\geq$50%) [65]. In addition, a recent study in a small cohort of heart transplant patients suggested that the absolute value of GLS and the gradient between endocardial and epicardial longitudinal strain values could be important non-invasive predictors of CAV [66].

In patients who cannot undergo repeated coronary examinations (e.g., patients with advanced renal failure), the latest ISHLT guidelines recommend the use of dobutamine stress echocardiography or treadmill stress echocardiography for CAV detection [4]. However, in HTRs, exercise may not be an adequate cardiovascular stressor due to denervation of the allograft and altered chronotropic response [67]. Therefore, in this patient population, stress echocardiography with pharmacological agents seems more favorable when this technique is indicated. Although some studies have demonstrated good sensitivity and specificity of exercise echocardiography with dipyridamole in detecting CAV [68,69], dobutamine is still the first choice. However, notably, although the use of dobutamine detects significant CAV with a sensitivity of 70–80%, it identifies mild CAV with low sensitivity [70]. The accuracy of exercise echocardiography may improve when combined with other techniques, such as myocardial deformation analysis and the use of contrast agents. For example, strain analysis may increase the sensitivity of dobutamine stress echocardiography from 63 to 88% in the detection of CAV [71], representing a promising tool warranting additional investigation.

6. Conclusions

Echocardiography is the first-line imaging modality of choice for the initial assessment of HTRs (Figure 5).

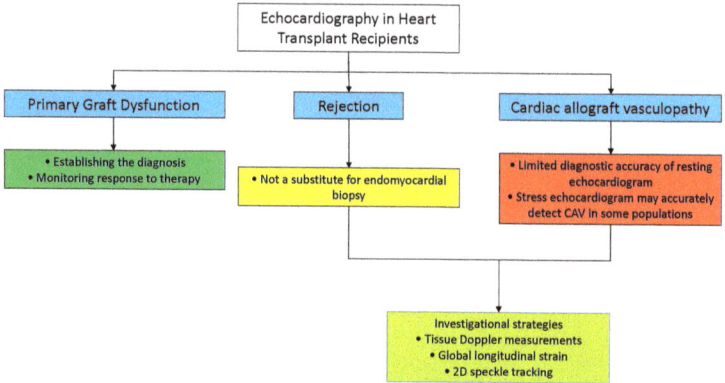

Figure 5. Role of echocardiography in HTRs. CAV: cardiac allograft vasculopathy.

It is a versatile tool that provides comprehensive evaluation of the structure and function of the allograft. Echocardiographic examinations can be easily performed at the bedside in the hours after transplantation and can be serially repeated without risk or discomfort for the patient. For the identification of PGD, echocardiography is an indispensable method of documenting biventricular systolic dysfunction, required for the diagnosis of PGD, and for monitoring the effectiveness of therapy. In detecting acute rejection, traditional echocardiography, in conjunction with new echocardiographic technologies, may offer complementary insight, though it is not currently a substitute for endomyocardial biopsy. In detecting CAV, stress echocardiography has the same diagnostic accuracy as coronarography in some populations, and a normal surveillance stress echocardiogram may allow deferment of invasive coronary angiogram. More data regarding the use of innovative sophisticated tools (3D echography and myocardial work) could enhance the future role of echocardiography in the management of HTRs.

Author Contributions: Conceptualization, D.M. and G.P.; writing—original draft preparation, D.M., R.G., and F.V.; writing—review and editing, M.K. and A.P. All authors have read and agreed to the published version of the manuscript.

Funding: This research received no external funding.

Institutional Review Board Statement: Not applicable.

Informed Consent Statement: Not applicable.

Data Availability Statement: Not applicable.

Conflicts of Interest: The authors declare no conflict of interest.

References

1. McDonagh, T.A.; Metra, M.; Adamo, M.; Gardner, R.S.; Baumbach, A.; Böhm, M.; Burri, H.; Butler, J.; Čelutkienė, J.; Chioncel, O.; et al. 2021 ESC Guidelines for the diagnosis and treatment of acute and chronic heart failure: Developed by the Task Force for the diagnosis and treatment of acute and chronic heart failure of the European Society of Cardiology (ESC) With the special contribution of the Heart Failure Association (HFA) of the ESC. *Eur. Heart J.* **2021**, *42*, 3599–3726. [PubMed]
2. Kittleson, M.M.; Kobashigawa, J.A. Cardiac Transplantation: Current Outcomes and Contemporary Controversies. *JACC Heart Fail.* **2017**, *5*, 857–868. [CrossRef] [PubMed]
3. Olympios, M.; Kwiecinski, J.; Berman, D.S.; Kobashigawa, J.A. Imaging in Heart Transplant Patients. *JACC: Cardiovasc. Imaging* **2018**, *11*, 1514–1530. [CrossRef]
4. Costanzo, M.R.; Dipchand, A.; Starling, R.; Anderson, A.; Chan, M.; Desai, S.; Fedson, S.; Fisher, P.; Gonzales-Stawinski, G.; Martinelli, L.; et al. The International Society of Heart and Lung Transplantation Guidelines for the care of heart transplant recipients. *J Heart Lung Transplant.* **2010**, *29*, 914–956.
5. Thorn, E.M.; de Filippi, C.R. Echocardiography in the cardiac transplant recipient. *Heart Fail Clin.* **2007**, *3*, 51–67. [CrossRef] [PubMed]
6. Wilhelmi, M.; Pethig, K.; Wilhelmi, M.; Nguyen, H.; Strüber, M.; Haverich, A. Heart transplantation: Echocardiographic assessment of morphology and function after more than 10 years of follow-up. *Ann. Thorac. Surg.* **2002**, *74*, 1075–1079. [CrossRef]
7. Okada, D.R.; Molina, M.R.; Kohari, M.; Vorovich, E.E.; Owens, A.T.; Han, Y. Clinical echocardiographic indices of left ventricular diastolic function correlate poorly with pulmonary capillary wedge pressure at 1 year following heart transplantation. *Int. J. Cardiovasc. Imaging* **2015**, *31*, 783–794. [CrossRef] [PubMed]
8. Nagueh, S.F.; Smiseth, O.A.; Appleton, C.P.; Gillebert, T.C.; Marino, P.N.; Oh, J.K.; Waggoner, A.D.; Flachskampf, F.A.; Pellikka, P.A.; Evangelisa, A. Recommendations for the evaluation of left ventricular diastolic function by echocardiography. *Eur. J. Echocardiogr.* **2016**, *29*, 277–314.25. [CrossRef] [PubMed]
9. Sundereswaran, L.; Nagueh, S.F.; Vardan, S.; Middleton, K.J.; Zoghbi, W.A.; Quiñones, M.A.; Torre-Amione, G. Estimation of left and right ventricular filling pressures after heart transplantation by tissue Doppler imaging. *Am. J. Cardiol.* **1998**, *82*, 352–357. [CrossRef]
10. Rustad, L.A.; Nytrøen, K.; Andreassen, A.; Geiran, O.; Endresen, K.; Gullestad, L.; Aakhus, S.; Amundsen, B.H. Heart transplant systolic and diastolic function is impaired by prolonged pretransplant graft ischaemic time and high donor age: An echocardiographic study. *Eur. J. Cardio-Thoracic Surg.* **2013**, *44*, e97–e104. [CrossRef]
11. Tallaj, J.A.; Kirklin, J.K.; Brown, R.N.; Rayburn, B.K.; Bourge, R.C.; Benza, R.L.; Pinderski, L.; Pamboukian, S.; McGiffin, D.C.; Naftel, D.C. Post-heart transplant diastolic dysfunction is a risk factor for mortality. *J Am Coll Cardiol.* **2007**, *50*, 1064–1069. [CrossRef] [PubMed]
12. Bhatia, S.J.; Kirshenbaum, J.M.; Shemin, R.J.; Cohn, L.H.; Collins, J.J.; Di Sesa, V.J.; Young, P.J.; Mudge, G.H., Jr.; Sutton, M.G. Time course of resolution of pulmonary hypertension and right ventricular re-modeling after orthotopic cardiac transplantation. *Circulation* **1987**, *76*, 819–826. [CrossRef] [PubMed]
13. Dandel, M.; Hummel, M.; Muller, J.; Wellnhofer, E.; Meyer, R.; Solowjowa, N.; Ewert, R.; Hetzer, R. Reliability of tissue Doppler wall motion monitoring after heart transplantation for replacement of invasive routine screenings by optimally timed cardiac biopsies and catheterizations. *Circulation* **2001**, *104*, I184–I191. [CrossRef] [PubMed]
14. Clemmensen, T.S.; Eiskjaer, H.; Logstrup, B.B.; Andersen, M.J.; Mellemkjær, S.; Poulsen, S.H. Echocardiographic assessment of right heart function in heart transplant re-cipients and the relation to exercise hemodynamics. *Transpl. Int.* **2016**, *29*, 909–920. [CrossRef] [PubMed]
15. Haddad, F.; Doyle, R.; Murphy, D.J.; Hunt, S.A. Right ventricular function in cardiovascular disease, part II: Pathophysiology, clinical importance, and management of right ventricular failure. *Circulation* **2008**, *117*, 1717–1731. [CrossRef]
16. Traversi, E.; Pozzoli, M.; Grande, A.; Forni, G.; Assandri, J.; Vigano, M.; Tavazzi, L. The bicaval anastomosis technique for orthotopic heart transplantation yields better atrial function than the standard technique: An echocardiographic automatic boundary detection study. *J. Heart Lung Transplant.* **1998**, *17*, 1065–1074.
17. Bech-Hanssen, O.; Pergola, V.; Al-Admawi, M.; Fadel, B.M.; Di Salvo, G. Atrial function in heart transplant recipients operated with the bicaval technique. *Scand. Cardiovasc. J.* **2016**, *50*, 42–51. [CrossRef]

18. Mondillo, S.; Maccherini, M.; Galderisi, M. Usefulness and limitations of transthoracic echocardiography in heart transplantation recipients. *Cardiovasc. Ultrasound* **2008**, *6*, 2. [CrossRef]
19. Kwon, M.H.; Shemin, R.J. Tricuspid valve regurgitation after heart transplantation. *Ann. Cardiothorac. Surg.* **2017**, *6*, 270–274. [CrossRef]
20. Stevenson, L.; Dadourian, B.J.; Kobashigawa, J.; Child, J.S.; Clark, S.H.; Laks, H. Mitral regurgitation after cardiac transplantation. *Am. J. Cardiol.* **1987**, *60*, 119–122. [CrossRef]
21. Bishawi, M.; Zanotti, G.; Shaw, L.; MacKenzie, M.; Castleberry, A.; Bartels, K.; Schroder, J.; Velazquez, E.; Swaminathan, M.; Rogers, J.; et al. Tricuspid Valve Regurgitation Immediately After Heart Transplant and Long-Term Outcomes. *Ann. Thorac. Surg.* **2019**, *107*, 1348–1355. [CrossRef]
22. Nguyen, V.; Cantarovich, M.; Cecere, R.; Giannetti, N. Tricuspid regurgitation after cardiac transplantation: How many biopsies are too many? *J. Heart Lung Transplant.* **2005**, *24* (Suppl. 7), S227–S231. [CrossRef]
23. Wong, R.C.; Abrahams, Z.; Hanna, M.; Pangrace, J.; Gonzalez-Stawinski, G.; Starling, R.; Taylor, D. Tricuspid regurgitation after car-diac transplantation: An old problem revisited. *J. Heart Lung Transplant.* **2008**, *27*, 247–252. [CrossRef]
24. Vandenberg, B.F.; Mohanty, P.K.; Craddock, K.J.; Barnhart, G.; Hanrahan, J.; Szentpetery, S.; Lower, R.R. Clinical significance of peri-cardial effusion after heart transplantation. *J. Heart Transplant.* **1988**, *7*, 128–134. [PubMed]
25. Ciliberto, G.; Anjos, M.C.; Gronda, E.; Bonacina, E.; Danzi, G.; Colombo, P.; Mangiavacchi, M.; Alberti, A.; Frigerio, M.; De Vita, C. Significance of pericardial effusion after heart transplantation. *Am. J. Cardiol.* **1995**, *76*, 297–300. [CrossRef]
26. Quin, J.A.; Tauriainen, M.; Huber, L.M.; McIntire, D.D.; Kaiser, P.A.; Ring, W.; Jessen, M.E. Predictors of pericardial effusion after orthotopic heart transplantation. *J. Thorac. Cardiovasc. Surg.* **2002**, *124*, 979–983. [CrossRef]
27. Chew, H.C.; Kumarasinghe, G.; Iyer, A.; Hicks, M.; Gao, L.; Doyle, A.; Jabbour, A.; Dhital, K.; Granger, E.; Jansz, P.; et al. Primary Graft Dysfunction After Heart Transplantation. *Curr. Transplant. Rep.* **2014**, *1*, 257–265. [CrossRef]
28. Kobashigawa, J.; Zuckermann, A.; Macdonald, P.; Leprince, P.; Esmailian, F.; Luu, M.; Mancini, D.; Patel, J.; Razi, R.; Reichen-spurner, H.; et al. Consensus Conference participants. Report from a consensus conference on primary graft dysfunction after cardiac transplantation. *J. Heart Lung Transplant.* **2014**, *33*, 327–340. [CrossRef]
29. Subramani, S.; Aldrich, A.; Dwarakanath, S.; Sugawara, A.; Hanada, S. Early Graft Dysfunction Following Heart Transplant: Prevention and Management. *Semin. Cardiothorac. Vasc. Anesthesia* **2020**, *24*, 24–33. [CrossRef]
30. Singh, S.S.A.; Dalzell, J.R.; Berry, C.; Al-Attar, N. Primary graft dysfunction after heart transplantation: A thorn amongst the roses. *Heart Fail Rev.* **2019**, *24*, 805–820. [CrossRef] [PubMed]
31. DePasquale, E.C.; Ardehali, A. Primary graft dysfunction in heart transplantation. *Curr. Opin. Organ Transplant.* **2018**, *23*, 286–294. [CrossRef]
32. Lund, L.H.; Edwards, L.B.; Kucheryavaya, A.Y.; Benden, C.; Christie, J.D.; Dipchand, A.I.; Dobbels, F.; Goldfarb, S.B.; Levvey, B.J.; Meiser, B.; et al. International Society of Heart and Lung Transplantation. The Registry of the International Society for Heart and Lung Transplantation: Thirty-first Official Adult Heart Transplant Report—2014; Focus Theme: Retransplantation. *J. Heart Lung Transplant.* **2014**, *33*, 996–1008. [CrossRef]
33. Khush, K.K.; Hsich, E.; Potena, L.; Cherikh, W.S.; Chambers, D.C.; Harhay, M.O.; Hayes, D., Jr.; Perch, M.; Sadavarte, A.; Toll, A.; et al. The International Thoracic Organ Transplant Registry of the International Society for Heart and Lung Transplantation: Thirty-eighth adult heart trans-plantation report-2021; Focus on recipient characteristics. *J. Heart Lung Transplant.* **2021**, *40*, 1035–1049. [CrossRef] [PubMed]
34. Crespo-Leiro, M.G.; Barge-Caballero, G.; Couto-Mallon, D. Noninvasive monitoring of acute and chronic rejection in heart transplantation. *Curr. Opin. Cardiol.* **2017**, *32*, 308–315. [CrossRef] [PubMed]
35. McManigle, W.; Pavlisko, E.; Martinu, T. Acute Cellular and Antibody-Mediated Allograft Rejection. *Semin. Respir. Crit. Care Med.* **2013**, *34*, 320–335. [CrossRef] [PubMed]
36. Alegre, M.-L.; Florquin, S.; Goldman, M. Cellular mechanisms underlying acute graft rejection: Time for reassessment. *Curr. Opin. Immunol.* **2007**, *19*, 563–568. [CrossRef] [PubMed]
37. Welch, T.S.; Mrisc, Z.; Sula, M. Monitoring for Rejection. In *Contemporary Heart Transplantation*, 1st ed.; Bogar, L., Otero, A.S., Eds.; Elsevier: New York, NY, USA; p. 10010.
38. Saraiva, F.; Matos, V.; Gonçalves, L.; Antunes, M.; Providência, L. Complications of Endomyocardial Biopsy in Heart Transplant Patients: A Retrospective Study of 2117 Consecutive Procedures. *Transplant. Proc.* **2011**, *43*, 1908–1912. [CrossRef]
39. Tang, Z.; Kobashigawa, J.; Rafiei, M.; Stern, L.K.; Hamilton, M. The natural history of biopsy-negative rejection after heart trans-plantation. *J. Transplant.* **2013**, *2013*, 236720.
40. Badano, L.P.; Miglioranza, M.H.; Edvardsen, T.; Colafranceschi, A.S.; Muraru, D.; Bacal, F.; Nieman, K.; Zoppellaro, G.; Braga, F.G.M.; Binder, T.; et al. Document reviewers. Document reviewers. European Association of Cardiovascular Imag-ing/Cardiovascular Imaging Department of the Brazilian Society of Cardiology recommendations for the use of cardiac imaging to assess and follow patients after heart transplantation. *Eur. Heart J. Cardiovasc. Imaging* **2015**, *16*, 919–948.
41. Sagar, K.B.; Hastillo, A.; Wolfgang, T.C.; Lower, R.R.; Hess, M.L. Left ventricular mass by M-mode echocardiography in cardiac transplant patients with acute rejection. *Circulation* **1981**, *64*, II217–II220.
42. Valantine, H.A.; Hunt, S.A.; Gibbons, R.; Billingham, M.E.; Stinson, E.B.; Popp, R.L. Increasing pericardial effusion in cardiac transplant recipients. *Circulation* **1989**, *79*, 603–609. [CrossRef]

43. Valantine, H.A.; Appleton, C.P.; Hatle, L.K.; Hunt, S.A.; Billingham, M.E.; Shumway, N.E.; Stinson, E.B.; Popp, R.L. A hemodynamic and Doppler echocardiographic study of ventricular function in long-term cardiac allograft recipients: Etiology and prognosis of restrictive-constrictive physiology. *Circulation* **1989**, *79*, 66–75. [CrossRef]
44. Yun, K.L.; Niczyporuk, A.M.; Daughters, G.T.; Ingels, N.B., Jr.; Stinson, E.B.; Alderman, E.L.; Hansen, E.D.; Miller, D.C. Alterations in left ventricular diastolic twist mechanics during acute human cardiac allograft rejection. *Circulation* **1991**, *83*, 962–973. [CrossRef] [PubMed]
45. Kato, T.S.; Homma, S.; Mancini, D. Novel echocardiographic strategies for rejection diagnosis. *Curr. Opin. Organ Transplant.* **2013**, *18*, 573–580. [CrossRef]
46. Mena, C.; Wencker, D.; Krumholz, H.M.; McNamara, R.L. Detection of Heart Transplant Rejection in Adults by Echocardiographic Diastolic Indices: A Systematic Review of the Literature. *J. Am. Soc. Echocardiogr.* **2006**, *19*, 1295–1300. [CrossRef] [PubMed]
47. Marciniak, A.; Eroglu, E.; Marciniak, M.; Sirbu, C.; Herbots, L.; Droogne, W.; Claus, P.; D'Hooge, J.; Bijnens, B.; Vanhaecke, J.; et al. The potential clinical role of ultrasonic strain and strain rate imaging in diagnosing acute rejection after heart transplantation. *Eur. J. Echocardiogr.* **2007**, *8*, 213–221. [CrossRef] [PubMed]
48. Kato, T.-S.; Oda, N.; Hashimura, K.; Hashimoto, S.; Nakatani, T.; Ueda, H.-I.; Shishido, T.; Komamura, K. Strain rate imaging would predict sub-clinical acute rejection in heart transplant recipients. *Eur. J. Cardio-Thoracic Surg.* **2010**, *37*, 1104–1110. [CrossRef]
49. Yuda, S. Current clinical applications of speckle tracking echocardiography for assessment of left atrial function. *J. Echocardiogr.* **2021**, *19*, 129–140. [CrossRef] [PubMed]
50. Sato, T.; Kato, T.S.; Kamamura, K.; Hashimoto, S.; Shishido, T.; Mano, A.; Oda, N.; Takahashi, A.; Ishibashi-Ueda, H.; Nakatani, T.; et al. Utility of left ventricular systolic torsion derived from 2-dimensional speckle-tracking echocardiography in monitoring acute cellular rejection in heart transplant recipients. *J. Heart Lung Transplant.* **2011**, *30*, 536–543. [CrossRef]
51. Mingo-Santos, S.; Moñivas-Palomero, V.; Garcia-Lunar, I.; Mitroi, C.D.; Goirigolzarri-Artaza, J.; Rivero, B.; Oteo, J.F.; Castedo, E.; González-Mirelis, J.; Cavero, M.A.; et al. Usefulness of Two-Dimensional Strain Parameters to Diagnose Acute Rejection after Heart Transplantation. *J. Am. Soc. Echocardiogr.* **2015**, *28*, 1149–1156. [CrossRef]
52. Aranda, J.M.; Hill, J. Cardiac transplant vasculopathy. *Chest* **2000**, *118*, 1792–1800. [CrossRef]
53. Schmauss, D.; Weis, M. Cardiac allograft vasculopathy: Recent developments. *Circulation* **2008**, *117*, 2131–2141. [CrossRef]
54. Lee, M.S.; Finch, W.; Weisz, G.; Kirtane, A.J. Cardiac allograft vasculopathy. *Rev. Cardiovasc. Med.* **2011**, *12*, 143–152.
55. Zimmer, R.J.; Lee, M.S. Transplant coronary artery disease. *JACC Cardiovasc. Interv.* **2010**, *3*, 367–377. [CrossRef]
56. Ortega-Legaspi, J.M.; Bravo, P.E. Diagnosis and management of cardiac allograft vasculopathy. *Heart* **2021**. [CrossRef] [PubMed]
57. Wu, H.A.; Kolias, T.J. Cardiac Transplantation: Pretransplant and Posttransplant Evaluation. In *The Practice of Clinical Echocardiography*, 6th ed.; Otto, C.M., Ed.; Elsevier: New York, NY, USA, 2021; pp. 585–596.
58. Smart, F.W.; Balantyne, C.M.; Cocanougher, B.; Farmer, J.A.; Sekela, M.E.; Noon, G.P.; Young, J.B. Insensitivity of noninvasive tests to detect coronary artery vasculopathy after after heart transplant. *Am. J. Cardiol.* **2011**, *67*, 243–247. [CrossRef]
59. Störk, S.; Behr, T.; Birk, M.; Überfuhr, P.; Klauss, V.; Spes, C.; Angermann, C. Assessment of Cardiac Allograft Vasculopathy Late After Heart Transplantation: When Is Coronary Angiography Necessary? *J. Heart Lung Transplant.* **2006**, *25*, 1103–1108. [CrossRef] [PubMed]
60. Lunze, F.I.; Colan, S.D.; Gauvreau, K.; Perez-Atayde, A.R.; Smith, R.N.; Blume, E.D.; Singh, T.P. Tissue Doppler imaging for rejection surveillance in pediatric heart transplant recipients. *J. Heart Lung Transplant.* **2013**, *32*, 1027–1033. [CrossRef]
61. Sciaccaluga, C.; Ghionzoli, N.; Mandoli, G.; Sisti, N.; D'Ascenzi, F.; Focardi, M.; Bernazzali, S.; Vergaro, G.; Emdin, M.; Valente, S.; et al. The role of non-invasive imaging modalities in cardiac allograft vasculopathy: An updated focus on current evidences. *Heart Fail. Rev.* **2021**, 1–12. [CrossRef] [PubMed]
62. Dandel, M.; Hummel, M.; Meyer, R.; Müller, J.; Kapell, S.; Ewert, R.; Hetzer, R. Left ventricular dysfunction during cardiac allograft rejection: Early diagnosis, relationship to the histological severity grade, and therapeutic implications. *Transplant. Proc.* **2002**, *34*, 2169–2173. [CrossRef]
63. Hummel, M.; Dandel, M.; Knollmann, F.; Müller, J.; Knosalla, C.; Ewert, R.; Grauhan, O.; Meyer, R.; Hetzer, R. Long-term surveillance of heart-transplanted patients: Noninvasive monitoring of acute rejection episodes and transplant vasculopathy. *Transplant. Proc.* **2001**, *33*, 3539–3542. [CrossRef]
64. Clemmensen, T.S.; Løgstrup, B.B.; Eiskjær, H.; Poulsen, S.H. Evaluation of longitudinal myocardial deformation by 2-dimensional speckle-tracking echocardiography in heart transplant recipients: Relation to coronary allograft vasculopathy. *J. Heart Lung Transplant.* **2015**, *34*, 195–203. [CrossRef] [PubMed]
65. Dandel, M.; Hetzer, R. Post-transplant surveillance for acute rejection and allograft vasculopathy by echocardiography: Usefulness of myocardial velocity and deformation imaging. *J. Heart Lung Transplant.* **2017**, *36*, 117–131. [CrossRef]
66. Sciaccaluga, C.; Mandoli, G.E.; Sisti, N.; Natali, M.B.; Ibrahim, A.; Menci, D.; D'Errico, A.; Donati, G.; Benfari, G.; Valente, S.; et al. Detection of cardiac allograft vasculopathy by multi-layer left ventricular longitudinal strain in heart transplant recipients. *Int. J. Cardiovasc. Imaging* **2021**, *37*, 1621–1628. [CrossRef]
67. Collings, A.C.; Pinto, F.J.; Valantine, H.A.; Popylisen, S.; Puryear, J.V.; Schnittger, I. Exercise echocardiography in heart transplant recipients: A comparison with angiography and intracoronary ultrasonography. *J. Heart Lung Transplant.* **1994**, *13*, 604–613. [PubMed]

68. Ciliberto, G.R.; Parodi, O.; Cataldo, G.; Mangiavacchi, M.; Alberti, A.; Parolini, M.; Frigerio, M. Prognostic value of contractile response during high-dose dipyridamole echo-cardiography test in heart transplant recipients. *J. Heart Lung Transplant.* **2003**, *22*, 526–532. [CrossRef]
69. Ciliberto, G.; Massa, D.; Mangiavacchi, M.; Danzi, G.B.; Pirelli, S.; Faletra, F.; Frigerio, M.; Gronda, E.; De Vita, C. High-dose dipyridamole echocardiography test in coronary artery disease after heart transplantation. *Eur. Heart J.* **1993**, *14*, 48–52. [CrossRef]
70. Clerkin, K.J.; Farr, M.A.; Restaino, S.W.; Ali, Z.A.; Mancini, D.M. Dobutamine stress echocardiography is inadequate to detect early cardiac allograft vasculopathy. *J. Heart Lung Transpl.* **2016**, *35*, 1040. [CrossRef]
71. Eroglu, E.; D'Hooge, J.; Sutherland, G.R.; Marciniak, A.; Thijs, D.; Droogne, W.; Herbots, L.; Van Cleemput, J.; Claus, P.; Bijnens, B.; et al. Quantitative dobutamine stress echocardiography for the early detection of cardiac allograft vasculopathy in heart transplant recipients. *Heart* **2008**, *94*, e3. [CrossRef]

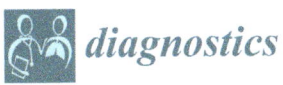

Article

Diagnostic Performance of Serum Biomarkers Fibroblast Growth Factor 21, Galectin-3 and Copeptin for Heart Failure with Preserved Ejection Fraction in a Sample of Patients with Type 2 Diabetes Mellitus

Raluca D. Ianoș [1], Călin Pop [2,3,*], Mihaela Iancu [4,*], Rodica Rahaian [5], Angela Cozma [6] and Lucia M. Procopciuc [7]

1. Department of Cardiology, Iuliu Hațieganu University of Medicine and Pharmacy, 400001 Cluj-Napoca, Romania; ralu_yannosh@yahoo.com
2. Department of Cardiology, Emergency County Hospital, 430031 Baia Mare, Romania
3. Faculty of Medicine Arad, "Vasile Goldiș" Western University, 310045 Arad, Romania
4. Department of Medical Informatics and Biostatistics, Iuliu Hațieganu University of Medicine and Pharmacy, 400349 Cluj-Napoca, Romania
5. Department of Immunology, Emergency County Hospital, 400006 Cluj-Napoca, Romania; rodicarahaian@gmail.com
6. Department of Internal Medicine, Iuliu Hațieganu University of Medicine and Pharmacy, 400015 Cluj-Napoca, Romania; angelacozma@yahoo.com
7. Department of Medical Biochemistry, Iuliu Hațieganu University of Medicine and Pharmacy, 400349 Cluj-Napoca, Romania; luciamariaprocopciuc@yahoo.com
* Correspondence: medicbm@yahoo.com (C.P.); miancu@umfcluj.ro (M.I.)

Abstract: More than half of the patients with heart failure have preserved ejection fraction (HFpEF), however evidence shows a mortality rate comparable to those with reduced ejection fraction. The aim of this study was to evaluate whether FGF21, galectin-3 and copeptin can be used as biomarkers to identify HFpEF in patients with confirmed type 2 diabetes mellitus (DM). Sixty-nine diabetic patients were enrolled and divided into two groups: patients with HFpEF (*n* = 40) and those without HFpEF (*n* = 29). The ability of the studied biomarkers to discriminate HFpEF cases from non-HFpEF subjects were evaluated by the area under the Receiver Operating Characteristics (ROC) curve and the 95% confidence interval (CI). Compared to patients without heart failure, those with HFpEF had significantly higher levels of FGF21 (mean 146.79 pg/mL vs. 298.98 pg/mL). The AUC value of FGF21 was 0.88, 95% CI: [0.80, 0.96], Se = 85% [70.2, 94.3], Sp = 79.3% [60.3, 92.0], at an optimal cut-off value of 217.40 pg/mL. There was no statistical significance associated with galectin-3 and copeptin between patient cohorts. In conclusion, galectin-3 and copeptin levels were not effective for detecting HFpEF, while FGF21 is a promising biomarker for diagnosing HFpEF in DM patients.

Keywords: biomarkers; heart failure; preserved ejection fraction; type 2 diabetes mellitus

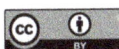

1. Introduction

Diabetes mellitus (DM) is an important risk factor for cardiovascular disease, representing a frequent cause of microvascular and macrovascular complications, cardiac damage including ischemic coronary artery disease diabetic cardiomyopa-thy, heart failure (HF) and autonomic neuropathy, with a cardiovascular mortality rate twice that of non-diabetic patients [1]. Mortality due to cardiomyopathy on account of DM is relatively high, diabetic cardiomyopathy (DCM) being evident in 60% of type 2 diabetic cases. It has been estimated that the prevalence of DM worldwide will increase from 2.8% in 2000 to 4.4% in 2030 [2].

Among patients with signs and symptoms of HF, approximately 50% have preserved left ventricular ejection fraction (HFpEF) [3]. Multiple comorbidities are common in both types of HF (preserved and reduced EF), but slightly more severe in HFpEF, in which approximately half of the patients have at least five major comorbidities [3]. In patients with HFpEF, a high proportion of deaths are due to cardiovascular events, but the proportion of non-cardiovascular deaths is higher in HFpEF than HFrEF. HFpEF incidence has increased from 47.8% to 52.3% between 2000 and 2010. The majority of observational studies have shown a similar risk of mortality in HFpEF compared to HFrEF, suggesting the importance of this pathology [3]. HFpEF develops from a combination of risk factors and comorbidities, including advanced age, female gender, obesity, systemic arterial hypertension and DM [4]. According to the European Heart Failure Management Guidelines, no treatment has so far been shown to reduce morbidity and mortality in HFpEF or intermediate ejection fraction [5,6]. The metabolic disturbances present in diabetic patients are often accompanied by cardiac changes consisting of local inflammation, oxidative stress, myocardial fibrosis and cardiomyocyte apoptosis. It is of great interest and utility to discover specific biomarkers that integrate these processes, in order to detect DCM at an early stage and evaluate their potential role in the introduction of targeted therapies to prevent progression of the disease to severe HF [7].

B-type natriuretic peptides (BNP and NT-proBNP) are diagnostic and prognostic biomarkers for congestive HF [6]. However, there are studies which indicate a limitation in the use of NT-proBNP for diagnosing HFpEF [8–10]. Therefore, new biomarkers and diagnostic strategies are needed to detect HFpEF.

Fibroblast growth factor 21 (FGF21), galectin-3 and copeptin [2,11] have been proposed as biomarker candidates to detect the early stages of cardiomyopathy.

In the literature, the role of galectin-3 (a beta-galactosidase binding lectin) is emphasized in the process of fibrosis, inflammation and cardiac remodeling [7]. At the cardiac level, its expression is low, but during cardiac injury, it is rapidly induced [7]. Although intracellular levels of galectin-3 correlate with tissue repair, its uncontrolled expression contributes to sustained activation of macrophages and myo-fibroblasts by dependent and independent transforming growth factor beta (TGF-β) pathways resulting in tissue fibrosis [7]. Galectin-3 is locally secreted by activated fibroblasts and macrophages, exerting its pro-fibrotic function by augmenting pro-liferation of myofibroblasts, extracellular matrix accumulation, macrophage infiltration and cardiac hypertrophy by stimulating TGF-β signaling pathways [7]. Plasma levels of galectin-3 have been proposed as a good biomarker for prediction and prognosis of left ventricular systolic dysfunction and HF in diabetic patients. Galectin-3 may be of therapeutic interest, since its inhibition prevents pro-inflammatory and pro-fibrotic mechanisms [7,12].

It is well known that hyperglycemia initiates DCM and contributes to various pathological processes of this disease. FGF21 is a polypeptide that plays a role in regulating glucose homeostasis and lipid metabolism, by reducing plasma glucose levels and lowering triglyceride levels in the liver and serum [13]. Recent clinical and subclinical studies have found that increased serum FGF21 is closely associated with DCM [14] and can be considered a potential biomarker. There is evidence that myocytes secrete FGF21 as an autocrine factor, to protect the heart from adverse cardiac remodeling [7,15]. However, whether an increased level of serum FGF21 is the basis of DCM pathogenesis or a key molecule involved in repairing the damage from DCM is so far unclear [13]. This biomarker has significant positive correlation with hypertension, DM, severity of HF, ischemic coronary artery disease and peripheral arterial disease [15–17]. There is indirect evidence that FGF21 is involved in cardiac remodeling and can be a therapeutic target in both metabolic and cardiovascular diseases [15].

Vasopressin secreted by the posterior pituitary gland is involved in osmoregulation with an important role in the pathophysiology of cardiac failure. In HF, the arginine vasopressin system contributes to the progression of left ventricular dysfunction by directly stimulating left ventricular hypertrophy and myocardial remodeling. Since vasopressin is unstable in plasma and has a low half-life, copeptin (C-terminal portion of pro-arginine vasopressin) was introduced as a vasopressin surrogate marker [18,19] and was investigated across the spectrum of cardiovascular diseases (including HF) as a prognostic marker [18]. A high copeptin level is independently associated with the incidence of DM, albuminuria and abdominal obesity [20–22].

The objectives of the present study were: (i) to evaluate whether FGF21 (an adiponectin with a role in regulating glucose and lipid homeostasis), copeptin (a precursor of pro-arginine vasopressin and a marker of neurohormonal activation) and galectin-3 (a marker of inflammation and fibrosis) can be used as biomarkers for the diagnosis of HFpEF in patients with type 2 DM; (ii) to determine the levels of biomarkers in patients with type 2 DM; and (iii) to assess the correlations between these biomarkers and echocardiographic parameters in the same population

2. Materials and Methods

2.1. Study Design and Characteristics

Between February 2019 and November 2020, 86 patients with DM were evaluated for inclusion in the study at the Nicolae Stăncioiu Heart Institute Cluj-Napoca, Romania, and at the Dr Constantin Opriș Emergency County Hospital, Baia Mare, Romania.

Institutional Review Board Statement: The study was conducted according to the guidelines of the Declaration of Helsinki, and approved by the Ethics Committee of Iuliu Hatieganu University of Medicine and Pharmacy, Cluj-Napoca, Romania (protocol code 48/11 March 2019) and Emergency County Hospital Baia Mare, Romania (no. 6361/28 February 2020). An informed consent was obtained from all subjects involved in the study.

The inclusion criteria consisted of the presence of DM under treatment, a left ventricular (LV) ejection fraction (EF) $\geq$ 50% and age over 18 years old. The exclusion criteria were recent hospitalization due to HF decompensation for patients with HF, severe valvular disease, hypertrophic or infiltrative cardiomyopathy, congenital heart disease, chronic obstructive pulmonary disease stage GOLD 3 or 4, pericardial disease, atrial fibrillation with high ventricular response > 100 bpm, severe renal failure (eGFR by CKD-EPI < 30 mL/min/1.73 m^2), severe anemia (hemoglobin < 7 g/dL) and neoplasia. After excluding subjects with intermediate LVEF (between 40–49%), we enrolled in our study 69 diabetic patients who fulfilled the inclusion criteria and we divided them into two groups: patients fulfilling the criteria for a diagnosis of HFpEF and patients without HF. We defined HFpEF according to a consensus recommendation from the Heart Failure Association of the European Society of Cardiology, using the HFA-PEFF diagnosis algorithm [4] based on clinical assessment revealing signs and symptoms of HF [4,23], echocardiographic measurements of function and morphology [4,24–27] and the level of natriuretic peptides. A HFA-PEFF score $\geq$ 5 points defines HFpEF. The score includes three domains (morphological, functional and biomarker) with major (2 points) and minor criteria (1point). The major criteria include septal e' < 7 cm/s, or lateral e' < 10 cm/s, or average E/e' $\geq$ 15 or TR velocity > 2.8 m/s (PASP > 35 mmHg), left atrial volume index > 34 mL/m^2 or left ventricular mass index $\geq$ 149 g/m^2 in men or $\geq$122 g/m^2 in women and relative wall thickness > 0.42, NT-proBNP > 220 pg/mL in sinus rhythm or >660 pg/mL in atrial fibrillation. The minor criteria are average E/e' 9–14 or GLS < 16%, left atrial volume index 29–34 mL/m^2 or relative wall thickness > 0.42, NT-proBNP 125–220 pg/mL in sinus rhythm or 365–660 pg/mL in atrial fibrillation.

2.2. Biomarkers

At the time of admission, blood samples were collected in serum separator tubes with clot activator (BD Vacutainer CAT) and allowed to clot at room temperature for no more than 2 h before centrifugation for 15 min at 1000$\times$ g to obtain serum. The samples were separated into Eppendorf tubes and stored at -80 °C until analysis. The NT-proBNP analysis was performed by an electrochemiluminescent immunoassay (Roche Diagnostics, Mannheim, Germany). We evaluated the seric concentration of the biomarkers through quantitative enzyme-linked immunosorbent assay (ELISA): FGF21(Catalog No E-EL-H0074, sensitivity 18.75 pg/mL, detection range: 31.25–2000 pg/mL, ElabscienceBiotechnology

Inc., Houston, TX, USA), Galectin-3 (Catalog No E-El-H1470, sensitivity 0.1 ng/mL, detection range 0.16–10 ng/mL, Elascience Biotechnology Inc., Houston, TX, USA), Copeptin (Catalog No E-EL-H0851, sensitivity 18.75 pg/mL, detectionrange 31.25–2000 pg/mL, Elabscience Biotechnology Inc., Houston, TX, USA).

2.3. Echocardiographic Assessment

All subjects underwent a complete two-dimensional transthoracic echocardi-ography (Philips CX 50, xMATRIX, Philips Ultrasound Inc., Bothell, WA, USA) examination prior to inclusion in the study protocol, using the cardiology software application. LVEF was obtained by using Simpson's method, with LV end-diastolic (EDV) and end-systolic volumes (ESV) acquired in the apical 4-chamber. Transmitral inflow, the peak velocities of early filling (E) and the deceleration time of E were evaluated by pulsed wave blood flow Doppler at the mitral valve leaflet tips in apical 4-chamber view. The early peak diastolic mitral annulus velocity (e′) was obtained by pulsed wave tissue Doppler in the LV septum and lateral wall. Pulmonary arterial systolic pressure was calculated using the modified Bernoulli equation as 4 × peak tricuspid regurgitation (TR) velocity adding the estimated right atrial pressure.

2.4. Statistical Analysis

Clinical features, laboratory and echocardiographic data were described as arithmetic mean (standard deviation), or as counts (percentage) for categorical variables. Patients were divided into two groups according to the presence or absence of HFpEF. The continuous variables were checked for univariate normal distribution through kurtosis-skewness analysis and Anderson-Darling test. The serum biomarkers FGF21, NT-proBNP and copeptin were consistent with log-normal distributions and were modeled using a natural logarithmic transformation. The log-transformed data were reported using geometric mean as a measure of central tendency and geometric standard deviation as a measure of log-normal dispersion. The comparisons between the studied groups concerning the serum biomarker values were performed based on their log-transformed data using Student-t test with equal variances or Welch's *t*-test. For continuous variables with deviations from normal distribution, we used the Mann-Whitney U test for comparisons between the studied groups. The associations between nominal variables and HF in patients with type 2 DM were tested using Chi-square or Fisher's exact test. Pearson or Spearman rank correlation coefficients were used to assess the correlation between the log-transformed biomarker values and clinical, laboratory and echocardiographic variables. The Pearson correlation coefficient was used to quantify the strength of a linear correlation between two quantitative variables assuming that each of the variables followed a normal distribution; otherwise, the Spearman coefficient was used.

The ability of biomarkers FGF21, copeptin and galectin-3 to distinguish HFpEF cases from non-HFpEF subjects was evaluated by the area under the Receiver Operating Characteristics (ROC) curve and the 95% confidence interval (CI), percentage of correct predictions (PCP) with their 95% CI, sensitivity and specificity (95% CI). A PCP value close to 1 denoted that the tested model had a good discrimination for HF The optimum cut-off point was obtained using the Youden index. All inferential analyses were performed using two-sided tests with statistical significance set at an estimated p-value < 0.05. All statistical analyses were performed in R software version 4.0.4 (R Foundation for Statistical Computing, Vienna, Austria).

3. Results

3.1. Baseline Characteristics of the Sample of Patients with Type 2 DM

Eighty-six consecutively selected patients were evaluated for inclusion in the study. Considering the inclusion and exclusion criteria, the studied sample consisted of 69 patients with type 2 DM divided into 2 groups: patients with HFpEF (n = 40, LVEF $\geq$ 50%) and those without HFpEF (n = 29). The distributions of baseline characteristics in each group are described in Table 1.

Table 1. Demographic, clinical and para-clinical characteristics of patients with type 2 DM.

	All DM Samples (n = 69)	DM without HFpEF (n_1 = 29)	DM with HFpEF (n_2 = 40)	p-Value
Age, years [a]	64.65 ± 9.83	63.83 ± 7.70	65.25 ± 11.17	0.557
Male [b]	37 (53.62)	18 (62.07)	19 (47.50)	0.231
Body mass index, kg/m² [a]	32.43 ± 6.69	30.94 ± 7.25	33.50 ± 6.11	0.117
Body Surface Area [a]	1.99 ± 0.21	2.00 ± 0.24	1.99 ± 0.18	0.866
SBP, mmHg [a]	138.40 ± 19.68	136.60 ± 18.57	139.70 ± 20.59	0.519
DBP, mmHg [a]	79.67 ± 10.96	77.45 ± 10.20	81.28 ± 11.33	0.153
Smoking [b]	15 (21.74)	8 (27.59)	7 (17.50)	0.316
Medical history [b]				
Hypertension	60 (86.96)	27 (93.10)	33 (82.50)	0.285
Atrial fibrillation	9 (13.04)	1 (3.45)	8 (20.00)	0.069
Paroxysmal atrial fibrillation	3 (4.35)	0 (0.00)	3 (7.50)	0.258
Previous stroke	2 (2.90)	0 (0.00)	2 (5.00)	0.506
Previous MI	32 (46.38)	10 (34.48)	22 (55.00)	0.092
COPD	3 (5.80)	1 (3.45)	3 (7.69)	0.631
PAD	5 (7.25)	5 (17.86)	0 (0.0)	0.009
Medication [b]				0.765
Insulin	30 (43.48)	12 (41.38)	18 (45.00)	
Oral antidiabetic drugs [b]	39 (56.52)	17 (58.62)	22 (55.00)	
Laboratory data [a]				
HbA1C, %	7.65 [7.20, 9.25]	7.42 [6.90, 7.69]	8.84 [7.30, 9.96]	0.008 *
Fasting blood glucose, mg/dL	187.50 ± 74.12	171.50 ± 58.59	199.10 ± 82.38	0.128
Total cholesterol, mg/dL	166.60 ± 46.16	156.60 ± 41.67	173.80 ± 48.37	0.127
LDL cholesterol, mg/dL	93.66 ± 38.42	88.13 ± 38.97	97.66 ± 38.01	0.313
HDL cholesterol, mg/dL	38.74 ± 9.19	37.32 ± 8.44	39.77 ± 9.68	0.277
Triglycerides, mg/dL	155.20 [112.40, 204.00]	156.40 [124.00, 181.10]	150.50 [107.20, 224.00]	0.918
eGFR, mL/min/1.73 m² by CKD-EPI	73.69 ± 24.49	78.07 ± 21.70	70.53 ± 26.14	0.209
Hemoglobin, g/dL	13.38 ± 1.71	13.73 ± 1.76	13.13 ± 1.65	0.152
Uric acid mg/dL	6.36 ± 1.88	5.92 ± 1.06	6.68 ± 2.26	0.070
Coronary angiography #, [b]				0.031 *
Absent	4 (5.80)	4 (16.00)	0 (0.00)	
Monovessel CAD	15 (21.74)	4 (16.00)	11 (32.35)	
Multivessel CAD	40 (57.97)	17 (68.00)	23 (67.65)	

[a] Data are presented as arithmetic mean ± sample standard deviation or median [25th percentile; 75th percentile], [b] absolute frequencies (relative frequencies, %). p-values were obtained by Student-t test with equal variances, Welch's t-test, Chi-square test or Fisher's exact test, * significant results ($p < 0.05$); # complete case data n = 59; HFpEF = heart failure with preserved ejection fraction, SBP = systolic blood pressure, DBP = diastolic blood pressure, NYHA = New York Heart Association, MI = myocardial infarction, COPD = chronic obstructive pulmonary disease, PAD = peripheral arterial disease, HbA1c = glycated hemoglobin, eGFR = estimated glomerular filtration rate; CKD-EPI = Chronic Kidney Disease Epidemiology Collaboration, CAD = coronary artery disease.

Patients with HFpEF had significantly different HbA1c values than patients without HF ($p = 0.008$). Concerning NYHA classification, we noticed that stages II and III were more frequent in patients with HFpEF (90% of cases). The presence of multivessel coronary artery disease was more frequent in patients with HFpEF compared to patients without HF ($p = 0.031$).

3.2. Comparisons of Serum FGF21, Galectin-3, Copeptin and Echocardiographic Parameters in Patients with Type 2 Diabetes Mellitus Grouped by Heart Failure

The NT-proBNP level was significantly higher in DM patients with HFpEF compared to patients without HEpEF (1279.83 ± 3.08 vs. 153.26 ± 2.75, $p < 0.001$). Similarly, there were significant differences between the two groups regarding the FGF21 level ($p < 0.001$).

There was no statistical difference in galectin-3 and copeptin concentrations between the two studied groups (Table 2). Echocardiographic parameters such as LVEF ($p = 0.003$), LVESV, $p = 0.014$) and E/e, left atrial (LA) surface, TR velocity ($p < 0.001$) were significantly different between DM patients with HFpEF and those without HFpEF.

Table 2. Comparison of FGF21, galectin-3, copeptin and echocardiographic parameters between the studied groups.

	All DM Samples ($n = 69$)	DM without HFpEF ($n_1 = 29$)	DM with HFpEF ($n_2 = 40$)	p-Value
FGF21, pg/mL [a]	221.72 ± 2.01	146.79 ± 1.76	298.98 ± 1.90	<0.001 *,[d]
Gal-3, ng/mL [b]	11.91 ± 1.52	11.66 ± 1.71	12.10 ± 1.36	0.239
Copeptin, pg/mL [a]	321.04 ± 2.55	348.35 ± 2.84	302.59 ± 2.36	0.541 [d]
LV ejection fraction, % [b]	54 [51, 59]	57 [54, 61]	53 [50, 55]	0.001 *
LV EDV, ml [c]	108 [90, 126]	103 [89, 112]	116 [94.25, 138.20]	0.061
LV ESV, ml [b]	50.4 ± 20.6	43.4 ± 17.2	55.5 ± 21.6	0.014 *
LVDd, mm [b]	49.8 ± 5.1	50.3 ± 4.6	49.5 ± 5.5	0.539
LVSd, mm [b]	29.0 ± 6.4	28.3 ± 6.2	29.6 ± 6.6	0.425
IVST, mm [b]	12.3 ± 1.7	12.2 ± 1.7	12.3 ± 1.6	0.886
PWT, mm [b]	12.0 ± 1.6	11.8 ± 1.8	12.1 ± 1.5	0.355
LA volume index, mL/m^2 [c]	30.0 [25.6, 35.0]	27.3 [24.0, 29.8]	32.31 [28.1, 41.3]	0.001 *
LA surface, cm^2 [b]	22.9 ± 6.8	19.3 ± 4.3	25.5 ± 7.2	<0.001 *
E wave velocity, m/s [b]	0.8 ± 0.3	0.7 ± 0.2	0.9 ± 0.3	0.002 *
A wave velocity, m/s [b]	0.8 ± 0.2	0.8 ± 0.2	0.9 ± 0.2	0.111
Mitral E/A ratio [b]	0.9 ± 0.3	0.9 ± 0.4	0.9 ± 0.3	0.722
TDE, msec [b]	217.8 ± 39.9	230.8 ± 33.5	208.4 ± 41.9	0.020 *
Septal e' velocity, cm/s [b]	7.2 ± 1.4	7.9 ± 1.3	6.7 ± 1.2	<0.001 *
Lateral e' velocity, cm/s [b]	8.6 ± 1.9	9.8 ± 1.5	7.7 ± 1.6	<0.001 *
E/e' mean ratio [b]	10.7 ± 3.9	8.2 ± 2.5	12.37 ± 3.9	<0.001 *
Relative wall thickness [b]	0.48 ± 0.1	0.46 ± 0.06	0.49 ± 0.08	0.058
TR velocity, m/s [b]	2.4 ± 0.6	2.06 ± 0.42	2.69 ± 0.61	<0.001 *
PASP, mmHg [b]	30.6 ± 15.6	21.7 ± 7.9	37.1 ± 16.6	<0.001 *

Data are presented as [a] geometric mean ± geometric standard deviation or [b] arithmetic mean ± sample standard deviation or [c] median [25th percentile; 75th percentile], p-values were obtained from Student-t tests for independent groups or Mann-Whitney U test; [d] Student-t test applied on log-transformed data; * significant results ($p < 0.05$); DM = type 2 diabetes mellitus; LVEDV = left ventricular end-diastolic volume, LVESV = left ventricular end-systolic volume. LVEDP = left ventricular end-diastolic pressure, LA = left atrial, IVST interventricular septum thickness s, PWT = posterior wall thickness, LV = left ventricular, LVDd = left ventricular end-diastolic dimension, LVSd = left ventricular end-systolic dimension, TDE = deceleration time, TR velocity = tricuspid regurgitation peak velocity, PASP= pulmonary artery systolic pressure FGF21-fibroblast growth factor; Gal-3 = galectin-3; HFpEF = heart failure with preserved ejection fraction.

3.3. Evaluation of FGF21, Copeptin and Gal-3 as Markers of HFpEF in Patients with Type 2 DM

Binomial logistic regression was performed to evaluate the association betweenFGF21, copeptin and galectin-3 and the odds of HFpEF (Table 3). In the univariable regression analysis, there was no statistical evidence of a significant association of galectin-3 and copeptin with the odds of HFpEF in patients with type 2 DM ($p = 0.240$ for galectin-3 and $p = 0.628$ for copeptin), but the biomarker FGF21 ($p = 0.001$) was significantly associated with the odds of HFpEF.

At the FGF21 optimal cut-off value of 217.40 pg/mL, 29 out of 40 HFpEF patients were identified as patients with HF. The ROC curve of FGF21 is presented in Figure 1 with an AUC value of 0.81, 95% CI: [0.70, 0.91]. After adjusting for demographic and clinical covariates such as age, gender, body mass index, diastolic blood pressure, HbA1c and previous myocardial infarction, the biomarker FGF21 remained in a significant association with the odds of HF ($p = 0.001$). The explanatory multivariable model demonstrated a good distinction between HFpEF and non-HFpEF patients with type 2 DM (AUC = 0.88, 95% CI: [0.80, 0.96], PCP = 81.16%, 95% PCP: [71.93, 90.39], Se = 85% [70.2, 94.3], Sp = 79.3% [60.3, 92.0].

Table 3. Logistic regression analysis of factors used to separate patients with diabetes and heart failure from those without heart failure.

Variables	Univariable Model Crude OR [95% CI]	p-Value	Multivariable Model Adjusted OR [95% CI]	p-Value
FGF21 (pg/mL)	5.16 [2.19, 15.47]	0.001 *	8.80 [2.95, 36.30]	0.001 *
Age (years)	1.16 [0.71, 1.90]	0.551	2.52 [1.12; 6.68]	0.039 *
Gender [a]	0.55 [0.20, 1.45]	0.233	0.67 [0.16, 2.72]	0.574
BMI (kg/m^2)	1.50 [0.91, 2.55]	0.118	0.69 [0.31, 1.44]	0.340
DBP (mmHG)	1.45 [0.88, 2.50]	0.157	1.20 [0.64, 2.38]	0.573
HbA1c (%)	1.99 [1.14, 3.93]	0.0267 *	2.27 [1.19, 5.13]	0.025 *
Previous MI	2.32 [0.88, 6.40]	0.094	3.81 [0.99, 17.19]	0.061

FGF21 = fibroblast growth factor 21, BMI = body mass index, DBP = diastolic blood pressure, HbA1c = glycated hemoglobin; MI = myocardial infarction; * statistical significance: $p < 0.05$; Multivariable Model: FGF21 adjusted for demographic and clinical covariates; OR = odds ratio; [a] Reference category: Gender = F.

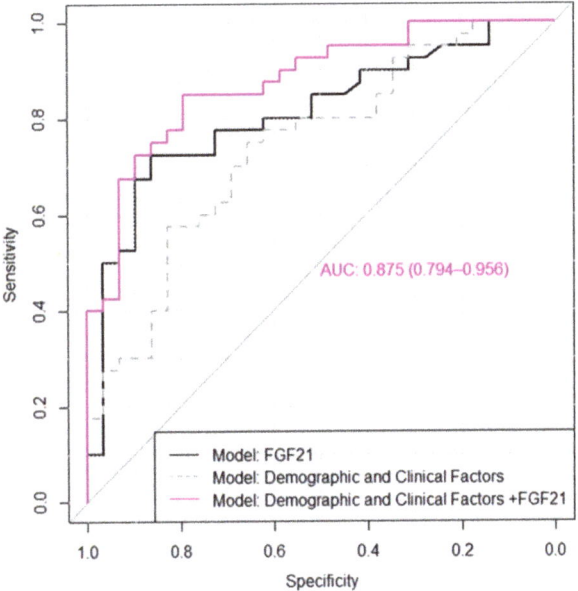

Figure 1. The ROC curves for distinction between type 2 diabetes mellitus patients with heart failure with preserved ejection fraction from those without heart failure. The demographic and clinical factors included in the tested model were age, gender, BMI, DBP, HbA1c and previous MI (See Table 3).

Although the addition of covariates (demographic and clinical factors) provided a greater model ability to discriminate between HFpEF and non-HFpEF patients with type 2 DM, the results showed only a tendency towards statistical significance: DeLong's test: $\Delta AUC = 0.07, p = 0.109$ (Figure 1).

3.4. Correlations among FGF21, Galectin-3, and Copeptin with Clinical, Laboratory Data and Echocardiographic Variables in All Samples of Patients with Type 2 DM

In bivariate correlation analysis between the studied biomarkers and echocardiographic characteristics (Table 4), there was a significant positive correlation of FGF21 with LVEDV (Spearman's correlation coefficient, $\rho = 0.32, p = 0.008$), LVESV (Pearson's correlation coefficient, $r = 0.39, p < 0.001$), LA surface (Pearson's correlation coefficient, $r = 0.26, p = 0.028$) and LA volume (Spearman's correlation coefficient, $\rho = 0.29, p = 0.017$).

Table 4. Matrix of correlation coefficients (95% CI) between FGF21, galectin-3 and copeptin with echocardiographic variables.

Variables	Log FGF21	Log Copeptin	Gal-3
	Correlation Coefficient (95% CI)	Correlation Coefficient (95% CI)	Correlation Coefficient (95% CI)
LV EF, %	−0.26 [−0.47, 0.02] (b)	0.20 [−0.05, 0.42] (b)	−0.14 [−0.37, 0.11] (b)
LV EDV, ml	0.32 [0.08, 0.52] (b),*	−0.30 [−0.50, −0.06] (b),*	0.21 [−0.03, 0.43] (b)
LV ESV, ml	0.39 [0.17, 0.57] (a),*	−0.31 [−0.51, −0.08] (a),*	0.20 [−0.04, 0.42] (a)
LA volume index, mL/m²	0.29 [0.05, 0.49] (b),*	−0.09 [−0.33, 0.15] (b)	0.25 [0.01, 0.47] (b),*
LA surface, cm²	0.26 [0.03, 0.47] (a),*	−0.05 [−0.29, 0.19] (a)	0.12 [−0.12, 0.34] (a)
E wave velocity, m/s	0.20 [−0.04, 0.41] (a)	0.25 [0.02, 0.46] (a),*	0.03 [−0.20, 0.27] (a)
A wave velocity, m/s	−0.01 [−0.26, 0.24] (a)	0.11 [−0.14, 0.35] (a)	0.01 [−0.23, 0.26] (a)
Mitral E/A ratio	0.19 [−0.06, 0.42] (a)	0.25 [0.00, 0.47] (a)	<0.01 [−0.25, 0.24] (a)
TDE, msec	−0.16 [−0.38, 0.08] (a)	−0.12 [−0.35, 0.12] (a)	<0.01 [−0.23, 0.24] (a)
Septal e' velocity, cm/s	−0.19 [−0.41, 0.05] (a)	−0.03 [−0.27, 0.21] (a)	−0.07 [−0.30, 0.17] (a)
Lateral e' velocity, cm/s	−0.21 [−0.42, 0.03] (a)	−0.01 [−0.25, 0.23] (a)	0.03 [−0.21, 0.26] (a)
E/e' mean ratio	0.23 [−0.01, 0.44] (a)	0.24 [0.00, 0.45] (a)	0.06 [−0.18, 0.29] (a)
Relative wall thickness	0.09 [−0.15, 0.32] (a)	0.28 [0.04, 0.48] (a),*	0.20 [−0.04, 0.41] (a)
TR velocity, m/s	0.25 [0.02, 0.46] (a)	−0.17 [0.40, 0.06] (a)	0.25 [0.02, 0.46] (a),*
PASP, mmHg	0.26 [0.03, 0.47] (a),*	−0.16 [−0.38, 0.08] (a)	0.27 [0.03, 0.48] (a),*

(a) Pearson (r), (b) Spearman (ρ)'s correlation coefficient, 95% CI = 95% Confidence Interval; * statistical significance: 95% CI did not contain 0; LVEDV = left ventricular end-diastolic volume, LVESV = left ventricular end-systolic volume. LVEDP = left ventricular end-diastolic pressure, LA = left atrial, IVST interventricular septum thickness, PWT = posterior wall thickness, LV = left ventricular, LVDd = left ventricular end-diastolic dimension, LVSd = left ventricular end-systolic dimension, TDE = deceleration time, TR velocity = tricuspid regurgitation peak velocity, PASP = pulmonary artery systolic pressure.

Copeptin had a negative correlation with LVEDV (ρ = −0.30, p = 0.014) and LSESV (r = −0.31, p = 0.008), and a linear positive correlation with E wave velocity (r = 0.25, p = 0.036). Galectin-3 was positively correlated only with LA volume index, TR velocity and pulmonary artery systolic pressure (Table 4).

4. Discussion

Patients with HFpEF represent nearly 50% of the HF population and is associated with a decreased life expectancy [26,28]. This impaired prognosis, however, is not fully explained by the associated comorbidities such as hypertension, diabetes mellitus, atrial fibrillation and obesity, as higher mortality rates have been reported in patients with HFpEF than in those with similar comorbidities but without HF [28]. Regarding NT-ProBNP, which has a high specificity but a lower sensitivity for the diagnosis of HFpEF, new biomarkers need to be investigated.

In this study, we demonstrated the utility of FGF21 in diagnosing HFpEF in diabetic patients, with a high sensitivity and specificity at a cut-off value of 217.4 pg/mL. FGF21 had a significant association with the odds of HF (p = 0.001), even after adjusting for demographic and studied clinical covariates. FGF21, in combination with demographic and clinical factors, had a better ability to distinguish between diabetic HFpEF and non-HF patients, but the results were not statistically significant, only showing a trend towards significance, possibly due to the small number of patients included.

These results are in accordance with the first study conducted by Ruey-Hsing in 2016 [6], which demonstrated the association between elevated levels of FGF21 and diastolic dysfunction in adult humans.

In recent years, there has been a lot of evidence to suggest that that increased serum FGF21 levels are found in obese, insulin-resistant patients, and those with metabolic syndrome [29]. Additionally, serum FGF21 levels were higher in diabetic patients with low urinary glucose excretion compared to those with high urinary glucose excretion (pg/mL, 429.4 vs. 263.5, p = 0.002) [30]. Elevated levels of FGF21 in serum during the early stages of various metabolic diseases are considered a compensatory response by the organism. Therefore, FGF21 is regarded as a hormone in response to stress and an early diagnostic marker of disease [13]. The results in our study also demonstrated a significant correlation between FGF21 levels and obesity, BMI, body surface area, total cholesterol and LDL cholesterol.

FGF21 binds to the FGF receptor (FGFR) in the presence of the co-factor ß-Klotho, acts as an adipokine in order to determine glucose uptake in adipocytes and further, increases insulin sensitivity [13,31,32]. In a recent review, the protective role of FGF21 was highlighted, especially in pathological processes such as suppressing apoptosis in the myocardium, reducing inflammation in cardiomyocytes and oxidative stress, and promoting fatty acid oxidation [13]. It is suggested that DCM can be delayed through the application of injectable exogenous FGF21, providing possible therapeutic targets in this disease [13]. Studies performed on mice suggest that exogenous FGF21 protects people from heart injury in DCM by antagonizing oxidative stress, but the quantity of exogenous FGF21 administered in these studies was considerably higher than that in normal physiological conditions [13,33]. Expression of FGF21 in the heart is under the control of the protein deacetylase Sirt1 (sirtuin1). In an environment with high levels of sugar and fat, activation of the Sirt1 pathway generates cardiac secretion of FGF21, which acts in an autocrine manner to prevent oxidative stress in cardiomyocytes, by promoting the expression of certain antioxidant genes (Ucp2, Ucp3, or Sod2) [34]. In conclusion, FGF21 performs a role in suppressing apoptosis in myocardial cells induced by oxidative damage both in vitro and in vivo, protection occurring through modulation of apoptosis-related genes and the oxidoreductase system. However, these findings are based on animal studies, with a lack of research data from clinical studies, requiring further investigations [13].

The diagnostic value of galectin-3, a biomarker of myocardial fibrosis and inflammation, has not been extensively studied. Van Kimmenade et al. found that galectin-3 values were significantly higher in subjects with HF, compared to those without HF. At a cut-off value of 6.88 ng/mL, galectin-3 had a sensitivity of 80% and a specificity of 52% in the diagnosis of HF as the etiology of dyspnea, with a receiver operating characteristic [ROC] curve analysis of 0.72 [35].

Another study conducted by Trippel et al. in a population with cardiovascular risk factors, found that at a cut-off value of 13.57 ng/mL, galectin-3 had a sensitivity of 61% and a specificity of 73% for diagnosis of HFpEF. The AUC of Gal-3 was 0.71. Furthermore, patients with galectin-3 $\geq$ 13.4 ng/mL developed incident HFpEF significantly more often than patients with galectin-3 < 13.4 ng/mL [36].

In the COACH study (de Boer et al.), higher levels of galectin-3 were associated with higher rates of re-hospitalization and death in HFpEF, but not in patients with HFrEF [37].

A systematic review and meta-analysis [24] which investigated the diagnostic potential of biomarkers in HFpEF found that the studies investigating galectin-3 as a diagnostic biomarker of HFpEF were conducted in Asia, with cut-off values of 9.55 ng/mL, 17.8 ng/mL, 20.12 ng/mL [28,38–40].

The study conducted by Salman et al. revealed that galectin-3 levels were 15.1 ng/mL in patients with type 2 DM and macroalbuminuria, 8.3 ng/mL in patients with type 2 DM and normoalbuminuria, and 9.8 ng/mL in patients with type 2 DM and normoalbuminuria, the results being statistically significant ($p = 0.01$ and $p = 0.05$, respectively). They also found a negative correlation between the galectin-3 level and eGFR [41].

A Chinese study on 284 diabetic patients (Jin Qi-hui et al.) demonstrated that the mean galectin-3 level was 27.4 ng/mL in patients with DM. At a serum galectin level > 25 ng/mL, they demonstrated that galectin-3 was a risk factor for HF [42].

The study conducted by Edelman et al. revealed that galectin-3 was associated with HFpEF and fibrosis [43]. Pecherina et al. investigated the serum galectin-3 levels in patients with ST-segment elevation myocardial infarction (STEMI) and preserved LVEF (HFpEF) compared to those with HFrEF, and found that this biomarker correlated with the parameters reflecting diastolic dysfunction in patients with HFpEF, and with LVEF and left ventricular end-systolic volume/diameter in patients with HFrEF [44]. The TOPCAT trial investigated the biomarker profiles of patients with diabetes and HFpEF compared to patients without DM. The authors reported levels of 22.0 ng/mL for galectin-3 in patients with DM with HFpEF, higher than in patients without diabetes, 20.0 ng/mL [45].

In our study, there was no statistically significant difference in galectin-3 concentrations between the studied groups; thus, we did not find a possible association with the risk of HF. The mean value of galectin-3 in our studied sample of diabetic patients was 11.9 ng/mL, lower than the value obtained by Jin Qi-hui et al. [42] in a Chinese population, and also lower than the value reported by the TOPCAT trial [45]. To our knowledge, studies enrolling Caucasian subjects with type 2 DM for evaluating the diagnostic performance of galectin in HFpEF are lacking. Schill et al. analyzed copeptin levels in 5297 individuals without prevalent HF from the Malmö Preventive Project and found that in older adults this biomarker could predict the development of HF [46]. Noor et al. published their results regarding the relationship of copeptin with DM progressing towards diabetic nephropathy and found significantly higher copeptin levels in subjects with a positive family history of DM compared to those with no history of DM (pg/mL, 243.77 vs. 165.2, $p = 0.025$). The same study found that the level of copeptin was negatively correlated with eGFR and there was no correlation between the level of copeptin and the level of HbA1c [47].

The copeptin level is higher and has a prognostic value in patients with HFrEF, but its role in HFpEF is still underexplored [11,48]. In acute HF, copeptin has been shown to be a prognostic predictor of HF hospitalization and mortality [49,50]. In a report from the prospective KaRen study, Hage C. et al. found that copeptin levels did not differ between patients with and without diastolic dysfunction [11]. Our results confirmed those of Hage C. et al.

FGF21 significantly correlated with echocardiographic parameters such as the left atrial volume, left atrial surface and pulmonary artery systolic pressure and had a borderline correlation with E/e' ratio, with results comparable to those obtained by Ruey-Hsing et al. in 2016 [6]. On the other hand, we did not find an association between the other biomarkers (galectin-3 and copeptin) and echocardiographic measurements of diastolic dysfunction.

In the present study, there was a significant difference in HbA1c levels among diabetic patients with and without HFpEF. The levels of HbA1c were significantly higher in diabetic patients with HFpEF compared to diabetic patients without HFpEF ($p = 0.008$). In our study, multivariate analysis confirmed that Hb1Ac is an independent risk factor for HF in diabetic patients ($p = 0.025$). Other studies have evaluated the association between Hb1Ac levels and the risk of HF in patients with diabetes. The study performed by Pazin Filho found that HbA1c is an independent risk factor for HF in patients with diabetes with or without cardiovascular diseases [51] and Zhao confirmed these results in African American and white patients with diabetes [52].

Moreover, Lind suggested that the risk of hospitalization increased in diabetic patients with poor glycemic control (HbA1c) > 7%) [53], and Erqou revealed that a higher HbA1c level was associated with a significantly increased risk for congestive heart failure [54]. Poor glycemic control is associated with a 1.56-fold increased risk of HF among adult patients with diabetes according to the results presented by Iribarren [55].

As far as we know, this is the first study conducted in a Caucasian population to evaluate for HFpEF in diabetic patients the diagnostic performance of three specific biomarkers that are involved in different types of pathological mechanisms of HF (FGF21 regulates glucose and lipid homeostasis, copeptin is involved in neurohormonal activation and galectin-3 promotes inflammation and fibrosis). FGF21 is a stress inducible hormone that plays important roles in regulating energy balance and glucose and lipid homeostasis [56] and there are studies demonstrating that myocytes secrete FGF21 as an autocrine factor, in order to protect the heart from adverse cardiac remodeling [7,15]. Studies conducted on rodents or on primates demonstrated that the administration of FGF21 brings considerable pharmacological benefits on a cluster of obesity-related metabolic complications, including a reduction in fat mass and alleviation of hyperglycemia, insulin resistance, dyslipidemia, cardiovascular disorders and non- alcoholic steatohepatitis (NASH).

Because native FGF21 is not suitable for clinical use due to its poor pharmacokinetic and biophysical properties, there has developed a large number of long-acting FGF21 analogues–ß-and agonistic monoclonal antibodies for theFGFR1–ß-klotho receptor complexes [56]. The clinical trials including patients with obesity, DM type 2 and nonalcoholic steatohepatitis, demonstrated substantial improvements in dyslipidemia, hepatic fat fractions and serum markers of liver fibrosis, whereas the primary end points of glycemic control have not been met [56]. In this context, several current drugs used for treatment inDM type 2 are highly effective for glucose lowering, but lack the considerable therapeutic effects of FGF21 on dyslipidemia. An association of FGF21- based pharmacotherapy with these glucose- lowering agents to treat multiple obesity- related metabolic complications might constitute a promising strategy that worth further exploration [56]. In our study we showed that FGF21 can represent a novel candidate biomarker for diagnosis in HFpEF in diabetic patients, facilitating its early detection, but further studies are needed to confirm our finding, with a larger number of patients. Furthermore, the utility of this biomarker is enhanced by the fact that FGF21 could be used in the future as a target therapy in metabolic and cardiovascular disease.

The main limitation of the present study was the relatively small sample size, which also restricted the testing of a multivariable model containing other known covariates such as coronary artery disease or NYHA class. The biomarker levels were measured only at the time of admission, and we do not have data about the change in their concentration at the time of readmission. Further assessment of these biomarkers (FGF21, galectin-3, copeptin) for HF diagnosis in patients with HFpEF should be conducted with a larger study cohort.

5. Conclusions

Neither galectin-3 nor copeptin showed promise as a biomarker in diagnosing HFpEF. In contrast with the negative findings related to galectin-3 and copeptin, fibroblast growth factor 21 may be a novel candidate biomarker for the diagnosis of HFpEF in diabetic patients. Further studies are needed with a larger sample of patients.

Author Contributions: Conceptualization, R.D.I.; Data curation, R.D.I. and R.R.; Formal analysis, M.I.; Investigation, R.D.I. and C.P.; Methodology, A.C. and L.M.P.; Project administration, L.M.P.; Resources, R.D.I., C.P., R.R. and A.C.; Software, M.I.; Supervision, C.P. and L.M.P.; Validation, M.I. and L.M.P.; Visualization, C.P. and L.M.P.; Writing—original draft, R.D.I. and M.I.; Writing—review & editing, C.P. and L.M.P. All authors have read and agreed to the published version of the manuscript. All authors had equal contributions to this article.

Funding: This research was funded by Iuliu Hatieganu University of Medicine and Pharmacy, Cluj-Napoca, Romania, grant number 1529/18 January 2019.

Institutional Review Board Statement: The study was conducted according to the guidelines of the Declaration of Helsinki, and approved by the Ethics Committee of Iuliu Hatieganu University of Medicine and Pharmacy, Cluj-Napoca, Romania (protocol code 48/11 March 2019) and Emergency County Hospital Baia Mare, Romania (no. 6361/28 February 2020).

Informed Consent Statement: An informed consent was obtained from all subjects involved in the study.

Data Availability Statement: The raw data involved in this study can be obtained upon reasonable request addressed to Lucia M. Procopciuc (luciamariaprocopciuc@yahoo.com).

Conflicts of Interest: The authors declare no conflict of interest.

References

1. Seshasai, S.R.S.; Kaptoge, S.S. Emerging Risk Factors Collaboration. Diabetes mellitus, fasting glucose, and risk of cause specific death. *N. Engl. J. Med.* **2011**, *364*, 829–841.
2. Yuvashree, M.; Pragasam, V. Diabetic Cardiomyopathy: A New Perspective of Mechanistic Approach. *J. Diabetes Metab.* **2015**, *6*, 605. [CrossRef]

3. Dunlay, S.M.; Roger, V.L.; Redfield, M.M. Epidemiology of heart failure with preserved ejection fraction. *Nat. Rev. Cardiol.* **2017**, *14*, 591–602. [CrossRef]
4. Pieske, B.; Tschöpe, C.; de Boer, R.A.; Fraser, A.G.; Anker, S.D.; Donal, E.; Edelmann, F. How to diagnose heart failure with preserved ejection fraction: The HFA–PEFF diagnostic algorithm: A consensus recommendation from the Heart Failure Association (HFA) of the European Society of Cardiology (ESC). *Eur. Heart J.* **2019**, *40*, 3297–3317. [CrossRef]
5. Zheng, S.L.; Chan, F.T.; Nabeebaccus, A.A.; Shah, A.M.; McDonagh, T.; Okonko, D.O. Drug treatment effects on outcomes in heart failure with preserved ejection fraction: A systematic review and meta-analysis. *Heart* **2018**, *104*, 407–415. [CrossRef]
6. Chou, R.H.; Huang, P.H.; Hsu, C.Y. Circulating Fibroblast Growth Factor 21 is Associated with Diastolic Dysfunction in Heart Failure Patients with Preserved Ejection Fraction. *Sci. Rep.* **2016**, *6*, 33953. [CrossRef] [PubMed]
7. Palomer, C.X.; Delgado, J.P.; Vazquez-Carrera, M. Emerging Actors in Diabetic Cardiomyopathy: Heartbreaker Biomarkers or Therapeutic Targets? *Trends Pharmacol. Sci.* **2018**, *39*, 452–467. [CrossRef]
8. Anjan, V.Y.; Loftus, T.M.; Burke, M.A.; Akhter, N.; Fonarow, G.C.; Gheorghiade, M.; Shah, S.J. Prevalence, clinical phenotype, and outcomes associated with normal B-type natriuretic peptide levels in heart failure with preserved ejection fraction. *Am. J. Cardiol.* **2012**, *110*, 870–876. [CrossRef]
9. Borlaug, B.A.; Nishimura, R.A.; Sorajja, P.; Lam, C.S.; Redfield, M.M. Exercise hemodynamics enhance diagnosis of early heart failure with preserved ejection fraction. *Circ. Heart Fail.* **2010**, *3*, 588–595. [CrossRef]
10. Meijers, W.C.; Hoekstra, T.; Jaarsma, T.; van Veldhuisen, D.J. Patients with heart failure with preserved ejection fraction and low levels of natriuretic peptides. *Neth. Heart J.* **2016**, *24*, 287–295. [CrossRef]
11. Hage, C.; Lund, L.H.; Donal, E. Copeptin in patients with heart failure and preserved ejection fraction: A report from the prospective KaRen-study. *Open Heart* **2015**, *2*, e000260. [CrossRef] [PubMed]
12. Pugliese, G.P.; Iacobini, C.I. Galectin-3 in diabetic patients. *Clin. Chem. Lab. Med.* **2014**, *52*, 1413. [CrossRef] [PubMed]
13. Zhang, X.; Yang, L.; Xu, X.; Tang, F.; Yi, P.; Qiu, B.; Hao, Y. A review of fibroblast growth factor 21 in diabetic cardiomyopathy. *Heart Fail. Rev.* **2019**, *24*, 1005–1017. [CrossRef] [PubMed]
14. Shao, M.; Yu, L.; Zhang, F.; Lu, X.; Li, X.; Cheng, P.; Lin, X.; He, L. Additive protection by LDR and FGF21 treatment against diabetic nephropathy in type 2 diabetes model. *Am. J. Physiol. Endocrinol. Metab.* **2015**, *309*, E45–E54. [CrossRef]
15. Yafei, S.; Elsewy, F.; Youssef, E.; Ayman, M.; El-Shafei, M. Fibroblast growth factor 21 association with subclinical atherosclerosis and arterial stiffness in type 2 diabetes. *Diabetes Metab. Syndr.* **2019**, *13*, 882–888. [CrossRef]
16. Zhang, W.; Chu, S.; Ding, W.; Wang, F. Serum Level of Fibroblast Growth Factor 21 Is Independently Associated with Acute Myocardial Infarction. *PLoS ONE* **2015**, *10*, e0129791. [CrossRef]
17. Jia, G.; Hill, M.A.; Sowers, J.R. Diabetic Cardiomyopathy. An Update of Mechanisms Contributing to This Clinical Entity. *Circ. Res.* **2018**, *122*, 624–638. [CrossRef]
18. Morgenthaler, N.G.; Struck, J.; Alonso, C.; Bergmann, A. Assay for the measurement of copeptin, a stable peptide derived from the precursor of vasopressin. *Clin. Chem.* **2006**, *52*, 112. [CrossRef]
19. Enhörning, S.; Bo Hedblad, B.; Nilsson, P.M.; Engstrom, G. Copeptin is an independent predictor of diabetic heart disease and death. *Am. Heart J.* **2015**, *169*, 549–556. [CrossRef]
20. Enhörning, S.; Wang, T.J.; Nilsson, P.M.; Almgren, P.; Hedblad, B.; Berglund, G. Plasma copeptin and the risk of diabetes mellitus. *Circulation* **2010**, *121*, 2102–2108. [CrossRef]
21. Enhörning, S.; Bankir, L.; Bouby, N.; Struck, J.; Hedblad, B.; Persson, M.; Morgenthaler, N.G. Copeptin, a marker of vasopressin, in abdominal obesity, diabetes and microalbuminuria: The prospective Malmö Diet and Cancer Study cardiovascular cohort. *Int. J. Obes.* **2013**, *37*, 598–603. [CrossRef] [PubMed]
22. Owan, T.E.; Hodge, D.O.; Herges, R.M.; Jacobsen, S.J. Trends in prevalence and outcome of heart failure with preserved ejection fraction. *N. Engl. J. Med.* **2006**, *355*, 251–259. [CrossRef] [PubMed]
23. Mant, J.; Doust, J.; Roalfe, A.; Barton, P.; Cowie, M.R.; Glasziou, P.; Mant, D. Systematic review and individual patient data meta-analysis of diagnosis of heart failure, with modelling of implications of different diagnostic strategies in primary care. *Health Technol. Assess.* **2009**, *13*, 1–207. [CrossRef] [PubMed]
24. Reddy, Y.N.V.; Carter, R.E.; Obokata, M.; Redfield, M.M.; Borlaug, B.A. A simple, evidence-based approach to help guide diagnosis of heart failure with preserved ejection fraction. *Circulation* **2018**, *138*, 861–870. [CrossRef] [PubMed]
25. Obokata, M.; Kane, G.C.; Reddy, Y.N.; Olson, T.P.; Melenovsky, V.; Borlaug, B.A. Role of Diastolic Stress Testing in the Evaluation for Heart Failure with Preserved Ejection Fraction: A Simultaneous Invasive-Echocardiographic Study. *Circulation* **2017**, *135*, 825–838. [CrossRef] [PubMed]
26. Campbell, R.T.; Jhund, P.S.; Castagno, D.; Hawkins, N.M.; Petrie, M.C.; McMurray, J.J. What have we learned about patients with heart failure and preserved ejection fraction from DIG-PEF, CHARM-preserved, and I-PRESERVE? *J. Am. Coll. Cardiol.* **2012**, *60*, 2349–2356. [CrossRef]
27. Shah, A.M.; Claggett, B.; Sweitzer, N.K.; Shah, S.J.; Anand, I.S.; O'Meara, E.; Desai, A.S.; Heitner, J.F.; Li, G.; Fang, J.; et al. Cardiac structure and function and prognosis in heart failure with preserved ejection fraction: Findings from the echocardiographic study of the Treatment of Preserved Cardiac Function Heart Failure Aldosterone Antagonist (TOPCAT) Trial. *Circ. Heart Fail.* **2014**, *5*, 740–751. [CrossRef]
28. Chen, H.; Chhor, M.; Rayner, B.; McGrath, K. Diagnostics and prognostic potential of current biomarkers in heart failure with preserved ejection fraction: A systematic review and meta-analysis. *medRxiv* **2020**, *4*, 18. [CrossRef]

29. Lee, Y.; Lim, S.; Hong, E.S.; Kim, J.H.; Moon, M.K.; Chun, E.J. Serum FGF21 concentration is associated with hypertriglyceridemia, hyperinsulinemia and pericardial fat accumulation, independently of obesity, but not with current coronary artery status. *Clin. Endocrinol.* **2014**, *80*, 57–64. [CrossRef]
30. Zhang, R.; Cai, X.; Du, Y.; Liu, L.; Han, X.; Liu, W.; Gong, S.; Zhou, X.; Wang, X. Association of serum fibroblast growth factor 21 and urinary glucose excretion in hospitalized patients with type 2 diabetes. *J. Diabetes Complicat.* **2021**, *35*, 107750. [CrossRef]
31. Kharitonenkov, A.; Shiyanova, T.L.; Koester, A.; Ford, A.M.; Micanovic, R.; Galbreath, E.J.; Sandusky, G.E.; Hammond, L.J.; Moyers, J.S. FGF21 as a novel metabolic regulator. *J. Clin. Investig.* **2005**, *115*, 1627–1635. [CrossRef]
32. Li, H.; Wu, G.; Fang, Q.; Zhang, M.; Hui, X.; Sheng, B.; Wu, L.; Bao, Y.; Li, P.; Xu, A. Fibroblast growth factor 21 increases insulin sensitivity through specific expansion of subcutaneous fat. *Nat. Commun.* **2018**, *9*, 272. [CrossRef]
33. Han, M.M.; Wang, W.F.; Liu, M.Y.; Li, D.S.; Zhou, B.; Yu, Y.H. FGF21 protects H9c2 cardiomyoblasts against hydrogen peroxide-induced oxidative stress injury. *Yao Xue Xue Bao* **2014**, *49*, 470–475.
34. Mäkelä, J.; Tselykh, T.V.; Maiorana, F.; Eriksson, O.; Do, H.T.; Mudò, G.; Korhonen, L.T.; Belluardo, N.; Lindholm, D. Fibroblast growth factor-21 enhances mitochondrial functions and increases the activity of PGC-1α in human dopaminergic neurons via Sirtuin-1. *Springerplus* **2014**, *3*, 2. [CrossRef]
35. Van Kimmenade, R.R.; Januzzi, J.L.; Ellinor, P.T.; Sharma, U.C.; Bakker, J.A. Utility of amino-terminal pro-brain natriuretic peptide, galectin-3, and apelin for the evaluation of patients with acute heart failure. *J. Am. Coll. Cardiol.* **2006**, *48*, 1217–1224. [CrossRef]
36. Trippel, T.D.; Mende, M.; Düngen, H.D.; Hashemi, D.; Petutschnigg, J.; Nolte, K.; Herrmann-Lingen, C. The diagnostic and prognostic value of galectin-3 in patients at risk for heart failure with preserved ejection fraction: Results from the DIAST-CHF study. *ESC Heart Fail.* **2021**, *8*, 829–841. [CrossRef] [PubMed]
37. De Boer, R.A.; Lok, D.J.; Jaarsma, T.; van der Meer, P.; Voors, A.A.; Hillege, H.L.; van Veldhuisen, D.J. Predictive value of plasma galectin-3 levels in heart failure with reduced and preserved ejection fraction. *Ann. Med.* **2011**, *43*, 60–68. [CrossRef]
38. Cui, Y.; Qi, X.; Huang, A.; Li, J.; Hou, W.; Liu, K. Differential and Predictive Value of Galectin-3 and Soluble Suppression of Tumorigenicity-2 (sST2) in Heart Failure with Preserved Ejection Fraction. *Med. Sci. Monit.* **2018**, *24*, 5139–5146. [CrossRef] [PubMed]
39. Yin, Q.S.; Shi, B.; Dong, L.; Bi, L. Comparative study of galectin-3 and B-type natriuretic peptide as biomarkers for the diagnosis of heart failure. *J. Geriatr. Cardiol.* **2014**, *11*, 79–82. [CrossRef] [PubMed]
40. Gurel, O.; Yilmaz, H. Galectin-3 as a new biomarker of diastolic dysfunction in hemodialysis patients. *Herz* **2015**, *40*, 788–794. [CrossRef]
41. Hussain, S.; Habib, A.; Hussain, M.S.; Najmi, A.K. Potential biomarkers for early detection of diabetic kidney disease. *Diabetes Res. Clin. Pract.* **2020**, *161*, 1–9. [CrossRef]
42. Jin, Q.H.; Lou, Y.F.; Li, T.L.; Chen, H.H.; Liu, Q.; He, X.J. Serum galectin-3: A risk factor for vascular complications in type 2 diabetes mellitus. *Chin. Med. J.* **2013**, *126*, 2109–2115.
43. Edelmann, F.; Holzendorf, V.; Wachter, R.; Nolte, K.; Schmidt, A.G.; Kraigher-Krainer, E.; Duvinage, A.; Unkelbach, I.; Düngen, H.D.; Tschöpe, C. Galectin-3 in patients with heart failure with preserved ejection fraction: Results from the Aldo-DHF trial. *Eur. J. Heart Fail.* **2015**, *17*, 214–223. [CrossRef] [PubMed]
44. Pecherina, T.; Kutikhin, A.; Kashtalap, V.; Karetnikova, V.; Gruzdeva, O.; Hryachkova, O.; Barbarash, O. Serum and Echocardiographic Markers May Synergistically Predict Adverse Cardiac Remodeling after ST-Segment Elevation Myocardial Infarction in Patients with Preserved Ejection Fraction. *Diagnostics* **2020**, *10*, 301. [CrossRef] [PubMed]
45. De Marco, C.; Claggett, B.L.; de Denus, S.; Zile, M.R.; Huynh, T.; Desai, A.S.; Sirois, M.G.; Solomon, S.D.; Pitt, B. Impact of diabetes on serum biomarkers in heart failure with preserved ejection fraction: Insights from the TOPCAT trial. *ESC Heart Fail.* **2021**, *8*, 1130–1138. [CrossRef] [PubMed]
46. Schill, F.; Timpka, S.; Nilsson, P.M.; Melander, O.; Enhörning, S. Copeptin as a predictive marker of incident heart failure. *ESC Heart Fail.* **2021**, *8*, 3180–3188. [CrossRef]
47. Noor, T.; Hanif, F.; Kiran, Z.; Rehman, R.; Khan, M.T.; Haque, Z.; Nankani, K. Relation of Copeptin with Diabetic and Renal Function Markers Among Patients with Diabetes Mellitus Progressing Towards Diabetic Nephropathy. *Arch. Med. Res.* **2020**, *51*, 548–555. [CrossRef]
48. Xu, L.; Liu, X.; Wu, S.; Gai, L. The clinical application value of the plasma copeptin level in the assessment of heart failure with reduced left ventricular ejection fraction a cross-sectional study. *Medicine* **2018**, *97*, e12610. [CrossRef]
49. Stoiser, B.; Mörtl, D.; Hülsmann, M.; Berger, R.; Struck, J.; Morgenthaler, N.G.; Bergmann, A.; Pacher, R. Copeptin, a fragment of the vasopressin precursor, as a novel predictor of outcome in heart failure. *Eur. J. Clin. Investig.* **2006**, *36*, 771–778. [CrossRef]
50. Maisel, A.; Xue, Y.; Shah, K.; Mueller, C.; Nowak, R.; Peacock, W.F.; Ponikowski, P.; Mockel, M.; Hogan, C. Increased 90-day mortality in patients with acute heart failure with elevated copeptin: Secondary results from the Biomarkers in Acute Heart Failure (BACH) study. *Circ. Heart Fail.* **2011**, *4*, 613–620. [CrossRef]
51. Pazin-Filho, A.; Kottgen, A.; Bertoni, A.G.; Russell, S.D.; Selvin, E.; Rosamond, W.D.; Coresh, J. HbA$_{1c}$ as a risk factor for heart failure in persons with diabetes: The Atherosclerosis Risk in Communities (ARIC) study. *Diabetologia* **2008**, *51*, 2197–2204. [CrossRef] [PubMed]
52. Zhao, W.; Katzmarzyk, P.T.; Horswell, R.; Wang, Y.; Johnson, J.; Hu, G. HbA1c and heart failure risk among diabetic patients. *J. Clin. Endocrinol. Metab.* **2014**, *99*, E263–E267. [CrossRef]

53. Lind, M.; Olsson, M.; Rosengren, A.; Svensson, A.M.; Bounias, I.; Gudbjörnsdottir, S. The relationship between glycaemic control and heart failure in 83,021 patients with type 2 diabetes. *Diabetologia* **2012**, *55*, 2946–2953. [CrossRef]
54. Erqou, S.; Lee, C.T.; Suffoletto, M.; Echouffo-Tcheugui, J.B.; de Boer, R.A.; van Melle, J.P.; Adler, A.I. Association between glycated haemoglobin and the risk of congestive heart failure in diabetes mellitus: Systematic review and meta-analysis. *Eur. J. Heart Fail.* **2013**, *15*, 185–193. [CrossRef] [PubMed]
55. Iribarren, C.; Karter, A.J.; Go, A.S.; Ferrara, A.; Liu, J.Y.; Sidney, S.; Selby, J.V. Glycemic Control and Heart Failure Among Adult Patients with Diabetes. *Circulation* **2001**, *103*, 2668–2673. [CrossRef] [PubMed]
56. Geng, L.; Lam, K.S.L.; Xu, A. The therapeutic potential of FGF21 in metabolic diseases: From bench to clinic. *Nat. Rev. Endocrinol.* **2020**, *16*, 654–667. [CrossRef] [PubMed]

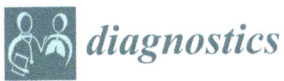

Review

Past, Present, and Future of Blood Biomarkers for the Diagnosis of Acute Myocardial Infarction—Promises and Challenges

Ioan Tilea [1,2], Andreea Varga [2,3,*] and Razvan Constantin Serban [4]

1. Department M4, Clinical Sciences, Faculty of Medicine, "G. E. Palade" University of Medicine, Pharmacy, Science and Technology of Targu Mures, 540142 Targu Mures, Romania; ioan.tilea@umfst.ro
2. Department of Cardiology II, Emergency Clinical County Hospital, 540042 Targu Mures, Romania
3. Department ME2, Faculty of Medicine in English, "G. E. Palade" University of Medicine, Pharmacy, Science and Technology of Targu Mures, 540142 Targu Mures, Romania
4. Cardiac Catheterization Laboratory, The Emergency Institute for Cardiovascular Diseases and Transplantation, 540136 Targu Mures, Romania; serbanrazvan1@gmail.com
* Correspondence: andreea.varga@umfst.ro; Tel.: +40-730808111

Abstract: Despite important advancements in acute myocardial infarction (AMI) management, it continues to represent a leading cause of mortality worldwide. Fast and reliable AMI diagnosis can significantly reduce mortality in this high-risk population. Diagnosis of AMI has relied on biomarker evaluation for more than 50 years. The upturn of high-sensitivity cardiac troponin testing provided extremely sensitive means to detect cardiac myocyte necrosis, but this increased sensitivity came at the cost of a decrease in diagnostic specificity. In addition, although cardiac troponins increase relatively early after the onset of AMI, they still leave a time gap between the onset of myocardial ischemia and our ability to detect it, thus precluding very early management of AMI. Newer biomarkers detected in processes such as inflammation, neurohormonal activation, or myocardial stress occur much earlier than myocyte necrosis and the diagnostic rise of cardiac troponins, allowing us to expand biomarker research in these areas. Increased understanding of the complex AMI pathophysiology has spurred the search of new biomarkers that could overcome these shortcomings, whereas multi-omic and multi-biomarker approaches promise to be game changers in AMI biomarker assessment. In this review, we discuss the evolution, current application, and emerging blood biomarkers for the diagnosis of AMI; we address their advantages and promises to improve patient care, as well as their challenges, limitations, and technical and diagnostic pitfalls. Questions that remain to be answered and hotspots for future research are also emphasized.

Keywords: acute myocardial infarction; blood biomarkers; diagnosis

1. Introduction

Cardiovascular diseases are responsible for almost half of all fatalities worldwide, causing more than four million deaths each year in Europe alone [1]. Among these, coronary artery disease is the leading cause of death, with acute myocardial infarction (AMI) accounting for most of the mortality related to coronary artery disease [2]. Changes in human lifestyle and behavior, particularly in developing countries, have led to a continuous, rapid increase in AMI incidence over recent decades, with annual growth rates of more than 3.5% [3]. About 10% of patients who present to emergency departments with chest pain every year are diagnosed with AMI [4].

Recognition that AMI most commonly occurs as a result of intracoronary thrombosis and that early opening of the occluded coronary artery significantly ameliorates outcomes in this high-risk population has reshaped AMI diagnosis over the years. Major interest emerged in developing strategies that would allow both early recognition and exclusion of AMI. The former would enable rapid, often life-saving interventions; the latter would allow rapid and safe patient discharge, considerably reducing healthcare costs. Diagnosis of AMI continues to be mainly driven by the occurrence of acute chest pain in the presence of typical ECG changes. However, approximately 90% of patients presenting with chest pain do not have AMI, and the sensitivity and specificity of ECG changes in AMI are rather low [4,5]. Moreover, there is a small, although non-negligible, proportion of patients that do not exhibit obvious symptoms and/or ECG changes. This context has emphasized the need for additional diagnostic criteria, and cardiac biomarkers have emerged as the most obvious approach.

Initially, serial, daily measurement of cardiac biomarkers served only as a strategy to retrospectively confirm AMI diagnosis. Since then, their role has become increasingly larger, and cardiac biomarker changes are now included as major diagnostic criteria in AMI (Figure 1) [6].

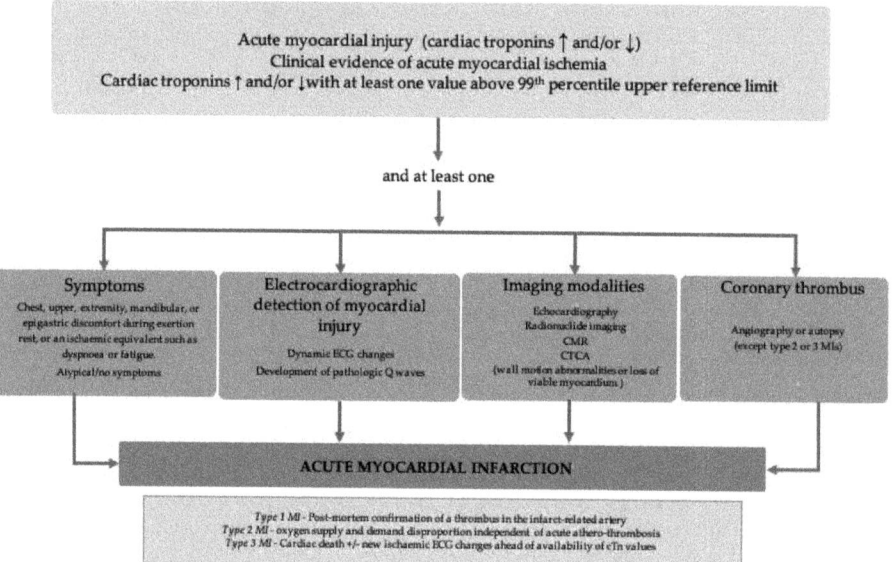

Figure 1. Schematic diagram of the universal definition of acute myocardial infarction, adapted from [7]: CMR—cardiac magnetic resonance; CTCA—computed tomographic angiography; MI—myocardial infarction; cTn—cardiac troponins.

This article reviews the evolution, current application, and emerging biomarkers for the diagnosis of AMI, addressing their advantages and promises to improve patient care, as well as their challenges, limitations, and technical and diagnostic pitfalls. Questions that remain to be answered and hotspots for future research are also emphasized.

2. Out-of-Date Biomarkers for Acute Myocardial Infarction Diagnosis

Severe myocardial ischemia and the consequent myocardial necrosis lead to the release of a plethora of cardiac enzymes into the circulation. Thus, markers such as myoglobin, lactate dehydrogenase (LDH), aspartate aminotransferase (AST), and creatine kinase (CK), including the concept of delta change, were introduced as initial indicators of AMI. Historically, AST and LDH were the first cardiac enzymes used for AMI diagnosis [8].

2.1. Aspartate Aminotransferase

Aspartate aminotransferase is a ubiquitous, soluble, intracellular enzyme critical in amino acid metabolism. The largest amounts of AST are expressed in the liver, the myocardium, the kidney, and the skeletal muscle. In 1954, Ladue et al. demonstrated a significant rise in AST 3–4 h after an AMI, beginning the age of enzyme-based AMI diagnosis [9]. Blood levels of AST increase within the first 12–24 h after AMI, reach a peak 1–2 days after the acute event, and return to baseline within 10–14 days after AMI (Table 1).

Table 1. Features of historical and current biomarkers used for acute myocardial infarction diagnosis.

Biomarker	TFPT (h)	TPL (h)	TRB	Sensitivity (%) *	Specificity (%) *	PPV (%) *	NPV (%) *
AST	12–24	24–48	10–14 days	75	71	75	71
LDH	6–12	24–72	8–14 days	82	70	76	77
Myoglobin	0.5–2	6–12	12–24 h	79	89	98	60
CK	3–8	12–24	48–72 h	95	68	30	99
CK-MB	4–8	12–24	48–72 h	92	90	98	83
cTn	3–6	10–24	5–10 days (TnI) 10–14 days (TnT)	97–100	94–97	98–99	88–100

TFPT—time to first positive test; h—hours; TPL—time to peak levels; TRB—time to return to baseline PPV—positive predictive value; NPV—negative predictive value; AST—aspartate aminotransferase; CK—creatine kinase; CK-MB—creatine kinase-myocardial band; cTn—cardiac troponins (i.e., T and I); LDH—lactate dehydrogenase. * Data reflect values obtained for serial measurement.

The ubiquitous expression of AST in a wide variety of tissues significantly affects its specificity for myocardial injury, limiting its use as a cardiac biomarker. Currently, AST is no longer used for AMI diagnosis.

2.2. Lactate Dehydrogenase

Only one year after the advent of AST as an AMI biomarker, LDH, an enzyme that reversibly converts lactate to pyruvate, emerged as a new promising indicator of AMI [10]. Blood levels of LDH typically increase within 6–12 h after the onset of AMI, peak within the following 1 to 3 days, and return to baseline within 8–14 days (Table 1). Similarly to AST, LDH is also expressed in a wide variety of tissues, including the liver, the kidney, the heart, the red blood cells, the lung, and particularly, the skeletal muscle, which makes LDH a marker with poor specificity for cardiac injury (Table 2).

Table 2. Most common non-acute myocardial infarction-related causes of cardiac biomarkers elevation.

Biomarker	Potential Causes of Elevation (Others Than Acute Myocardial Infarction)
AST	• Liver diseases (hepatitis, cirrhosis, carcinoma, liver necrosis, cholestasis); • Skeletal muscle injury (trauma, myopathy); • Hemolysis; • Infectious mononucleosis; • Shock, sepsis.
LDH	• Hemolytic anemia, hemolysis; • Liver diseases (hepatitis, cirrhosis, carcinoma, liver necrosis, cholestasis); • Stroke; • Pancreatitis; • Skeletal muscle injury (exhaustive exercise, muscle trauma, rhabdomyolysis, muscular dystrophy, polymyositis, alcohol myopathy, seizures); • Carcinomas, leukemia; • Hypothyroidism; • Lung diseases; • Shock, sepsis.
Myoglobin	• Skeletal muscle injury (exhaustive exercise, muscle trauma, rhabdomyolysis, muscular dystrophy, polymyositis, alcohol myopathy); • Surgery; • Shock, sepsis, burns; • Chronic kidney disease; • Carcinomas (colon, lung, prostate, endometrium).

Table 2. Cont.

Biomarker	Potential Causes of Elevation (Others Than Acute Myocardial Infarction)
CK-MB	• Significant skeletal muscle injury (trauma, rhabdomyolysis, convulsions, muscular dystrophy, intramuscular injections); • Cocaine abuse; • Shock, sepsis; • Malignancies; • Hypothyroidism; • Heart conditions (heart failure, myocarditis/pericarditis, aortic dissection, cardiac arrhythmias, cardiac trauma, cardiac surgery, cardioversion, cardiomyopathies, cardiotoxic drugs); • Chronic kidney disease.
cTn	• Heart conditions (heart failure, myocarditis/pericarditis, aortic dissection, cardiac arrhythmias, cardiac trauma, cardiac surgery, cardioversion, cardiomyopathies, cardiotoxic drugs); • Lung diseases (pulmonary embolism, severe pulmonary hypertension, chronic obstructive pulmonary disease); • Chronic kidney disease; • Significant skeletal muscle injury (trauma, rhabdomyolysis); • Sepsis; • Systemic inflammatory diseases.

AST—aspartate aminotransferase; CK-MB—creatine kinase-myocardial band; cTn—cardiac troponins (i.e., T and I); LDH—lactate dehydrogenase.

Of the five LDH izoenzymes, the heart expresses LDH-1 with four heart subunits (H_4); the isomeric form LDH-2 exists in a tetrameric combination of three heart and one muscle subunit (H_3M_1) [11]. Hence, an LDH-1/LDH-2 ratio >1 has been proposed as a specific AMI marker. The LDH-1 isoenzyme is not highly specific to the heart, however, and the LDH-1/LDH-2 ratio did not impose as a relevant AMI biomarker [12].

Nowadays, the only use of LDH is in distinguishing between acute and subacute AMI in the late stage of the ischemic event when other cardiac markers have already returned to their normal levels.

2.3. Myoglobin

Myoglobin is a low molecular weight iron- and oxygen-binding protein abundantly expressed in the myocardium and skeletal muscle. Myoglobin is rapidly released by the injured myocardium. Its blood levels start to increase within the first 30 min to 2 h after the onset of ischemia, which makes myoglobin an important marker for the early detection/exclusion of cardiac injury. Its levels increase during the first 6–10 h after AMI, reach a peak ≈12 h after the acute event, and return to baseline by 24 h after AMI (Table 1). Myoglobin is not found in any other tissue than the muscle, making it a sensitive marker for AMI, with high negative predictive value, and therefore is a useful test to rapidly rule out AMI in the emergency room. However, because myoglobin expression is not restricted to the myocardium (Table 2), its specificity and positive predictive value are rather low [13].

2.4. Creatine Kinase and Creatine Kinase Myocardial Band

Creatine kinase is an enzyme abundantly expressed in the myocardial cells, where it catalyzes reversible transfer of high-energy phosphate from ATP to creatine, producing creatine phosphate. Since the early 1970s, and particularly since the 1980s, with the advent of the ELISA technique, CK has become a crucial laboratory parameter for the identification of myocardial damage and AMI. The enzyme is present, however, in a large variety of other tissues (Table 2), strongly affecting its specificity as a biomarker of myocardial damage. This issue has been partly overcome by use of the CK-myocardial band (CK-MB) isoform, found in the heart, where it represents ≈20% of total CK, but also in the skeletal muscle, diaphragm, uterus, and several other issues [14]. With ≈91% sensitivity and specificity for the diagnosis of AMI during the first 6 h after symptoms onset, CK-MB has become widely used in emergency department settings [15]. Its levels start to increase 4–9 h after the onset of AMI, reach a peak within the first 24 h, and return to baseline during the next 48–72 h (Table 1). In patients with AMI, there is a strong correlation between CK and

CK-MB levels and infarct size, making these markers suitable for estimating the severity of AMI. Evaluation of CK-MB has, however, several major drawbacks. Firstly, due to its high molecular weight, CK-MB has limited ability to detect minor myocardial damage. Secondly, CK and CK-MB expression is not restricted to the heart. Hence, a number of other conditions can also lead to significant CK and CK-MB increases (Table 2), reducing their diagnostic specificity for AMI. Thirdly, cross reactivity can occur with other different compounds, including heterophilic antibodies such as rheumatoid factor. Due to these flaws, CK-MB evaluation is no longer recommended for AMI diagnosis, although it still has a role in estimating infarct size [7,16].

3. Cardiac Troponins—The Current Gold Standard in the Laboratory Diagnosis of Acute Myocardial Infarction

Along with the introduction of new myocardial injury biomarkers, the sensitivity for the diagnosis of AMI also recorded an important rise. However, because all previously identified markers were also expressed in a variety of other tissues, specificity continued to be problematic (see Table 2). Hence, numerous patients presenting with non-AMI and even non-cardiac chest pain syndromes continued to undergo extensive, costly, and often invasive evaluations. At the same time, traditional enzyme evaluation was largely incapable of detecting AMI patients with small amounts of cellular death. Introduction of cardiac troponins (cTn) as biomarkers of myocardial injury has radically changed the landscape of AMI diagnosis. At present, cTn are the most widely used, evidence-based, and guideline-endorsed biomarkers of AMI, manifesting a major and immediate impact on AMI patients' management [16].

Nevertheless, values above the upper reference limit of cardiac troponins can be detected in other circumstances unrelated to a thrombotic acute coronary event [17].

Patients with moderate chronic kidney disease or dialyzed patients present persistent elevated cTn values, associated with increased cardiac death and all-cause mortality [18]. In clinical and ECG features suggestive for an AMI, in an end-stage chronic kidney disease patient, dynamic changes higher or equal to 20% in cTn over 6 to 9 h should be interpreted as positive for an AMI [17].

However, the prognostic role of cardiac troponins in the assessment of other potential causes of elevation showed an important independent value, such as in acute heart failure. Serial measurements of troponin can be used for risk assessment in heart failure outpatients, because regular or persistent elevations of cTn are corelated with high risk of death or hospital readmission [19]. The cut off values of troponin T in predicting mortality in acute heart failure is variable in studies with different endpoints, varying from 0.01 ng/mL to cTn above URL or the 99th percentile. [20]

Elevated plasma troponin levels in acute phase of pulmonary embolism are defined as concentrations above upper reference limits; these limits are assay dependent [21].

The rule-in or rule-out of AMI diagnosis based entirely on positive values of troponins addresses challenges, and these values should be interpreted considering clinical presentation, serial ECGs, and other patient variables.

In the myocardium, troponin exists as a hetero-trimer composed of troponin I (TnI), T (TnT), and C (TnC) as subunits. The troponin complex interacts with tropomyosin as part of the thin filaments of the cardiac sarcomere, regulating the calcium-dependent interaction of actin and myosin in response to cytosolic calcium changes. TnC also exists in the striated muscle, rendering it unsuitable for AMI diagnosis, whereas TnT and TnI are specific to the heart and are therefore termed "cardiac troponins". Although TnI assays have generally been affected by more technical problems, this isoform has been shown to have greater early diagnostic accuracy and to be more specific for myocardial injury than TnT, which has also been shown to increase in settings such as skeletal muscle injury, kidney disease, malignancy, or sepsis [22,23]. In average, the amount of cTn per gram of myocardium is ≈13–15-fold higher than that of CK-MB, explaining the higher sensitivity of cTn in detecting early and/or minor myocardial damage [14]. Myocardial cells possess very small pools of cytosolic troponin, whereas the troponin bulk is located within the contractile apparatus of these cells. In contrast, circulating troponin levels are extremely low in the healthy individual. Hence, troponin plasma levels allow easy identification of even small myocyte injury. In patients with AMI, troponin release occurs initially from the cytosolic pool and later from the contractile apparatus of the damaged cells. This specific dynamic of release explains why cTn rises rapidly after the onset of myocardial ischemia, reaches a peak within the first 12–24 h, and remains high for 1–3 weeks after the acute event (Table 1).

With the advent of high-sensitivity cTn (hs-cTn) assays, sensitivity has become even higher, enabling the detection of troponin levels 10-fold lower than the initial values [24]. By definition, these assays must have an imprecision of less than 10% at the 99th percentile of a reference population and be able to measure cTn levels in at least 50% of a healthy reference population, although the most recent assays have been shown to detect troponin in >95% of healthy reference cohorts and to have an imprecision level in the range of 2–5% [16,25,26]. Overall, the added value of hs-cTn assays is not to identify more AMI cases, but rather to identify AMI more rapidly and to more quickly exclude those patients that do not have AMI [27]. Current rule-in and rule-out diagnostic algorithms rely on very low cTn cut-offs at the first presentation, and rapid, sequential measurements on admission and shortly (1–2 h) after, together with the calculation of delta troponin (i.e., rate of troponin change) [28]. Tables 3 and 4 present the specific cut-off levels of different hs-cTn T and hs-cTn I used in the current diagnosis of myocardial infarction, by each manufacturer.

Table 3. Troponin T assay specific cut-off levels in the rule-in or rule-out 0 h/1 h and 0 h/2 h algorithms in NSTEMI diagnosis; values are expressed in ng/L; adapted from [7].

Variation	Elecsys® Troponin T high-Sensitive Assay (Roche Diagnostics)	
	0 h/1 h	0 h/2 h
Very low	<5	<5
Low	<12	<14
No hΔ	<3	<4
High	≥52	≥52
hΔ	≥5	≥10

Table 4. Troponin I assay specific cut-off levels in the rule-in or rule-out 0 h/1 h and 0 h/2 h algorithms in NSTEMI diagnosis; values are expressed in ng/l; adapted from [7].

Variation	Assay/Manufacturer																			
	Architect/Abbott		Centaur/Siemens		Access/Beckman Coulter		Clarity/Singulex		Vitros/Clinical Diagnostics		Pathfast/LSI Medience		TriageTrue/Quidel	
	0 h/1 h	0 h/2 h	0 h/1 h	0 h/2 h	0 h/1 h	0 h/2 h	0 h/1 h	0 h/2 h	0 h/1 h	0 h/2 h	0 h/1 h	0 h/2 h	0 h/1 h	0 h/2 h
Very low	<4	<4	<3	<3	<4	<4	<1	<1	<1	<1	<3	<3	<4	<4
Low	<5	<6	<6	<8	<5	<5	<2	TBD	<2	TBD	<4	TBD	<5	TBD
No hΔ	<2	<2	<3	<7	<4	<5	<1	TBD	<1	TBD	<3	TBD	<3	TBD
High	≥64	≥64	≥120	≥120	≥50	≥50	≥30	≥30	≥40	≥40	≥90	≥60	≥60	≥60
hΔ	≥6	≥15	≥12	≥20	≥15	≥20	≥6	TBD	≥4	TBD	≥20	TBD	≥8	TBD

Mortality attributable to AMI has significantly declined over the years, mainly due to early recognition and rapid, effective, myocardial revascularization. Repeated testing by principal laboratories is a significant logistic challenge, however, that cannot be overcome by many of the diagnostic laboratories. Implementation of algorithms requiring fast decision-making thus had to be paralleled by earlier access to biomarkers, particularly troponin. Point-of-care tests (POCTs) for cTnI with diagnostic sensitivity comparable to that of central laboratory testing have become available, allowing markedly improved turnaround times and immediacy of results, along with improved therapeutic decision-making, patient flow and experience, and reduced costs [26]. Currently available hs-cTn POCT systems only provide diagnostic sensitivity comparable to that of central laboratory testing ≈6 h after admission, thus limiting their use. Randomized trials on the impact of

POCTs in patients presenting with chest pain have also provided rather inconsistent results. However, in general, POCTs appeared to improve patient flow and decrease the length of stay in the emergency departments, while increasing hospital and coronary care unit admissions [26].

4. Newer Biomarkers for Laboratory Diagnosis of Acute Myocardial Infarction

The introduction of cTn testing has dramatically changed the diagnosis of AMI, allowing earlier therapeutic interventions in AMI patients and the more rapid discharge of patients without AMI. Although clearly superior to earlier AMI biomarkers in detecting myocardial ischemia, cTn are far from ideal. The level of oxidation/reduction of the troponin molecule, phosphorylation, fibrin strands, and heterophilic antibodies have the potential to interfere with TnI assays [29]. Circulating troponin levels increase as early as 2–4 h after the onset of AMI, but still leave a "troponin gap" that prevents earlier detection of AMI, which could further improve prognosis in these high-risk patients. Finally, whereas the use of hs-cTn testing has massively increased diagnostic sensitivity, this has come at the cost of a decrease in diagnostic specificity. Indeed, several cardiac and non-cardiac factors (Table 2) have been shown to affect troponin levels [30]. Even mild increases in troponin levels, regardless of the underlying cause, have been shown to predict adverse prognoses. This makes troponin assessment in the emergency department an excellent test to reliably rule out low-risk individuals. However, based solely on troponin levels, many individuals will continue to undergo further evaluations, potentially delaying therapy for other, non-cardiac causes of troponin elevation [31]. Moreover, the high sensitivity of new generation hs-cTn assays could increase emergency department workload by blurring the line between health and disease (i.e., designating "healthy" individuals as being "ill") and, by including such patients in the AMI category, could also lead to an apparent improvement in AMI outcomes [32].

The continuous progress in the treatment of cardiac diseases and the introduction of new therapeutic approaches has imposed the rapid and continuous development of new laboratory assays [33]. The wide use of percutaneous coronary interventions, the introduction of newer generation antiplatelet agents, and recognition that in AMI, such strategies need to be applied as early as possible, have spurred the search of novel AMI biomarkers. These possible key tools can improve AMI diagnostic accuracy or enable the instant ruling out of AMI without the need for serial measurement (i.e., increase specificity) and enable faster detection of AMI (i.e., increase sensitivity). To accomplish these goals, novel biomarkers will have to meet two crucial criteria: accuracy and speed [34]. Any new AMI biomarker will therefore have to be specifically expressed in the myocardial tissue, at relatively high levels, and be released into the bloodstream rapidly after symptom onset. Several novel biomarkers that promise to fulfil at least part of these needs have been recently identified (Figure 2) [7,35–38].

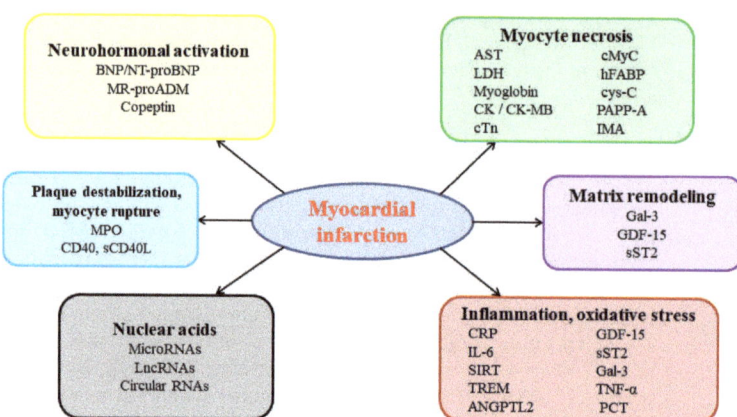

Figure 2. Pathophysiological pathways in acute myocardial infarction and examples of associated candidate circulating biomarkers; ANGPTL2—angiopoietin-like 2; BNP—B-type natriuretic peptide; CD40—cluster of differentiation 40; cMyC—cardiac myosin-binding protein C; CRP—C-reactive protein; cys-C—cystatin C; Gal-3—galectin-3; GDF-15—growth differentiation factor 15; hFABP—heart-type fatty acid binding protein; IL-6—interleukin 6; IMA—ischemia-modified albumin; LncRNAs—long non-coding ribonucleic acids; MPO—myeloperoxidase; MR-proADM—midregional proadrenomedullin; NT-proBNP—N-terminal fragment of the B-type natriuretic peptide precursor; PAPP-A—pregnancy-associated plasma protein-A; PCT—procalcitonin; RNA—ribonucleic acids; sCD40L—soluble ligand of cluster of differentiation 40; SIRT—sirtuins; sST2—soluble suppression of tumorigenicity factor 2; TNF-α—tumor necrosis factor α.

4.1. Biomarkers of Myocardial Necrosis

Recent studies have supplemented the set of classic biomarkers of myocardial necrosis with a number of additional biomarkers, including the heart-type fatty acid binding protein (hFABP), the ischemia-modified albumin (IMA), and the sarcomeric cardiac myosin-binding protein C (cMyC).

Similarly to myoglobin, hFABP, a low-molecular-weight, non-enzymatic protein involved in the intracellular buffering and transport of long-chain fatty acids, is rapidly (i.e., within ≈3 h) released into the circulation after the onset of myocardial injury, its levels returning to baseline 12–24 h after the acute ischemic event [39]. Although hFABP appears to add incremental value to cTn, increasing diagnostic accuracy and accelerating clinical diagnostic decisions, hFABP is also expressed in the kidney and skeletal muscle, and its elimination is highly dependent on kidney function [40]. Thus, its value as a diagnostic marker of AMI remains controversial.

Acute myocardial ischemia induces major protein changes, including alterations of the N-terminus of albumin, leading to the formation of IMA. In the same manner to myoglobin and hFABP, IMA levels also increase rapidly (i.e., within 3 h) after AMI onset. A combined approach, using IMA and TnT at presentation for chest pain, appeared to increase AMI diagnostic accuracy compared with TnT alone [41]. However, when used alone, IMA displays sensitivity too low (i.e., 70%) to allow useful clinical decision-making, and its specificity is significantly affected by the fact that IMA levels also increase in a large variety of other medical conditions, as well as infections, liver, and advanced kidney diseases, cancer, or brain ischemia [42].

Sarcomeric cMyC is one of the most promising novel myocardial necrosis biomarkers. This myosin-binding protein isoform is exclusively expressed at the level of the heart, making it a specific marker of myocardial injury; it is more rapidly released into the bloodstream as a result of myocardial necrosis than troponin, allowing earlier detection of myocardial injury and disease [43]. The cardiac myosin-binding protein C myocardial concentration is almost twice that of cTn, which makes cMyC a more sensitive AMI biomarker than troponin, and the addition of cMyC to high-sensitive cardiac troponin T provides supplementary AMI-related diagnostic information [44].

Over the years, cardiovascular medicine has seen numerous, often major, paradigm changes. In atherosclerosis, concepts have moved from a purely lipid-related, to a more complex, lipid-inflammatory pathophysiology [45]. In atrial fibrillation, concepts have moved from a purely electrical disease to a more tangled combination of electrical, structural, autonomic, and molecular underlying changes [46–48]. In AMI, for years, biomarkers have been focused on the concept of myocardial necrosis. However, recent years have brought a major paradigm change in AMI biomarker research, and studies focusing on other ischemia-related mechanisms including neurohormonal activation, inflammation, plaque instability, and myocyte membrane rupture have started to emerge. With the extend of newer, more complex molecular techniques, multi-omic approaches have also started to be used for improvement of AMI diagnosis.

4.2. Biomarkers of Neurohormonal Activation

The observation that neurohormonal activation is a major change occurring in AMI patients has drawn attention to potentially novel AMI biomarkers, including the B-type natriuretic peptide (BNP) and the N-terminal fragment of its precursor (NT-proBNP), copeptin, and the midregional proadrenomedullin (MR-proADM).

Secreted by the ventricular myocytes in response to stretch, the proBNP precursor is cleaved into BNP and the inactive fragment NT-proBNP. Once released, BNP exerts vasodilating, natriuretic, hypocoagulative, inotropic, antiarrhythmic, and anti-renin–angiotensin–aldosterone and sympathoadrenal system effects, while promoting cell differentiation and tissue repair and supporting immunity, metabolic responses, and inflammation [49]. In patients with AMI, BNP and NT-proBNP levels have been associated with infarct size [50]. However, both BNP and NT-proBNP increase in a large variety of non-AMI-related settings, including some that may be accompanied by clinical symptoms comparable with AMI, such as acute heart failure and pulmonary embolism, as well as in kidney dysfunction, hypertension, chronic heart failure, myocarditis, cardiac arrhythmias, electrical cardioversion, or sepsis, precluding the use of these peptides as diagnostic AMI biomarkers, although they remain crucial for prognostic assessment in these patients [51]. According to 2020 ESC Guidelines for the management of acute coronary syndromes in patients presenting without persistent ST-segment elevation, the BNP and NT-proBNP plasma concentrations should be considered to contribute to patient's prognosis (death, acute heart failure) [7].

Copeptin, a stable glycopeptide derived from the C-terminal fragment of the vasopressin prohormone, has been shown to be co-released with arginine vasopressin within the first 4 h after AMI. Circulating copeptin levels have been shown to exhibit linear correlation with those of arginine vasopressin, a key regulator of water homeostasis and plasma osmolality [52]. This makes copeptin an excellent surrogate marker of arginine vasopressin secretion, which has a very short half-life. When combined with cTn, copeptin has been shown to improve sensitivity and easily rules out AMI early [53]. However, copeptin is not a specific cardiac marker, neither is it recommended to routinely measure it for constant risk or prognosis judgement [7]. Other conditions, including kidney disease, heart failure, or sepsis, can also influence copeptin levels, and its levels have been shown to be affected by gender, body mass, hydration status, blood pressure, and glomerular filtration rate [51], thus precluding its use as a stand-alone diagnostic AMI biomarker.

Adrenomedullin is a stress hormone expressed in a large variety of tissues, including the brain, kidney, vasculature, and adrenal medulla, involved in diuresis and natriuresis, vasodilation, and inotropism regulation. Adrenomedullin is generated from its more stable precursor MR-proADM. In clinical studies, MR-proADM has been shown to significantly increase in AMI patients, particularly in those developing post-AMI heart failure, and high MR-proADM levels have been associated with significant increases in short- and long-term mortality and hospitalization for heart failure following AMI [54,55]. Increased MR-proADM levels have even been proposed as a rule-in criteria for AMI, but its exact value as a diagnostic biomarker in addition to the already established criteria remains to be evaluated.

Immediately after the onset of AMI, the renin–angiotensin–aldosterone system (RAAS) is activated, and this phenomenon is linked with an unfavorable prognosis [56]. High levels of angiotensin II aggravate myocardial ischemia-mediated vasoconstriction. In hypertensive women who experience an AMI, the renin–angiotensin–aldosterone axis is suggested to be upregulated [57].

Heightened RAAS activity demonstrates a determining implication not only within the pathogenesis of AMI, but also as an estimated model with 5 years post-AMI mortality, as revealed by the RAAS polymorphisms in the presence of AGT CC genotype and ACE allele, individual or in association [58].

Increased plasma renin activity (PRA) values were detected in both hypertensive and normotensive patients, in whom the diagnosis of AMI was ruled in; these were independently associated with a poor prognosis in AMI patients [59,60]. In the myocardium, increased aldosterone synthesis is induced by an acute coronary event, triggering ventricular fibrosis post-AMI [61].

4.3. Biomarkers of Inflammation

Myocardial inflammation is a critical process occurring in the setting of AMI that has been related to a variety of deleterious consequences, including electrical instability and increased risk of cardiac arrhythmias, autonomic dysfunction, and fibrosis development [48,62–64]. A wide variety of pro-inflammatory cytokines have been shown to increase in the setting of AMI and to predict prognosis in this population. This is particularly the case for C-reactive protein (CRP), interleukin- (IL-) 6, and procalcitonin (PCT).

Increased CRP levels have been linked with the extent of myocardial injury and with poorer prognosis in AMI patients. In animal studies, CRP removal was able to significantly reduce infarct size and improve outcomes [65]. Ries et al., in a pilot study in humans with AMI (CAMI-1 study), reported that CRP apheresis managed to reduce circulating CRP levels and a loss of correlation between CRP levels and infarct size, although CRP reduction was not associated with a significant reduction in infarct size [66]. However, because CRP increases in a wide variety of other settings, its levels are not sufficiently specific to qualify it as a reliable marker of AMI.

In the setting of AMI, increased IL-6 levels favor activation and recruitment of inflammatory cells, promote CRP release, and exert cardiac negative inotropic effects, predicting poor prognosis in this population [67]. Meanwhile, the IL-6 receptor blockade has been shown to reduce the inflammatory response and cTn release in patients with non-STE segment elevation AMI, suggesting that, similarly with CRP, IL-6 could emerge as not only a diagnostic AMI biomarker, but also as a potentially new therapeutic target in AMI [68]. However, the low specificity of IL-6 and the lack of large confirmatory studies limit IL-6 use as a diagnostic AMI biomarker.

The peptide precursor of the hormone calcitonin, PCT, has also been shown to increase in inflammatory settings, including AMI, and to have prognostic value in ischemic heart disease [69].

The potential role in the development of atherosclerosis and acute coronary syndromes of a group of zinc-dependent endopeptidases, namely, matrix metalloproteinases (MMPs), was investigated in previous studies [70–72].

The increased circulating levels of MMP 2, 3, 9 and 28 in AMI do not distinguish between atherothrombotic and non-atherothrombotic events. [70,73].

Due to matrix metalloproteinase-9 linking with plaque rupture and myocardial necrosis, MMP-9 has demonstrated its position as an early-stage biomarker of AMI [70]. It was also suggested that the value of MMP-28 correlates with GRACE score and could be a predictor of short-term prognoses in AMI cases [72].

Other inflammatory biomarkers, including IL-1β, IL-37, and angiopoietin-like protein 2, have also been shown to increase in AMI patients, but further studies are needed before drawing a definitive conclusion in their regard [35].

4.4. Biomarkers of Plaque Destabilization and Myocyte Rupture

Myeloperoxidase (MPO), a component of neutrophil granules, is abundantly released from unstable atherosclerotic plaques and plays a critical role in myocardial inflammation and oxidative stress. When used alone, MPO does not seem to be appropriate for AMI diagnosis [74]. However, when combined with TnI and CK-MB, MPO appears to improve the early diagnostic accuracy of AMI [75].

Cluster of differentiation 40 protein, CD40, and its soluble ligand, sCD40L, are expressed by a wide variety of cell types and have been shown to be released during cardiac myocyte rupture. Both molecules are involved in inflammation and thrombosis and have been proposed as diagnostic AMI biomarkers [76]. However, their exact value remains to be established [35].

Biomarkers, including lipid markers (lipoprotein A, apolipoproteins A and B), endothelial cells- (endocan) and platelet- (mean platelet volume, mean platelet volume-to-platelet count ratio, beta-thromboglobulin, platelet miR-126) related markers have been proposed as AMI biomarkers [14,51]. Further enhanced studies are required to establish the additional value in AMI diagnosis for other biomarkers such as the degree of mobilization of mononuclear and endothelial progenitor cells, triggering receptors expressed on myeloid cells 1 and 4, cystatin C, pregnancy-associated plasma protein-A, class II phosphatidylinositol 3-phosphate kinase, sirtuins, arginine methyltransferase 5, and chitinase-3-like protein 1 [30].

The main characteristics of newer biomarkers potentially used in the diagnosis of AMI are depicted in Table 5.

Table 5. Characteristics of newer biomarkers used in the diagnosis of acute myocardial infarction.

Biomarker.	Value	TFPT (h)	TPL (h)	TRB (h)	Sensitivity (%)	Specificity (%)	PPV (%)	NPV (%)	References
hFABP	7 µg/L (cut-off)	3 h	-	12–14	81.8%	100.0%	55%	66.7%	[35,77]
IMA	88.2–111.8 U/mL (reference interval)	3 h	6	24	70%	80%	96%	91%	[78]
cMyC	10 ng/L	<60 min	2	-	100%	41.3%	27.3%	100%	[79]
Copeptin	2.18–2.35 ng/mL reference interval	0–1 h	0–1 h	12–36 h	79.41–87.80%	60.38–62.73%	40.91–46.15%	89.93–98.17%	[53,80]

TFPT—time to first positive test; h—hours; TPL—time to peak levels; TRB—time to return to baseline PPV—positive predictive value; NPV—negative predictive value.

Studies about other newer biomarkers, such as CRP, IL-6, procalcitonin, CD40, myeloperoxydase, and sCD40L, could be valuable in the diagnosis and prognosis of AMI, although further studies are needed [14,35]. Guidelines recommend the use of BNP/NTproBNP in the setting of different situations, especially in patients with suspected heart failure, as a prognostic indicator against AMI diagnosis biomarker and supporting the risk stratification of adverse outcomes [81].

5. A Glimpse into the Future—Emerging Molecular Candidate Biomarkers for Acute Myocardial Infarction

The development of new, high-technology laboratory methods continues to improve therapy monitoring, as well as diagnostic and prognostic accuracy in cardiovascular medicine [36,82]. With the advent of novel molecular biology techniques, evaluation of the entire molecular chain, from DNA to RNA, proteins, and metabolites has become possible. Multi-omic approaches based on genomic, transcriptomic, proteomic, and metabolomic studies that allow the evaluation of RNAs, peptides and proteins, and metabolites using whole blood, plasma, or serum, or even selected circulating cell types or extracellular vesicles, promise to be a game changer in AMI assessment.

5.1. Novel Peptide, Protein, and Enzyme Candidates for Acute Myocardial Infarction Diagnosis

Growth differentiation factor 15 (GDF-15), galectin-3 (Gal-3), and soluble suppression of tumorigenicity factor 2 (sST2) appear to be among the most promising novel AMI biomarkers and have been extensively studied over the past years.

Circulating levels of GDF-15, a member of the transforming growth factor beta cytokine superfamily expressed in a wide variety of cardiovascular and non-cardiovascular cells, have been shown to increase in inflammatory and high oxidative stress states and tissue injury, including AMI, and to predict prognosis in this population [83]. Galectin-3 has also been shown to participate in inflammation, cardiac fibrosis and repair, and maladaptive ventricular remodeling, as well as in atherosclerotic plaques formation, destabilization, and rupture. Increased Gal-3 levels have been reported in AMI patients, in whom Gal-3 has also been proposed as a valuable predictive marker [84]. Moreover, experimental data suggest that whereas Gal-3 could initially contribute to myocardial repair and the preservation of cardiac geometry and function, over the long term, Gal-3 activation could promote myocardial fibrosis and adverse ventricular remodeling [85]. Likewise, sST2, a member of the IL-1 receptor family, has been shown to increase in AMI patients and to predict prognosis in this setting [86]. However, due to insufficient specificity, sST2 is unlikely to enter clinical practice as a diagnostic AMI biomarker. Other potential peptide and protein biomarkers, including glycogen phosphorylase isoenzyme BB, involved in myocardial carbohydrate metabolism regulation and released rapidly after myocardial injury; S100A, a class of small-molecule calcium-binding proteins involved in cell division and metabolism regulation and highly sensitive in depicting myocardial injury; irisin, a recently identified hormone that facilitates glucose uptake and improves cardiac muscle activity; and adropin, a secretory protein involved in regulation of energy metabolism and insulin resistance, are currently under evaluation [14]. Several of them have been proposed as independent predictors of post-AMI outcomes, but none has demonstrated clear advantage over cTn in AMI diagnosis to date.

5.2. Metabolomics—Emerging Targets for Acute Myocardial Infarction Diagnosis

By allowing rapid assessment of various products of cell metabolism, including during acute events, metabolomics has emerged as a promising new source of highly specific diagnostic AMI biomarkers. Studies in patients with septal ablation-induced AMI identified several myocardial cells metabolites released very early (i.e., within 10 min) after AMI onset [87]. These include molecules involved in the pentose phosphate, pyrimidine, and tricarboxylic acid pathways. However, the exact value of these new biomarkers in AMI diagnosis in addition to or instead of cTn remains to be established.

5.3. Circulating Ribonucleic Acids as Potential Diagnostic Biomarkers of Acute Myocardial Infarction

Non-coding RNAs, including microRNAs (miRNAs), circular RNAs, and long non-coding RNAs (lncRNAs), act as strong, tissue- and cell-specific epigenetic regulators of cardiac gene expression, homeostasis, and function, and have recently emerged as promising biomarkers in a wide variety of cardiovascular diseases. These molecules circulate in the peripheral blood, either bound to transport proteins or packaged in microparticles, thus being stably transported in the blood, protected from degradation, and detectable in blood samples. A number of these circulating non-coding RNAs have been or are currently under investigation as potential diagnostic AMI biomarkers.

MicroRNAs are small, single-stranded RNA molecules that work as post-transcriptional protein synthesis suppressors via gene silencing. Four miRNAs—miR-1, miR-133a/b, miR-208b, and miR-499, the latter two being expressed solely in the cardiac myocytes—have been consistently reported to increase in AMI patients, although controversies still remain regarding the value of individual miRNAs as AMI biomarkers [68]. With 78% sensitivity and 82% specificity, total miRNA levels appear to be suitable diagnostic biomarkers of AMI, with miR-499 appearing to be among the most significantly associated with AMI, increasing very early (i.e., within few hours after AMI onset), to very high (i.e., up to 3×10^5) levels, and returning to baseline within hours or days after the acute event, while also reaching high (i.e., 88% and 87%) sensitivity and specificity [88]. Other miRNAs, including miR-21, miR-92a, miR-122, miR-181a, miR-320a, miR-328, and miR-375, have also been shown to increase in the peripheral blood in the setting of AMI [89]. Certain miRNAs appear to be highly specific for AMI and to display faster release kinetics than cTn. Moreover, studies have suggested that the miRNA signature could even distinguish between ST and non-ST segment elevation myocardial infarction [90]. In addition, in rats with experimental AMI, antagonizing certain miRNAs, such as miR-31, managed to reduce infarct size and post-AMI ventricular remodeling, preserving cardiac structure and function [91]. Several lncRNAs, namely, myocardial infarction-associated transcript (MIAT), H19, and metastasis-associated lung adenocarcinoma transcript 1 (MALAT1), have also been reported to be altered in AMI patients, but studies in this regard are still in their infancy [92–95].

6. Gaps in Knowledge and Future Research

The widespread use of cTn has revolutionized AMI diagnosis. Particularly, with the advent of hs-cTn, we can confidently say that sensitivity is no longer an issue in AMI diagnosis. However, two problems remain to be solved. Firstly, the increased sensitivity provided by hs-cTn assays came with a cost—an inevitable decrease in diagnostic specificity. Secondly, although cTn increase relatively early after the onset of AMI, they still leave a time gap between the onset of myocardial ischemia and our ability to detect it, thus precluding very early management of AMI. Historical markers, such as myoglobin, increase much faster than cTn, but they do not provide sufficient diagnostic specificity.

To date, all AMI biomarkers have focused on molecules released by the cardiac myocytes as a result of myocardial necrosis. More recently, understanding of the complex AMI pathophysiology has opened the way for new biomarker identification. Acknowledgment that processes such as inflammation, neurohormonal activation, or myocardial stress occur much earlier than myocyte necrosis has allowed us to expand biomarker research in these areas (Figure 1). Although most of the emerging biomarkers are not specific enough to impose as stand-alone AMI biomarkers, and are therefore unlikely to replace cTn in the foreseeable future, they could bring additional value for AMI diagnosis when included in multi-biomarker approaches. Including tissue-specific markers, such as certain miRNAs, could also be of invaluable help.

Multi-omic approaches hold great promise for more accurate and faster AMI diagnosis. MicroRNAs appear to be particularly promising in this regard, given that myocyte stress induced by anoxia, acidosis, and/or edema precedes myocardial necrosis in AMI patients and is rapidly reflected in circulating miRNAs levels. The rapid progress in molecular biomarker research must be matched, however, by similar progresses in laboratory techniques. Indeed, bioluminescence, solution-phase bioluminescence, and high-throughput sequencing methods have been developed for miRNA detection, but improvement is still necessary to provide instruments that can accurately, conveniently, inexpensively, and rapidly quantify circulating miRNAs in a large number of hospital laboratories. Integrated interpretation of multi-omics data also remains rather difficult at present, and may require machine learning to transform this approach into a clinically useful diagnostic tool.

Multi-biomarker strategies that reflect several AMI-related pathophysiological processes and include several enzymatic, non-enzymatic, and/or molecular markers may provide the solution for obtaining highly sensitive, highly specific, and very rapid AMI diagnoses. Such an approach was already shown to be superior to individual marker assessment for predicting post-AMI outcomes [96]. In a pilot study, a multi-marker panel termed "plaque disruption index" has been shown to present higher diagnostic accuracy for type 1 AMI than coronary angiography [97]. However, large clinical trials are still required before drawing definitive conclusions in this regard.

Regardless of future AMI diagnoses relying on single- or multi-marker approaches, any new approach will have to provide more readily available, more affordable, and more clinically relevant information than the strategies currently used in clinical practice, while also complying with high standards of precision and accuracy. Markers that do not fulfill these requirements will most likely not find their place in clinical practice. The ideal AMI biomarker, which is exclusively expressed in the myocardial tissue and whose plasma levels are not affected by any other pathology, remains to be identified. MicroRNAs could prove of invaluable help in this regard. It is unlikely that a single miRNA will prove superior to the traditional markers for AMI diagnosis. However, a combination of miRNAs, reflecting cardiomyocyte stress, inflammation, endothelial cells, and fibroblast damage, and/or other AMI-related pathophysiological processes, could change the future of AMI diagnosis. Moreover, miRNA-based therapies have the potential to modulate an entire pathway by regulating multiple genes at the same time. The advent of such therapies, and particularly of anti-miRNA strategies, is therefore expected to spur further research in this area.

The massive number of emerging biomarkers and the impressive progress achieved over the past decades in AMI diagnosis were spurred by a revolutionary paradigm shift—one that has drawn AMI diagnosis out of the 'myocardial necrosis box'. Further understanding of AMI pathophysiology is expected to open new directions of research and enable the identification of even better diagnostic AMI biomarkers. Laboratory techniques will have to parallel this effort and ideally provide POCT systems able to detect single analytes as well as panels of circulating markers, and thus to enable accurate and rapid AMI diagnosis, including during patient transport to hospital. This would allow further cutting down time in AMI management, which in turn is expected to result in considerable improvement in AMI outcomes, both over the short and the long term.

7. Conclusions

Circulating biomarkers are key to AMI diagnosis. With their increased specificity, cTn have revolutionized the diagnosis, as well as the management of AMI. The advent of hs-cTn covered an unmet need and boosted diagnostic sensitivity, allowing more rapid therapeutic interventions. Unfortunately, this increased sensitivity was accompanied by a drop in specificity, not for the analyte, but for the diagnosis of AMI. Up to two-thirds of patients presenting with cTn levels that overtly exceed the threshold for AMI diagnosis do not have AMI and undergo costly, time-consuming, often invasive, although completely futile investigations. Further advancement in AMI diagnosis is therefore required. Traditional markers have all been focused on detecting myocardial necrosis. Acknowledgment that other processes, such as inflammation, neurohormonal activation, or myocardial stress, occur much earlier than myocyte necrosis, has opened the way for new approaches in AMI biomarker research. The ideal biomarker, that would allow rapid and reliable AMI rule in and rule out, is still to be discovered. However, biomarker research in AMI has massively advanced over the past years, and a solution to this problem is expected to be found in the near future, most likely in the form of multi-marker assessment, based on a combination of biomarkers that reflect several axes involved in the natural evolution of AMI. Future clinical trials, with large sample sizes, will have to confirm the utility of biomarkers that are currently under investigation, to identify novel potential biomarkers, and to validate the clinical impact of multi-biomarker-based AMI diagnosis.

Author Contributions: Conceptualization, I.T., A.V. and R.C.S.; methodology, I.T., A.V. and R.C.S.; software, I.T., A.V. and R.C.S.; validation, I.T., A.V. and R.C.S.; formal analysis, I.T., A.V. and R.C.S.; resources, I.T., A.V. and R.C.S.; data curation, I.T., A.V. and R.C.S.; writing—original draft preparation, I.T., A.V. and R.C.S.; writing—review and editing, I.T., A.V. and R.C.S.; visualization, I.T., A.V. and R.C.S.; supervision, I.T., A.V. and R.C.S.; project administration, I.T., A.V. and R.C.S.; funding acquisition, I.T. All authors have read and agreed to the published version of the manuscript.

Funding: This work was supported by a grant of the Romanian Ministry of Education and Research, CNCS-UEFISCDI, project number PN-III-P1-1.1-PD-2019-0181, within PNCDI III.

Acknowledgments: The authors would like to thank Alina Scridon from "G.E. Palade" University of Medicine, Pharmacy, Science and Technology of Targu Mures, Romania for critically revising the manuscript and for her helpful suggestions.

Conflicts of Interest: The authors declare no conflict of interest.

References

1. Townsend, N.; Nichols, M.; Scarborough, P.; Rayner, M. Cardiovascular disease in Europe 2015: Epidemiological update. *Eur. Heart J.* **2015**, *36*, 2673–2674. [CrossRef]
2. Mendis, S.; Puska, P.; Norrving, B. *Global Atlas on Cardiovascular Disease Prevention and Control*; World Health Organization: Geneva, Switzerland, 2011. Available online: https://apps.who.int/iris/handle/10665/44701 (accessed on 23 March 2021).
3. Benjamin, E.J.; Blaha, M.J.; Chiuve, S.E.; Cushman, M.; Das, S.R.; Deo, R.; de Ferranti, S.D.; Floyd, J.; Fornage, M.; Gillespie, C.; et al. Heart disease and stroke statistics-2017 update: A report from the American Heart Association. *Circulation* **2017**, *135*, e146–e603. [CrossRef]
4. Haasenritter, J.; Stanze, D.; Widera, G.; Wilimzig, C.; Abu Hani, M.; Sonnichsen, A.C.; Bosner, S.; Rochon, J.; Donner-Banzhoff, N. Does the patient with chest pain have a coronary heart disease? Diagnostic value of single symptoms and signs—A meta-analysis. *Croat. Med. J.* **2012**, *53*, 432–441. [CrossRef]
5. Wang, J.J.; Pahlm, O.; Warren, J.W.; Sapp, J.L.; Horáček, B.M. Criteria for ECG detection of acute myocardial ischemia: Sensitivity versus specificity. *J. Electrocardiol.* **2018**, *51*, S12–S17. [CrossRef] [PubMed]
6. Ibanez, B.; James, S.; Agewall, S.; Antunes, M.J.; Bucciarelli-Ducci, C.; Bueno, H.; Caforio, A.L.P.; Crea, F.; Goudevenos, J.A.; Halvorsen, S.; et al. 2017 ESC Guidelines for the management of acute myocardial infarction in patients presenting with ST-segment elevation: The Task Force for the management of acute myocardial infarction in patients presenting with ST-segment elevation of the European Society of Cardiology (ESC). *Eur. Heart J.* **2018**, *39*, 119–177.
7. Collet, J.P.; Thiele, H.; Barbato, E.; Barthélémy, O.; Bauersachs, J.; Bhatt, D.L.; Dendale, P.; Dorobantu, M.; Edvardsen, T.; Folliguet, T.; et al. 2020 ESC Guidelines for the management of acute coronary syndromes in patients presenting without persistent ST-segment elevation. *Eur. Heart J.* **2021**, *42*, 1289–1367. [CrossRef]
8. Parsanathan, R.; Jain, S.K. Novel invasive and noninvasive cardiac-specific biomarkers in obesity and cardiovascular diseases. *Metab. Syndr. Relat. Disord.* **2020**, *18*, 10–30. [CrossRef]
9. Ladue, J.S.; Wroblewski, F.; Karmen, A. Serum glutamic oxaloacetic transaminase activity in human acute transmural myocardial infarction. *Science* **1954**, *120*, 497–499. [CrossRef] [PubMed]
10. Wroblewski, F.; Ladue, J.S. Lactic dehydrogenase activity in blood. *Proc. Soc. Exp. Biol. Med.* **1955**, *90*, 210–213. [CrossRef] [PubMed]
11. Bishop, M.J.; Everse, J.; Kaplan, N.O. Identification of lactate dehydrogenase isoenzymes by rapid kinetics. *Proc. Natl. Acad. Sci. USA* **1972**, *69*, 1761–1765. [CrossRef] [PubMed]
12. Rotenberg, Z.; Davidson, E.; Weinberger, I.; Fuchs, J.; Sperling, O.; Agmon, J. The efficiency of lactate dehydrogenase isoenzyme determination for the diagnosis of acute myocardial infarction. *Arch. Pathol. Lab. Med.* **1988**, *112*, 895–897.
13. Malasky, B.R.; Alpert, J.S. Diagnosis of myocardial injury by biochemical markers: Problems and promises. *Cardiol. Rev.* **2002**, *10*, 306–317. [CrossRef]
14. Aydin, S.; Ugur, K.; Aydin, S.; Sahin, I.; Yardim, M. Biomarkers in acute myocardial infarction: Current perspectives. *Vasc. Health Risk Manag.* **2019**, *15*, 1–10. [CrossRef]
15. Keffer, J.H. Myocardial markers of injury. Evolution and insights. *Am. J. Clin. Pathol.* **1996**, *105*, 305–320. [CrossRef] [PubMed]
16. Thygesen, K.; Alpert, J.S.; Jaffe, A.S.; Chaitman, B.R.; Bax, J.J.; Morrow, D.A.; White, H.D. Executive Group on behalf of the Joint European Society of Cardiology (ESC)/American College of Cardiology (ACC)/American Heart Association (AHA)/World Heart Federation (WHF) Task Force for the Universal Definition of Myocardial Infarction. Fourth universal definition of myocardial infarction (2018). *Circulation* **2018**, *138*, e618–e651.
17. Newby, L.K.; Jesse, R.L.; Babb, J.D.; Christenson, R.H.; De Fer, T.M.; Diamond, G.A.; Fesmire, F.M.; Geraci, S.A.; Gersh, B.J.; Larsen, G.C.; et al. ACCF 2012 expert consensus document on practical clinical consid-erations in the interpretation of troponin elevations: A report of the American College of Cardiology Foundation task force on Clinical Expert Consensus Documents. *J. Am. Coll. Cardiol.* **2012**, *60*, 2427–2463. [CrossRef] [PubMed]
18. Nallet, O.; Gouffran, G.; Lavie Badie, Y. L'élévation de la troponine en dehors des syndromes coronariens aigus Troponin elevation in the absence of acute coronary syndrome. *Ann. Cardiol. Angeiol. (Paris)* **2016**, *65*, 340–345. [CrossRef]
19. Masson, S.; Latini, R.; Anand, I.S. An Update on Cardiac Troponins as Circulating Biomarkers in Heart Failure. *Curr. Hear. Fail. Rep.* **2010**, *7*, 15–21. [CrossRef]
20. Harrison, N.; Favot, M.; Levy, P. The Role of Troponin for Acute Heart Failure. *Curr. Hear. Fail. Rep.* **2019**, *16*, 21–31. [CrossRef]
21. Konstantinides, S.V.; Meyer, G.; Becattini, C.; Bueno, H.; Geersing, G.J.; Harjola, V.P.; Huisman, M.V.; Humbert, M.; Jennings, C.S.; Jiménez, D.; et al. 2019 ESC Guidelines for the diagnosis and management of acute pulmonary embolism developed in collaboration with the European Respiratory Society (ERS): The Task Force for the diagnosis and management of acute pulmonary embolism of the European Society of Cardiology (ESC). *Eur. Respir. J.* **2019**, *54*, 1901647. [PubMed]

22. Rubini Gimenez, M.; Twerenbold, R.; Reichlin, T.; Wildi, K.; Haaf, P.; Schaefer, M.; Zellweger, C.; Moehring, B.; Stallone, F.; Sou, S.M.; et al. Direct comparison of high-sensitivity-cardiac troponin I vs. T for the early diagnosis of acute myocardial infarction. *Eur. Heart J.* **2014**, *35*, 2303–2311. [CrossRef] [PubMed]
23. Lindner, G.; Pfortmueller, C.A.; Braun, C.T.; Exadaktylos, A.K. Non-acute myocardial infarction-related causes of elevated high-sensitive troponin T in the emergency room: A cross-sectional analysis. *Intern. Emerg. Med.* **2014**, *9*, 335–339. [CrossRef]
24. Shah, A.S.; McAllister, D.A.; Mills, R.; Lee, K.K.; Churchhouse, A.M.; Fleming, K.M.; Layden, E.; Anand, A.; Fersia, O.; Joshi, N.V.; et al. Sensitive troponin assay and the classification of myocardial infarction. *Am. J. Med.* **2015**, *128*, 493–501. [CrossRef]
25. Apple, F.S.; Collinson, P.O. Analytical characteristics of high-sensitivity cardiac troponin assays. *Clin. Chem.* **2012**, *58*, 54–61. [CrossRef] [PubMed]
26. Collinson, P. Cardiac biomarkers by point-of-care testing—Back to the future? *J. Lab. Med.* **2020**, *44*, 89–95. [CrossRef]
27. Twerenbold, R.; Jaeger, C.; Rubini Gimenez, M.; Wildi, K.; Reichlin, T.; Nestelberger, T.; Boeddinghaus, J.; Grimm, K.; Puelacher, C.; Moehring, B.; et al. Impact of high-sensitivity cardiac troponin on use of coronary angiography, cardiac stress testing, and time to discharge in suspected acute myocardial infarction. *Eur. Heart J.* **2016**, *37*, 3324–3332. [CrossRef]
28. Pickering, J.W.; Greenslade, J.H.; Cullen, L.; Flaws, D.; Parsonage, W.; Aldous, S.; George, P.; Worster, A.; Kavsak, P.A.; Than, M.P. Assessment of the European Society of Cardiology 0-hour/1-hour algorithm to rule-out and rule-in acute myocardial infarction. *Circulation* **2016**, *134*, 1532–1541. [CrossRef]
29. Thygesen, K.; Mair, J.; Giannitsis, E.; Mueller, C.; Lindahl, B.; Blankenberg, S.; Huber, K.; Plebani, M.; Biasucci, L.M.; Tubaro, M.; et al. How to use high-sensitivity cardiac troponins in acute cardiac care. *Eur. Heart J.* **2012**, *33*, 2252–2257. [CrossRef]
30. Eggers, K.M.; Lindahl, B. Application of cardiac troponin in cardiovascular diseases other than acute coronary syndrome. *Clin. Chem.* **2017**, *63*, 223–235. [CrossRef]
31. Kaier, T.E.; Alaour, B.; Marber, M. Cardiac myosin-binding protein c-from bench to improved diagnosis of acute myocardial infarction. *Cardiovasc. Drugs Ther.* **2019**, *33*, 221–230. [CrossRef]
32. McDonaugh, B.; Whyte, M.B. The evolution and future direction of the cardiac biomarker. *EMJ Cardiol.* **2020**, *8*, 97–106.
33. Scridon, A.; Serban, R.C. Laboratory monitoring—A turning point in the use of new oral anticoagulants. *Ther. Drug Monit.* **2016**, *38*, 12–21. [CrossRef] [PubMed]
34. Xu, W.; Wang, L.; Zhang, R.; Sun, X.; Huang, L.; Su, H.; Wei, X.; Chen, C.C.; Lou, J.; Dai, H.; et al. Diagnosis and prognosis of myocardial infarction on a plasmonic chip. *Nat. Commun.* **2020**, *11*, 1654. [CrossRef] [PubMed]
35. Wang, X.Y.; Zhang, F.; Zhang, C.; Zheng, L.R.; Yang, J. The biomarkers for acute myocardial infarction and heart failure. *Biomed. Res. Int.* **2020**, *2020*, 2018035. [CrossRef]
36. Richards, A.M. Future biomarkers in cardiology: My favourites. *Eur. J. Heart Fail Suppl.* **2018**, *20* (Suppl. G), G37–G44. [CrossRef]
37. Yang, F.; Ma, L.; Zhang, L.; Wang, Y.; Zhao, C.; Zhu, W.; Liang, W.; Liu, Q. Association between serum lipoprotein-associated phospholipase A2, ischemic modified albumin and acute coronary syndrome: A cross-sectional study. *Heart Vessel.* **2019**, *34*, 1608–1614. [CrossRef]
38. Cao, Y.; Li, R.; Zhang, F.; Guo, Z.; Tuo, S.; Li, Y. Correlation between angiopoietin-like proteins in inflammatory mediators in peripheral blood and severity of coronary arterial lesion in patients with acute myocardial infarction. *Exp. Ther. Med.* **2019**, *17*, 3495–3500. [CrossRef]
39. Kim, Y.; Kim, H.; Kim, S.Y.; Lee, H.K.; Kwon, H.J.; Kim, Y.G.; Lee, J.; Kim, H.M.; So, B.H. Automated heart-type fatty acid-binding protein assay for the early diagnosis of acute myocardial infarction. *Am. J. Clin. Pathol.* **2010**, *134*, 157–162. [CrossRef]
40. Dupuy, A.M.; Cristol, J.P.; Kuster, N.; Reynier, R.; Lefebvre, S.; Badiou, S.; Jreige, R.; Sebbane, M. Performances of the heart fatty acid protein assay for the rapid diagnosis of acute myocardial infarction in ED patients. *Am. J. Emerg. Med.* **2015**, *33*, 326–330. [CrossRef]
41. Mehta, M.D.; Marwah, S.A.; Ghosh, S.; Shah, H.N.; Trivedi, A.P.; Haridas, N. A synergistic role of ischemia modified albumin and high-sensitivity troponin T in the early diagnosis of acute coronary syndrome. *J. Fam. Med. Prim. Care* **2015**, *4*, 570–575. [CrossRef]
42. Manini, A.F.; Ilgen, J.; Noble, V.E.; Bamberg, F.; Koenig, W.; Bohan, J.S.; Hoffmann, U. Derivation and validation of a sensitive IMA cutpoint to predict cardiac events in patients with chest pain. *Emerg. Med. J.* **2009**, *26*, 791–796. [CrossRef]
43. Baker, J.O.; Tyther, R.; Liebetrau, C.; Clark, J.; Howarth, R.; Patterson, T.; Möllmann, H.; Nef, H.; Sicard, P.; Kailey, B.; et al. Cardiac myosin-binding protein C: A potential early biomarker of myocardial injury. *Basic Res. Cardiol.* **2015**, *110*, 23. [CrossRef] [PubMed]
44. Kaier, T.E.; Stengaard, C.; Marjot, J.; Sørensen, J.T.; Alaour, B.; Stavropoulou-Tatla, S.; Terkelsen, C.J.; Williams, L.; Thygesen, K.; Weber, E.; et al. Cardiac myosin-binding protein C to diagnose acute myocardial infarction in the pre-hospital setting. *J. Am. Heart Assoc.* **2019**, *8*, e013152. [CrossRef] [PubMed]
45. Shapiro, M.D.; Fazio, S. From lipids to inflammation: New approaches to reducing atherosclerotic risk. *Circ. Res.* **2016**, *118*, 732–749. [CrossRef] [PubMed]
46. Scridon, A.; Tabib, A.; Barrès, C.; Julien, C.; Chevalier, P. Left atrial endocardial fibrosis and intra-atrial thrombosis—Landmarks of left atrial remodeling in rats with spontaneous atrial tachyarrhythmias. *Rom. J. Morphol. Embryol.* **2013**, *54*, 405–411.
47. Scridon, A.; Fouilloux-Meugnier, E.; Loizon, E.; Perian, M.; Rome, S.; Julien, C.; Barrès, C.; Chevalier, P. Age-dependent myocardial transcriptomic changes in the rat. Novel insights into atrial and ventricular arrhythmias pathogenesis. *Rev. Romana Med. Lab.* **2014**, *22*, 9–23. [CrossRef]

48. Scridon, A.; Serban, R.C.; Chevalier, P. Atrial fibrillation—Neurogenic or myogenic? *Arch. Cardiovasc. Dis.* **2018**, *111*, 59–69. [CrossRef]
49. Volpe, M.; Carnovali, M.; Mastromarino, V. The natriuretic peptides system in the pathophysiology of heart failure: From molecular basis to treatment. *Clin. Sci.* **2016**, *130*, 57–77. [CrossRef]
50. Drewniak, W.; Szybka, W.; Bielecki, D.; Malinowski, M.; Kotlarska, J.; Krol-Jaskulska, A.; Popielarz-Grygalewicz, A.; Konwicka, A.; Dąbrowski, M. Prognostic significance of NT-proBNP levels in patients over 65 presenting acute myocardial infarction treated invasively or conservatively. *Biomed. Res. Int.* **2015**, *2015*, 782026. [CrossRef]
51. Berezin, A.E.; Berezin, A.A. Adverse cardiac remodeling after acute myocardial infarction: Old and new biomarkers. *Dis. Markers* **2020**, *2020*, 1215802. [CrossRef]
52. Dobsa, L.; Edozien, K.C. Copeptin and its potential role in diagnosis and prognosis of various diseases. *Biochem. Med.* **2013**, *23*, 172–190. [CrossRef]
53. Jeong, J.H.; Seo, Y.H.; Ahn, J.Y.; Kim, K.H.; Seo, J.Y.; Chun, K.Y.; Lim, Y.S.; Park, P.W. Performance of copeptin for early diagnosis of acute myocardial infarction in an emergency department setting. *Ann. Lab. Med.* **2020**, *40*, 7–14. [CrossRef] [PubMed]
54. Miyao, Y.; Nishikimi, T.; Goto, Y.; Miyazaki, S.; Daikoku, S.; Morii, I.; Matsumoto, T.; Takishita, S.; Miyata, A.; Matsuo, H.; et al. Increased plasma adrenomedullin levels in patients with acute myocardial infarction in proportion to the clinical severity. *Heart* **1998**, *79*, 39–44. [CrossRef] [PubMed]
55. Falkentoft, A.C.; Rørth, R.; Iversen, K.; Høfsten, D.E.; Kelbæk, H.; Holmvang, L.; Frydland, M.; Schoos, M.M.; Helqvist, S.; Axelsson, A.; et al. MR-proADM as a prognostic marker in patients with ST-segment-elevation myocardial infarction-DANAMI-3 (a Danish Study of Optimal Acute Treatment of Patients With STEMI) Substudy. *J. Am. Heart Assoc.* **2018**, *7*, e008123. [CrossRef] [PubMed]
56. Ma, T.K.W.; Kam, K.K.H.; Yan, B.P.; Lam, Y.-Y. Renin-angiotensin-aldosterone system blockade for cardiovascular diseases: Current status. *Br. J. Pharmacol.* **2010**, *160*, 1273–1292. [CrossRef]
57. Eggers, K.M.; Lindhagen, L.; Baron, T.; Erlinge, D.; Hjort, M.; Jernberg, T.; Johnston, N.; Marko-Varga, G.; Rezeli, M.; Spaak, J.; et al. Sex-differences in circulating biomarkers during acute myocardial infarction: An analysis from the SWEDEHEART registry. *PLoS ONE* **2021**, *16*, e0249830. [CrossRef] [PubMed]
58. Hara, M.; Sakata, Y.; Nakatani, D.; Suna, S.; Usami, M.; Matsumoto, S.; Sugitani, T.; Ozaki, K.; Nishino, M.; Sato, H.; et al. Renin-angiotensin-aldosterone system polymorphisms and 5-year mortality in survivors of acute myocardial infarction: A report from the Osaka Acute Coronary Insufficiency Study. *Int. Heart J.* **2014**, *55*, 190–196. [CrossRef] [PubMed]
59. Blumenfeld, J.D.; Sealey, J.E.; Alderman, M.H.; Cohen, H.; Lappin, R.; Catanzaro, D.F.; Laragh, J.H. Plasma renin activity in the emergency department and its independent association with acute myocardial infarction. *Am. J. Hypertens.* **2000**, *13*, 855–863. [CrossRef]
60. Kamon, D.; Okura, H.; Okamura, A.; Nakada, Y.; Hashimoto, Y.; Sugawara, Y.; Ueda, T.; Nishida, T.; Onoue, K.; Soeda, T.; et al. Plasma Renin Activity Is an Independent Prognosticator in Patients with Myocardial Infarction. *Circ. J.* **2019**, *83*, 1324–1329. [CrossRef]
61. Cohn, J.N.; Colucci, W. Cardiovascular Effects of Aldosterone and Post–Acute Myocardial Infarction Pathophysiology. *Am. J. Cardiol.* **2006**, *97*, 4–12. [CrossRef]
62. Marinković, G.; Koenis, D.S.; de Camp, L.; Jablonowski, R.; Graber, N.; de Waard, V.; de Vries, C.J.; Goncalves, I.; Nilsson, J.; Jovinge, S.; et al. S100A9 links inflammation and repair in myocardial Infarction. *Circ. Res.* **2020**, *127*, 664–676. [CrossRef] [PubMed]
63. Serban, R.C.; Balan, A.I.; Perian, M.; Pintilie, I.; Somkereki, C.; Huțanu, A.; Scridon, A. Atrial electrical remodeling induced by chronic ischemia and inflammation in patients with stable coronary artery disease. *Chin. J. Physiol.* **2019**, *62*, 11–16. [PubMed]
64. Scridon, A.; Dobreanu, D.; Chevalier, P.; Șerban, R.C. Inflammation, a link between obesity and atrial fibrillation. *Inflamm. Res.* **2015**, *64*, 383–393. [CrossRef]
65. Sheriff, A.; Schindler, R.; Vogt, B.; Abdel-Aty, H.; Unger, J.K.; Bock, C.; Gebauer, F.; Slagman, A.; Jerichow, T.; Mans, D.; et al. Selective apheresis of C-reactive protein: A new therapeutic option in myocardial infarction? *J. Clin. Apher.* **2015**, *30*, 15–21. [CrossRef] [PubMed]
66. Ries, W.; Torzewski, J.; Heigl, F.; Pfluecke, C.; Kelle, S.; Darius, H.; Ince, H.; Mitzner, S.; Nordbeck, P.; Butter, C.; et al. C-Reactive Protein apheresis as anti-inflammatory therapy in acute myocardial infarction: Results of the CAMI-1 study. *Front. Cardiovasc. Med.* **2021**, *8*, 591714. [CrossRef] [PubMed]
67. Fanola, C.L.; Morrow, D.A.; Cannon, C.P.; Jarolim, P.; Lukas, M.A.; Bode, C.; Hochman, J.S.; Goodrich, E.L.; Braunwald, E.; O'Donoghue, M.L. Interleukin-6 and the risk of adverse outcomes in patients after an acute coronary syndrome: Observations from the SOLID-TIMI 52 (Stabilization of Plaque Using Darapladib-Thrombolysis in Myocardial Infarction 52) Trial. *J. Am. Heart Assoc.* **2017**, *6*, e005637. [CrossRef] [PubMed]
68. Kleveland, O.; Kunszt, G.; Bratlie, M.; Ueland, T.; Broch, K.; Holte, E.; Michelsen, A.E.; Bendz, B.; Amundsen, B.H.; Espevik, T.; et al. Effect of a single dose of the interleukin-6 receptor antagonist tocilizumab on inflammation and troponin T release in patients with non-ST-elevation myocardial infarction: A double-blind, randomized, placebo-controlled phase 2. *Eur. Heart J.* **2016**, *37*, 2406–2413. [CrossRef]
69. Kelly, D.; Khan, S.Q.; Dhillon, O.; Quinn, P.; Struck, J.; Squire, I.B.; Davies, J.E.; Ng, L.L. Procalcitonin as a prognostic marker in patients with acute myocardial infarction. *Biomarkers* **2010**, *15*, 325–331. [CrossRef]

70. Landeaus, L.; Leskelä, J.; Winkelmann, A.; Tervahartiala, T.; Sorsa, T.; Pesonen, E.; Pussinen, P.J. Serum MMP-9 Diagnostics, Prognostics, and Activation in Acute Coronary Syndrome and Its Recurrence. *J. Cardiovasc. Transl. Res.* **2018**, *11*, 210–220. [CrossRef]
71. Zhang, Z.Q.; Ding, J.W.; Wang, X.A.; Luo, C.Y.; Yu, B.; Zheng, X.X.; Zhou, T.; Shang, B.X.; Tong, X.H.; Zhang, J. Abnormal circadian rhythms are associated with plaque instability in acute coronary syndrome patients. *Int. J. Clin. Exp. Pathol.* **2019**, *12*, 3761–3771.
72. Zhou, K.; Li, Y.; Xu, Y.; Guo, R. Circulating Matrix Metalloproteinase-28 Levels Are Related to GRACE Scores and Short-Term Outcomes in Patients with Acute Myocardial Infarction. *BioMed Res. Int.* **2020**, *2020*, 1–8. [CrossRef]
73. Owolabi, U.S.; Amraotkar, A.R.; Coulter, A.R.; Singam, N.S.V.; Aladili, B.N.; Singh, A.; Trainor, P.J.; Mitra, R.; DeFilippis, A.P. Change in matrix metalloproteinase 2, 3, and 9 levels at the time of and after acute atherothrombotic myocardial infarction. *J. Thromb. Thrombolysis* **2020**, *49*, 235–244. [CrossRef] [PubMed]
74. Hochholzer, W.; Morrow, D.A.; Giugliano, R.P. Novel biomarkers in cardiovascular disease: Update 2010. *Am. Heart J.* **2010**, *160*, 583–594. [CrossRef] [PubMed]
75. Omran, M.M.; Zahran, F.M.; Kadry, M.; Belal, A.A.M.; Emran, T.M. Role of myeloperoxidase in early diagnosis of acute myocardial infarction in patients admitted with chest pain. *J. Immunoass. Immunochem.* **2018**, *39*, 337–347. [CrossRef]
76. Tousoulis, D.; Antoniades, C.; Nikolopoulou, A.; Koniari, K.; Vasiliadou, C.; Marinou, K.; Koumallos, N.; Papageorgiou, N.; Stefanadi, E.; Siasos, G.; et al. Interaction between cytokines and sCD40L in patients with stable and unstable coronary syndromes. *Eur. J. Clin. Investig.* **2007**, *37*, 623–628. [CrossRef] [PubMed]
77. Xie, P.-Y.; Li, Y.-P.; Chan, C.P.-Y.; Cheung, K.-Y.; Cautherley, G.W.H.; Renneberg, R. A One-step immunotest for rapid detection of heart-type fatty acid-binding protein in patients with acute coronary syndromes. *J. Immunoass. Immunochem.* **2009**, *31*, 24–32. [CrossRef]
78. Gurumurthy, P.; Borra, S.K.; Yeruva, R.K.R.; Victor, D.; Babu, S.; Cherian, K.M. Estimation of Ischemia Modified Albumin (IMA) Levels in Patients with Acute Coronary Syndrome. *Indian J. Clin. Biochem.* **2013**, *29*, 367–371. [CrossRef]
79. Kaier, T.E.; Twerenbold, R.; Puelacher, C.; Marjot, J.; Imambaccus, N.; Boeddinghaus, J.; Nestelberger, T.; Badertscher, P.; Sabti, Z.; Giménez, M.R.; et al. Direct comparison of cardiac myosin-binding protein C with cardiac troponins for the early diagnosis of acute myocardial infarction. *Circulation* **2017**, *136*, 1495–1508. [CrossRef]
80. Slagman, A.; Searle, J.; Müller, C.; Möckel, M. Temporal Release Pattern of Copeptin and Troponin T in Patients with Suspected Acute Coronary Syndrome and Spontaneous Acute Myocardial Infarction. *Clin. Chem.* **2015**, *61*, 1273–1282. [CrossRef]
81. Ponikowski, P.; Voors, A.A.; Anker, S.D.; Bueno, H.; Cleland, J.G.; Coats, A.J.; Falk, V.; González-Juanatey, J.R.; Harjola, V.P.; Jankowska, E.A.; et al. 2016 ESC Guidelines for the diagnosis and treatment of acute and chronic heart failure: The Task Force for the diagnosis and treatment of acute and chronic heart failure of the European Society of Cardiology (ESC). Developed with the special contribution of the Heart Failure As-sociation (HFA) of the ESC. *Eur. J. Heart Fail.* **2016**, *18*, 891–975.
82. Varga, A.; Serban, R.C.; Muntean, D.L.; Tatar, C.M.; Farczadi, L.; Tilea, I. Rapid liquid chromatography tandem mass spectrometry determination of rivaroxaban levels in human plasma for therapeutic drug monitoring. *Rev. Romana Med. Lab.* **2017**, *25*, 145–155. [CrossRef]
83. Zhang, S.; Dai, D.; Wang, X.; Zhu, H.; Jin, H.; Zhao, R.; Jiang, L.; Lu, Q.; Yi, F.; Wan, X.; et al. Growth differentiation factor-15 predicts the prognoses of patients with acute coronary syndrome: A meta-analysis. *BMC Cardiovasc. Disord.* **2016**, *16*, 82. [CrossRef]
84. Lisowska, A.; Knapp, M.; Tycińska, A.; Motybel, E.; Kamiński, K.; Święcki, P.; Musiał, W.J.; Dymicka-Piekarska, V. Predictive value of Galectin-3 for the occurrence of coronary artery disease and prognosis after myocardial infarction and its association with carotid IMT values in these patients: A mid-term prospective cohort study. *Atherosclerosis* **2016**, *246*, 309–317. [CrossRef] [PubMed]
85. Sanchez-Mas, J.; Lax, A.; Asensio-Lopez, M.C.; Fernandez-Del Palacio, M.J.; Caballero, L.; Garrido, I.P.; Pastor, F.; Januzzi, J.L.; Pascual-Figal, D.A. Galectin-3 expression in cardiac remodeling after myocardial infarction. *Int. J. Cardiol.* **2014**, *172*, e98–e101. [CrossRef]
86. Schernthaner, C.; Lichtenauer, M.; Wernly, B.; Paar, V.; Pistulli, R.; Rohm, I.; Jung, C.; Figulla, H.R.; Yilmaz, A.; Cadamuro, J.; et al. Multibiomarker analysis in patients with acute myocardial infarction. *Eur. J. Clin. Investig.* **2017**, *47*, 638–648. [CrossRef]
87. Lewis, G.D.; Wei, R.; Liu, E.; Yang, E.; Shi, X.; Martinovic, M.; Farrell, L.; Asnani, A.; Cyrille, M.; Ramanathan, A.; et al. Metabolite profiling of blood from individuals undergoing planned myocardial infarction reveals early markers of myocardial injury. *J. Clin. Investig.* **2008**, *118*, 3503–3512. [CrossRef] [PubMed]
88. Cheng, C.; Wang, Q.; You, W.; Chen, M.; Xia, J. MiRNAs as biomarkers of myocardial infarction: A meta-analysis. *PLoS ONE* **2014**, *9*, e88566. [CrossRef] [PubMed]
89. D'Alessandra, Y.; Devanna, P.; Limana, F.; Straino, S.; Di Carlo, A.; Brambilla, P.G.; Rubino, M.; Carena, M.C.; Spazzafumo, L.; De Simone, M.; et al. Circulating microRNAs are new and sensitive biomarkers of myocardial infarction. *Eur. Heart J.* **2010**, *31*, 2765–2773. [CrossRef] [PubMed]
90. Devaux, Y.; Vausort, M.; Goretti, E.; Nazarov, P.V.; Azuaje, F.; Gilson, G.; Corsten, M.F.; Schroen, B.; Lair, M.L.; Heymans, S.; et al. Use of circulating microRNAs to diagnose acute myocardial infarction. *Clin. Chem.* **2012**, *58*, 559–567. [CrossRef]
91. Martinez, E.C.; Lilyanna, S.; Wang, P.; Vardy, L.A.; Jiang, X.; Armugam, A.; Jeyaseelan, K.; Richards, A.M. MicroRNA-31 promotes adverse cardiac remodeling and dysfunction in ischemic heart disease. *J. Mol. Cell. Cardiol.* **2017**, *112*, 27–39. [CrossRef]

92. Azat, M.; Huojiahemaiti, X.; Gao, R.; Peng, P. Long noncoding RNA MIAT: A potential role in the diagnosis and mediation of acute myocardial infarction. *Mol. Med. Rep.* **2019**, *20*, 5216–5222. [CrossRef]
93. Wang, X.M.; Li, X.M.; Song, N.; Zhai, H.; Gao, X.M.; Yang, Y.N. Long non-coding RNAs H19, MALAT1 and MIAT as potential novel biomarkers for diagnosis of acute myocardial infarction. *Biomed. Pharmacother.* **2019**, *118*, 109208s. [CrossRef]
94. Hu, H.; Wu, J.; Li, D.; Zhou, J.; Yu, H.; Ma, L. Knockdown of lncRNA MALAT1 attenuates acute myocardial infarction through miR-320-Pten axis. *Biomed. Pharmacother.* **2018**, *106*, 738–746. [CrossRef] [PubMed]
95. Uchida, S.; Dimmeler, S. Long noncoding RNAs in cardiovascular diseases. *Circ. Res.* **2015**, *116*, 737–750. [CrossRef]
96. Kim, H.; Yang, D.H.; Park, Y.; Han, J.; Lee, H.; Kang, H.; Park, H.S.; Cho, Y.; Chae, S.C.; Jun, J.E.; et al. Incremental prognostic value of C-reactive protein and N-terminal proB-type natriuretic peptide in acute coronary syndrome. *Circ. J.* **2006**, *70*, 1379–1384. [CrossRef] [PubMed]
97. Al-Mohaissen, M.A.; Carere, R.G.; Mancini, G.B.; Humphries, K.H.; Whalen, B.A.; Lee, T.; Scheuermeyer, F.X.; Ignaszewski, A.P. A plaque disruption index identifies patients with non-STE-type 1 myocardial infarction within 24 hours of troponin positivity. *PLoS ONE* **2016**, *11*, e0164315.

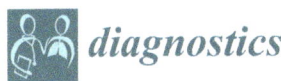

Article

Serum and Echocardiographic Markers May Synergistically Predict Adverse Cardiac Remodeling after ST-Segment Elevation Myocardial Infarction in Patients with Preserved Ejection Fraction

Tamara Pecherina, Anton Kutikhin *, Vasily Kashtalap, Victoria Karetnikova, Olga Gruzdeva, Oksana Hryachkova and Olga Barbarash

Research Institute for Complex Issues of Cardiovascular Diseases, 6 Sosnovy Boulevard, 650002 Kemerovo, Russia; pechtb@kemcardio.ru (T.P.); kashvv@kemcardio.ru (V.K.); karevn@kemcardio.ru (V.K.); gruzov@kemcardio.ru (O.G.); hryaon@kemcardio.ru (O.H.); barbol@kemcardio.ru (O.B.)
* Correspondence: kytiag@kemcardio.ru; Tel.: +7-384-960-907-7067

Received: 25 April 2020; Accepted: 13 May 2020; Published: 14 May 2020

Abstract: Improvement of risk scoring is particularly important for patients with preserved left ventricular ejection fraction (LVEF) who generally lack efficient monitoring of progressing heart failure. Here, we evaluated whether the combination of serum biomarkers and echocardiographic parameters may be useful to predict the remodeling-related outcomes in patients with ST-segment elevation myocardial infarction (STEMI) and preserved LVEF (HFpEF) as compared to those with reduced LVEF (HFrEF). Echocardiographic assessment and measurement of the serum levels of NT-proBNP, sST2, galectin-3, matrix metalloproteinases, and their inhibitors (MMP-1, MMP-2, MMP-3, TIMP-1) was performed at the time of admission (1st day) and on the 10th–12th day upon STEMI onset. We found a reduction in NT-proBNP, sST2, galectin-3, and TIMP-1 in both patient categories from hospital admission to the discharge, as well as numerous correlations between the indicated biomarkers and echocardiographic parameters, testifying to the ongoing ventricular remodeling. In patients with HFpEF, NT-proBNP, sST2, galectin-3, and MMP-3 correlated with the parameters reflecting the diastolic dysfunction, while in patients with HFrEF, these markers were mainly associated with LVEF and left ventricular end-systolic volume/diameter. Therefore, the combination of the mentioned serum biomarkers and echocardiographic parameters might be useful for the prediction of adverse cardiac remodeling in patients with HFpEF.

Keywords: biomarkers; ST-segment elevation myocardial infarction; preserved left ventricular ejection fraction; reduced left ventricular ejection fraction; heart failure; NT-proBNP; soluble ST2; galectin-3; matrix metalloproteinases; tissue inhibitors of metalloproteinases

1. Introduction

Despite cardiovascular mortality trending to decline worldwide in the recent decade [1], it is still unacceptably high in Russian Federation [2,3]. Advances in the diagnosis and treatment of coronary artery disease (CAD), particularly ST-segment elevation myocardial infarction (STEMI), considerably reduced in-hospital but not long-term mortality rates, even in patients with preserved (≥50%) left ventricular ejection fraction (LVEF) [4]. The main cause of adverse outcomes upon MI is ventricular remodeling—a deposition of a disorganized extracellular matrix governed by activated resident fibroblasts—which ultimately results in chronic heart failure (CHF) [5,6]. Timely diagnostics of ventricular remodeling requires sensitive and specific biomarkers, which should be detectable in the serum, permitting noninvasive sample collection [7]. Unfortunately, albeit serum biomarkers are routinely measurable and can be combined with other diagnostic and prognostic modalities, they generally provide little information on the actual state of ventricular remodeling, which restricts their implementation into its management [8].

Promising serum markers of ventricular remodeling include N-terminal pro-B-type natriuretic peptide (NT-proBNP, a protein released from cardiomyocytes at myocardial stretch), soluble suppression of tumorigenicity 2 (sST2, a cytokine-related protein and an established marker of inflammation, hemodynamic stress, and cardiomyocytes strain), galectin-3 (an inflammatory β-galactoside-binding lectin acting as a matricellular protein), matrix metalloproteinases (MMPs) and their tissue inhibitors (TIMPs) regulating the profibrotic remodeling [7,8], and exosomes enriched by pro-fibrotic miRNA (miR-1, -21, -34a, -133, -192, -194, -208a, -425, -744) [9], although none of them have been recommended for the specific assessment of ventricular remodeling progression so far [8]. Hence, the search for novel systemic markers of ventricular remodeling is ongoing, and various patient cohorts are involved.

Currently, >70% of patients with CHF aged >65 years have a preserved LVEF (HFpEF), and this proportion tends to increase together with the rising prevalence of associated underlying health conditions (obesity, metabolic syndrome, and diabetes mellitus) [10]. In contrast to CHF with a reduced (<50%) LVEF (HFrEF), which progression can be directly assessed in a noninvasive manner by echocardiography, efficient monitoring of the cardiac status in the patients with HFpEF is challenging [11], although a number of studies in this direction have been reported [12,13]. Taken together, these facts underscore the importance of finding the informative and routinely measurable biomarkers of ventricular remodeling in this patient category [14]. Ideally, the candidate molecules should be involved in the development of ventricular remodeling rather than simply reflecting the stiffness of the heart extracellular matrix. In addition, a panel of serum biomarkers can be combined with echocardiographic parameters, possibly correlating with each other and thereby reinforcing the association with ventricular remodeling.

Here, we evaluated whether the combination of serum biomarkers (NT-proBNP, sST2, galectin-3, MMP-1, MMP-2, MMP-3, and TIMP-1) and echocardiographic parameters may be useful to predict the ventricular remodeling-related outcomes in patients with HFpEF as compared to those with HFrEF.

2. Materials and Methods

In this prospective study, we enrolled 100 consecutive patients with HFpEF and 154 patients with HFrEF who have been admitted to Research Institute for Complex Issues of Cardiovascular Diseases (Kemerovo, Russian Federation) in 2015. The investigation was carried out in accordance with the Good Clinical Practice and the Declaration of Helsinki. The study protocol was approved (date of approval: 04 February 2015) by the Local Ethical Committee of Research Institute for Complex Issues of Cardiovascular Diseases (Protocol No. 20150204). All patients provided a written informed consent after receiving a full explanation of the study. Criteria of inclusion were: (1) STEMI diagnosed by means of the respective European Society of Cardiology guidelines [14]; (2) age between 18 and 75; (3) successful percutaneous coronary intervention (PCI). Patients with no clinical signs of heart failure (Killip class I) and LVEF ≥ 40% were assigned to HFpEF group while those with heart failure clinical signs (Killip class to II-IV) and LVEF <40% were considered as having HFrEF. Criteria of exclusion were: (1) Diagnosed acute/chronic liver or kidney failure, cancer, chronic obstructive pulmonary disease, autoimmune, endocrine, or mental disorders; (2) STEMI occurred as a result of unsuccessful PCI or coronary artery bypass graft surgery; (3) in-hospital death of the patient. The study design is represented in Figure 1.

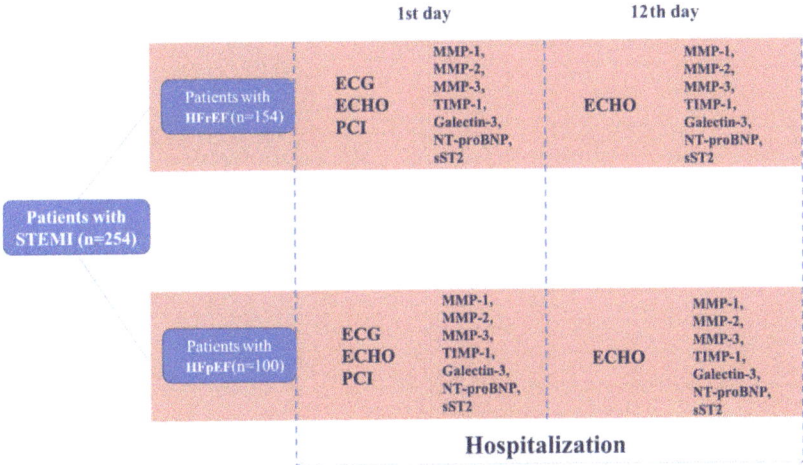

Figure 1. Study design. STEMI—ST-segment elevation myocardial infarction, HFpEF—STEMI with preserved ejection fraction, HFrEF—STEMI with reduced ejection fraction, ECG—electrocardiography, ECHO—echocardiography, PCI—percutaneous coronary intervention, MMP—matrix metalloproteinase, TIMP—tissue inhibitor of metalloproteinases, NT-proBNP—N-terminal pro-B-type natriuretic peptide, sST2—soluble suppression of tumorigenicity 2.

Thrombolytic therapy was applied in 11 (11%) patients. Biochemical profile and complete blood count were determined in all patients in addition to the collection of clinicopathological and demographic data from the case histories (Table 1).

Table 1. Clinicopathological features of the patients diagnosed with ST-segment elevation myocardial infarction with preserved ejection fraction (HFpEF, $n = 100$) and ST-segment elevation myocardial infarction with reduced ejection fraction (HFrEF, $n = 154$).

Features	Patients with HFpEF, n (%)	Patients with HFrEF, n (%)	p Value
Male gender	74 (74.0%)	102 (66.2%)	0.24
Past medical history of myocardial infarction	5 (5.0%)	70 (45.4%)	0.0001
Past medical history of percutaneous coronary intervention	3 (3.0%)	2 (1.3%)	0.62
Past medical history of coronary artery bypass graft surgery	0 (0.0%)	1 (0.6%)	1.0
Past medical history of angina pectoris	31 (31.0%)	108 (70.1%)	0.0001
Past medical history of atrial fibrillation	4 (4.0%)	28 (18.2%)	0.002
Past medical history of chronic heart failure	12 (12.0%)	101 (65.6%)	0.0001
Past medical history of stroke or transient ischemic attack	4 (4.0%)	18 (11.7%)	0.06
Peripheral artery disease	1 (1.0%)	10 (6.5%)	0.07
Arterial hypertension	70 (70.0%)	131 (85.1%)	0.006
Chronic kidney disease, stage 1–3	2 (2.0%)	15 (9.7%)	0.03
Type 2 diabetes mellitus	11 (11.0%)	30 (19.5%)	0.10
Glucose intolerance	2 (2.0%)	0 (0.0%)	0.15
Smoking	56 (56.0%)	57 (37.0%)	0.004
Hypercholesterolemia	22 (22.0%)	69 (44.8%)	0.0003
Overweight or obesity	71 (71.0%)	91 (59.1%)	0.07
Family history of coronary artery disease	3 (3.0%)	37 (24.0%)	<0.0001
Median (Interquartile Range)			
Age, years	57 (52; 63)	63 (56; 67)	<0.0001
Body mass index	26.9 (24.3; 29.8)	27.9 (25.1; 31.2)	0.0036
Duration of hospital stay	14 (12; 18)	15 (13; 19)	0.01

Prior to MI, cardiovascular drugs were rarely used in patients with HFpEF (Table 2).

Table 2. The list of medications used in patients with ST-segment elevation myocardial infarction with preserved ejection fraction (HFpEF).

Drug	Prior to Myocardial Infarction Number of Patients (Equal to the Proportion as $n = 100$)	During the Hospital Stay Number of Patients (Equal to the Proportion as $n = 100$)
Aspirin	9	99
Clopidogrel	0	83
Ticagrelor	0	25
Beta-blockers	11	97
ACE inhibitors	11	77
Statins	4	94

ACE—angiotensin-converting enzyme.

During the hospital stay, treatment was performed in accordance with the respective European Society of Cardiology guidelines [15]. Angina pectoris, chronic heart failure, atrial fibrillation, peripheral artery disease, arterial hypertension, diabetes mellitus/glucose intolerance, and hypercholesterolemia were diagnosed according to the respective ESC guidelines [16–22], while chronic kidney disease and overweight/obesity were defined as recommended in KDIGO [23] and NICE [24] guidelines. Past medical history of MI, stroke/transient ischemic attack, PCI or CABG surgery, smoking status, and family history of CAD were defined using the medical records. Coronary angiography was performed within the first hours after hospital admission using GE Healthcare Innova 3100 Cardiac Angiography System (General Electric Healthcare, Chicago, IL, USA). Although 26 out of 100 (26%) patients with HFpEF suffered from multivessel CAD and 17 out of 100 (17%) patients had complications during in-hospital stay, none of them died (Table 3).

Table 3. Coronary angiography features and in-hospital complications in patients with ST-segment elevation myocardial infarction with preserved ejection fraction (HFpEF).

Coronary Angiography Features	Number of Patients (Equal to the Proportion as $n = 100$)
>50% stenosis	41
Multivessel coronary artery disease (>3 affected arteries)	26
Complications during the hospital stay	
Arrhythmia or heart block	8
Pulmonary oedema	2
Radial artery bleeding	2
Coronary artery perforation	2
Early postoperative angina	1
Recurrent myocardial infarction	1
Cardiogenic shock	1
Death	0

Echocardiography (Sonos 2500 Diagnostic Ultrasound System, Hewlett Packard, Palo Alto, CA, USA) and enzyme-linked immunosorbent assay (ELISA) measurement of serum NT-proBNP (SK-1204, Biomedica, Vienna, Austria), sST2 (BC-1065X, Critical Diagnostics, San Diego, CA, USA), galectin-3 (BMS279/4, Thermo Fisher Scientific, Waltham, Massachusetts, MA, USA), matrix metalloproteinase (MMP)-1 (PDMP100, R&D Systems, Minneapolis, MN, USA), MMP-2 (PDMP200, R&D Systems, Minneapolis, MN, USA), MMP-3 (KAC1541, Thermo Fisher Scientific, Waltham, Massachusetts, MA, USA), and tissue inhibitor of metalloproteinases (TIMP-1, PDTM100, R&D Systems, Minneapolis, MN, USA) were performed on the 1st and 10th–12th day of hospitalization.

Statistical analysis was carried out utilizing Statistica 8.0 (Dell, Round Rock, TX, USA). Binary data (frequencies) were compared by Yates's chi-squared test. A sampling distribution was assessed by the Shapiro-Wilk test. Descriptive data were represented by median and interquartile range (25th and 75th percentiles). Unpaired and serial (before-after) measurements were compared by Mann-Whitney

U-test and Wilcoxon matched-pairs signed rank test, respectively. To assess the correlation, Spearman's rank correlation coefficient was employed. p values ≤ 0.05 were regarded as statistically significant.

3. Results

As compared to patients with HFrEF, patients with HFpEF had significantly lower prevalence of past medical history of myocardial infarction, angina pectoris, atrial fibrillation, chronic heart failure, arterial hypertension, and chronic kidney disease, as well as major cardiovascular risk factors such as smoking, hypercholesterolemia, and family history of coronary artery disease (Table 1).

In patients with HFpEF, serial echocardiographic examination revealed a significant increase in LVEF, stroke volume, early mitral filling velocity to early diastolic mitral annular velocity ratio, and early mitral inflow velocity, along with a concurrent decrease in left ventricular end-diastolic volume, left ventricular end-systolic volume, left ventricular end-systolic diameter, deceleration time, left ventricular ejection time, early diastolic myocardial velocity, early to late diastolic myocardial velocity ratio, and early diastolic myocardial velocity to early mitral inflow velocity ratio from the 1st to the 10th–12th day after STEMI onset (Table 4), suggesting moderate improvement of the cardiac function.

Table 4. Echocardiographic parameters in patients diagnosed with ST-segment elevation myocardial infarction with preserved ejection fraction (HFpEF, n = 100) at the time of admission and on 10th–12th day of hospital stay.

Parameter	1st Day after STEMI Onset Median (Interquartile Range)	10th–12th Day after STEMI Onset Median (Interquartile Range)	p Value
Left ventricular ejection fraction, %	56.0 (48.5; 61.0)	60.0 (52.0; 64.0)	0.015
Left ventricular end-diastolic volume, mL	126.0 (117.25; 142.25)	118.0 (98.0; 135.0)	0.003
Left ventricular end-systolic volume, mL	66.0 (54.0; 83.0)	62.0 (51.0; 74.0)	0.015
Left ventricular end-diastolic diameter, cm	5.5 (5.2; 5.7)	5.4 (5.23; 5.7)	0.861
Left ventricular end-systolic diameter, cm	3.9 (3.6; 4.3)	3.8 (3.5; 4.1)	0.038
Left ventricular end-diastolic volume/body surface area, mL/m2	10.88 (9.9; 11.84)	10.4 (9.44; 11.84)	0.875
Left ventricular end-systolic volume/body surface area, mL/m2	37.0 (28.0; 42.75)	32.0 (26.0; 39.0)	0.112
Pulmonary artery pressure, mmHg	25.0 (23.0; 27.5)	25.0 (23.0; 27.0)	0.086
Left ventricular end-diastolic pressure, mmHg	10.88 (9.9; 11.84)	10.4 (9.44; 11.84)	0.070
Stroke volume, mL	79.0 (70.25; 88.0)	81.0 (74.25; 90.0)	0.005
Left ventricular mass, g	241.0 (217.5; 271.0)	234.0 (213.0; 271.0)	0.141
Left ventricular mass/body surface area, g/m2	130.0 (122.0; 140.75)	124.0 (116.0; 142.0)	0.515
Left atrial diameter, cm	4.1 (3.9; 4.25)	4.1 (3.9; 4.3)	0.799
Right atrial diameter, cm	4.1 (3.9; 4.4)	4.2 (3.9; 4.4)	0.411
Right ventricular diameter, cm	1.8 (1.5; 1.9)	1.8 (1.5; 1.9)	0.855
Isovolumic relaxation time, ms	111.0 (104.0; 118.0)	110.0 (104.0; 118.0)	0.171
Early diastolic ventricular filling velocity (E, cm/sec)	57.0 (49.0; 70.0)	60.0 (47.0; 71.75)	0.662
Late diastolic ventricular filling velocity (A, cm/sec)	69.0 (59.0; 78.0)	69.5 (54.25; 78.75)	0.710
Early to late diastolic ventricular filling velocity ratio (E/A)	0.78 (0.71; 1.17)	0.79 (0.68; 1.24)	0.282
Deceleration time, ms	202.0 (170.0; 223.0)	195.0 (170.0; 221.75)	0.025
Acceleration time, ms	131.0 (114.5; 142.5)	131.0 (111.0; 137.0)	0.243

Table 4. *Cont.*

Parameter	1st Day after STEMI Onset Median (Interquartile Range)	10th–12th Day after STEMI Onset Median (Interquartile Range)	p Value
Left ventricular ejection time, ms	294.0 (279.5; 305.0)	287.0 (268.0; 300.0)	0.026
Early diastolic myocardial velocity, cm/sec	7.0 (6.0; 8.0)	6.0 (5.0; 8.0)	0.018
Late diastolic myocardial velocity, cm/sec	8.0 (6.9; 9.0)	7.95 (7.0; 9.0)	0.675
Early to late diastolic myocardial velocity ratio	0.83 (0.7; 1.14)	0.75 (0.67; 1.14)	0.009
Early mitral filling velocity to early diastolic mitral annular velocity ratio	8.59 (7.36; 10.23)	9.0 (7.67; 10.42)	0.038
Early mitral inflow velocity, cm/sec	37.0 (29.0; 45.0)	40.0 (32.0; 48.0)	0.001
Early diastolic myocardial velocity to early mitral inflow velocity ratio	1.56 (1.3; 2.0)	1.36 (1.03; 1.87)	0.001
Tei index (myocardial performance index)	0.7 (0.65; 0.77)	0.71 (0.65; 0.78)	0.758

In patients with HFpEF, serum levels of MMP-1, MMP-2, and MMP-3 did not exceed reference ranges at any of measured time points albeit augmented to the 10th–12th day after STEMI onset in comparison with the time of admission (Table 5). In contrast, TIMP-1 and galectin-3 were significantly higher at both of the time points, while NT-proBNP and sST2 demonstrated an increase exclusively on the first day of hospital stay (Table 5). Notably, serum concentrations of all elevated biomarkers (NT-proBNP, sST2, galectin-3, TIMP-1) were significantly reduced on the 10th–12th day after STEMI onset as compared with the time of admission (Table 5). The most pronounced decrease was documented for NT-proBNP and sST2 (3.8- and 1.8-fold, respectively).

Patients with HFrEF had normal levels of MMP-1, MMP-2, MMP-3, and TIMP-1 but elevated NT-proBNP, sST2, and galectin-3 at both of the time points, although the latter markers significantly reduced to the 10th–12th day after STEMI onset (Table 5). Notably, MMP-1, MMP-2, and MMP-3 increased to the 10th–12th day after STEMI onset, similar to the patients with HFpEF (Table 5).

In comparison with patients with HFrEF, those with HFpEF had significantly higher levels of NT-proBNP, sST2, galectin-3, MMP-2, and MMP-3 in conjunction with lower concentration of MMP-1 and TIMP-1 (Table 5).

Table 5. Serum concentrations of biomarkers in patients diagnosed with ST-segment elevation myocardial infarction with preserved ejection fraction (HFpEF, $n = 100$) and ST-segment elevation myocardial infarction with reduced ejection fraction (HFrEF, $n = 154$) at the time of admission and on 10th–12th day of hospital stay.

Parameter	Reference Range	1st Day after STEMI Onset Median (Interquartile Range)	10th–12th day after STEMI Onset Median (Interquartile Range)	p Value
Patients with HFpEF				
NT-proBNP, fmol/mL	5.0–12.0	17.84 (6.36; 60.4)	4.68 (2.5; 8.35)	0.0361
sST2, ng/mL	14.0–22.5	40.75 (26.98; 64.6)	22.19 (18.11; 25.3)	0.0001
Galectin-3, ng/mL	0.62–6.25	11.37 (9.49; 14.0)	9.05 (6.0; 10.41)	0.0001
MMP-1, ng/mL	0.91–9.34	2.14 (1.43; 5.39)	2.59 (1.72; 4.0)	0.2372
MMP-2, ng/mL	139.0–356.0	254.9 (217.2; 283.83)	295.2 (267.3; 326.65)	0.0003
MMP-3, ng/mL	2.0–36.6	7.22 (5.29; 10.6)	11.89 (8.99; 13.63)	0.0001
TIMP-1, ng/mL	11.0–743.0	899.25 (592.5; 1080.0)	853.5 (559.75; 1017.5)	0.7332

Table 5. Cont.

Parameter	Reference Range	1st Day after STEMI Onset Median (Interquartile Range)	10th–12th day after STEMI Onset Median (Interquartile Range)	p Value
		Patients with HFrEF		
NT-proBNP, fmol/mL	5.0–12.0	29.87 (10.65; 84.91)	18.69 (8.65; 42.76)	0.0265
sST2, ng/mL	14.0–22.5	56.45 (33.77; 75.88)	35.33 (22.79; 47.16)	0.0020
Galectin-3, ng/mL	0.62–6.25	14.59 (10.64; 16.45)	12.17 (9.12; 14.89)	0.0231
MMP-1, ng/mL	0.91–9.34	1.66 (0.73; 3.02)	2.20 (1.32; 4.51)	0.0001
MMP-2, ng/mL	139.0–356.0	289.3 (222.92; 315.31)	332.12 (297.7; 423.59)	0.0032
MMP-3, ng/mL	2.0–36.6	12.48 (10.19; 16.97)	14.67 (12.34; 17.93)	0.0035
TIMP-1, ng/mL	11.0–743.0	567.32 (412.9; 787.32)	414.22 (324.23; 668.45)	0.0039
		HFpEF vs. HFrEF (p Value)		
NT-proBNP, fmol/mL	5.0–12.0	0.0056	0.0001	
sST2, ng/mL	14.0–22.5	0.0001	0.0001	
Galectin-3, ng/mL	0.62–6.25	0.0001	0.0001	
MMP-1, ng/mL	0.91–9.34	0.0075	0.82	
MMP-2, ng/mL	139.0–356.0	0.0001	0.0001	
MMP-3, ng/mL	2.0–36.6	0.0001	0.0001	
TIMP-1, ng/mL	11.0–743.0	0.0001	0.0001	

HFpEF—ST-segment elevation myocardial infarction with preserved ejection fraction, HFrEF—ST-segment elevation myocardial infarction with reduced ejection fraction, NT-proBNP—N-terminal pro-B-type natriuretic peptide, sST2—soluble suppression of tumorigenicity 2, MMP—matrix metalloproteinase, TIMP—tissue inhibitor of metalloproteinases.

Correlation analysis performed in regards to the patients with HFpEF (Figure 2) demonstrated that, at the time of admission, the serum concentration of sST2 directly correlated with a number of echocardiographic parameters (left ventricular end-diastolic ($r = 0.42$, $p = 0.026$) and end-systolic volume ($r = 0.41$, $p = 0.030$), as well as pulmonary artery pressure ($r = 0.44$, $p = 0.001$)). Likewise, serum galectin-3 on the first day after STEMI onset positively correlated with a myocardial performance (Tei) index ($r = 0.41$, $p = 0.001$). Serum NT-proBNP negatively correlated with early to late diastolic myocardial velocity ratio ($r = -0.49$, $p = 0.001$) on the 1st day and with LVEF on the 10th–12th day of hospital stay ($r = -0.47$, $p = 0.007$) and positively correlated with left ventricular end-systolic volume ($r = 0.47$, $p = 0.002$) left ventricular end-systolic diameter ($r = 0.41$, $p = 0.020$), and left ventricular end-diastolic pressure ($r = 0.41$, $p = 0.030$) at the latter time point.

At the time of admission, serum MMP-1 correlated with left ventricular mass to body surface area index ($r = 0.46$, $p = 0.006$), yet on the 10th–12th day after STEMI onset, TIMP-1, but not MMPs, showed a significant correlation ($r = 0.56$, $p = 0.020$). MMP-3, determined at the time of admission, negatively correlated with LVEF on the 10th–12th day of hospital stay ($r = -0.68$, $p = 0.010$), while MMP-1 positively correlated with left ventricular end-diastolic volume/body surface area ($r = 0.57$, $p = 0.040$) and left ventricular end-systolic volume/body surface area ($r = 0.58$, $p = 0.030$) if both were measured at the latter time point.

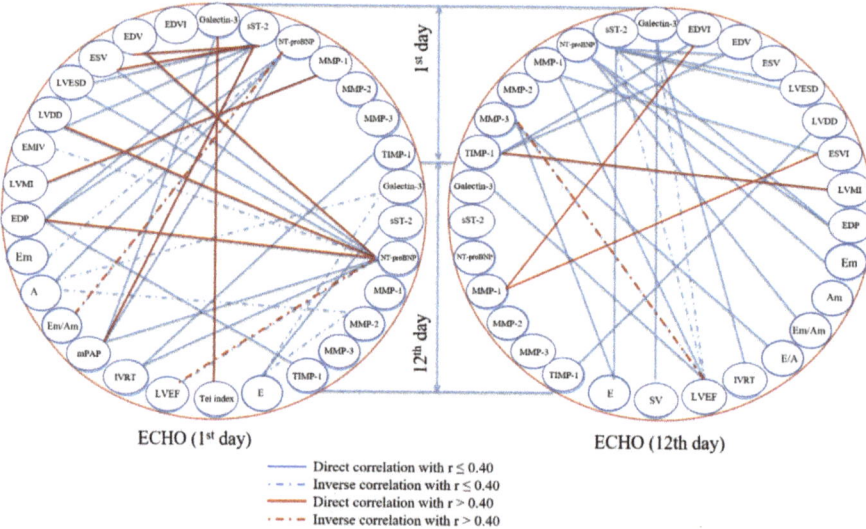

Figure 2. Correlation analysis of echocardiographic parameters and serum biomarkers in patients with ST-segment elevation myocardial infarction and preserved left ventricular ejection fraction (HFpEF, only statistically significant correlations with Spearman's rho > 0.4–0.7 are marked red). Abbreviations used: A—late diastolic ventricular filling velocity, Am—late diastolic myocardial velocity, E—early diastolic ventricular filling, E/A—early to late diastolic ventricular filling velocity ratio, Em—early diastolic myocardial velocity, Em/Am—early to late diastolic myocardial velocity ratio, EDP—left ventricular end-diastolic pressure, EDV—left ventricular end-diastolic volume, EDVI—end-diastolic volume index (left ventricular end-diastolic volume/body surface area), EMIV—early mitral inflow velocity, ESV—left ventricular end-systolic volume (ESV), ESVI—end-systolic volume index (left ventricular end-systolic volume/body surface area), IVRT—isovolumic relaxation time, LVDD—left ventricular end-diastolic diameter, LVEF—left ventricular ejection fraction, LVESD—left ventricular end-systolic diameter, LVMI—left ventricular mass index (left ventricular mass/body surface area), mPAP—pulmonary artery pressure, MMP—matrix metalloproteinase, NT-proBNP—N-terminal pro-B-type natriuretic peptide, sST2—soluble suppression of tumorigenicity 2, SV—stroke volume, TIMP—tissue inhibitor of metalloproteinases.

Patients with HFrEF generally had similar correlation trends (Figure 3). Serum NT-proBNP, sST2, galectin-3, and intriguingly, MMP-3, negatively correlated with LVEF at the time of admission ($r = -0.57$, $p = 0.0019$; $r = -0.44$, $p = 0.0032$; $r = -0.45$, $p = 0.0021$; $r = -0.43$, $p = 0.0010$, respectively), and similar trend was found regarding the hospital discharge. However, TIMP-1 directly correlated with LVEF ($r = 0.49$; $p = 0.0003$) and isovolumic relaxation time ($r = 0.41$; $p = 0.0012$) at the same time point.

Further, NT-proBNP and MMP-3 measured at the time of admission directly correlated with left ventricular end-systolic volume and diameter ($r = 0.47$, $p = 0.0017$ and $r = 0.42$, $p = 0.0234$, respectively, for NT-proBNP; $r = 0.41$, $p = 0.0138$ and $r = 0.43$, $p = 0.0085$, respectively, for MMP-3) at the 10th–12th day after STEMI onset. At the latter time point, MMP-3 also correlated with left ventricular end-systolic diameter ($r = 0.42$, $p = 0.0026$).

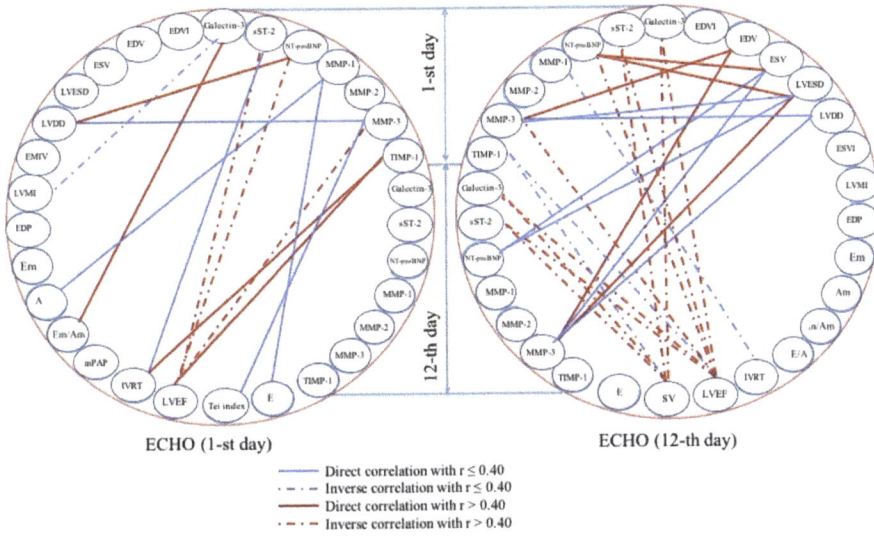

Figure 3. Correlation analysis of echocardiographic parameters and serum biomarkers in patients with ST-segment elevation myocardial infarction and reduced left ventricular ejection fraction (HFrEF, only statistically significant correlations with Spearman's rho > 0.4–0.7 are marked red). Abbreviations used: A—late diastolic ventricular filling velocity, Am—late diastolic myocardial velocity, E—early diastolic ventricular filling, E/A—early to late diastolic ventricular filling velocity ratio, Em—early diastolic myocardial velocity, Em/Am—early to late diastolic myocardial velocity ratio, EDP—left ventricular end-diastolic pressure, EDV—left ventricular end-diastolic volume, EDVI—end-diastolic volume index (left ventricular end-diastolic volume/body surface area), EMIV—early mitral inflow velocity, ESV—left ventricular end-systolic volume (ESV), ESVI—end-systolic volume index (left ventricular end-systolic volume/body surface area), IVRT—isovolumic relaxation time, LVDD—left ventricular end-diastolic diameter, LVEF—left ventricular ejection fraction, LVESD—left ventricular end-systolic diameter, LVMI—left ventricular mass index (left ventricular mass/body surface area), mPAP—pulmonary artery pressure, MMP—matrix metalloproteinase, NT-proBNP—N-terminal pro-B-type natriuretic peptide, sST2—soluble suppression of tumorigenicity 2, SV—stroke volume, TIMP—tissue inhibitor of metalloproteinases.

Therefore, serum markers well correlate with echocardiographic parameters at both of the studied time points in patients with both HFpEF and HFrEF are suggestive of a similar negative long-term prognosis in both of the groups despite better clinical symptoms in those with HFpEF in early HF stages. Hence, patients with HFpEF also have a high risk of adverse outcome.

4. Discussion

Unfortunately, preserved LVEF also does not guarantee the favorable outcome after STEMI and is frequently followed by CHF, arrhythmia, or heart block [25]. Multiple studies reported that patients with preserved LVEF after STEMI have similar prevalence of cardiovascular events as those with reduced LVEF [26], yet the data on available serum biomarkers informative of ventricular remodeling are still scarce [8]. Identification of patients with pathological cardiac remodeling and its sequelae is of crucial importance for the risk stratification.

Among the plethora of biomarkers, serum NT-proBNP is widely employed for the diagnostics of CHF, as well as control of treatment efficacy and prognostication in such patients [27]. Natriuretic peptides inhibit renin-angiotensin system and enhance sodium excretion, promoting peripheral vasodilation [28]. In our study, serum NT-proBNP was elevated at the time of admission and returned to the normal values to the 10th–12th day upon STEMI onset. In addition, we found a direct correlation of serum NT-proBNP with left ventricular end-systolic volume, left ventricular end-systolic diameter, and left ventricular end-diastolic pressure on 10th–12th day upon STEMI onset, along with the inverse correlation with early to late diastolic myocardial velocity ratio at the time of admission. Importantly, serum NT-proBNP also negatively correlated with LVEF on 10th–12th day upon STEMI onset. Previous studies well confirmed the role of serum NT-proBNP in predicting adverse cardiovascular outcome in patients with HFpEF [29,30].

The interleukin-1 receptor family member sST2 is considerably increased in response to the disrupted extracellular matrix homeostasis and subsequent cardiac remodeling [31,32]. In keeping with these data, serum sST2 declined from the 1st to the 10th–12th day after STEMI onset and directly correlated with left ventricular end-diastolic and end-systolic volume along with pulmonary artery pressure at the time of admission. In other studies, serum sST2 was elevated in patients with congestive heart failure, correlating with left ventricular end-diastolic pressure and serum NT-proBNP [33]. Hypertensive patients with HFpEF had elevated serum sST2 which demonstrated better predictive value as compared with NT-proBNP (AUC 0.8 and 0.7, respectively), with 13.5 ng/mL as a cutoff in multivariate analysis [34]. Predicting efficacy of serum sST2 in relation to the outcomes was higher for HFpEF as compared to the patients with reduced LVEF, indicating a positive association with all-cause death and repeated HF-related hospitalization [35].

Galectin-3 is a beta-galactoside-binding pleiotropic lectin released into the extracellular matrix by activated cardiac macrophages and regulating apoptosis, proliferation, inflammation, and fibrosis [36,37], being notable for its association with left ventricular remodeling [38], incident heart failure [39], and its severity [37]. In patients with HFpEF, serum galectin-3 was significantly elevated as compared to the control subjects and strongly correlated with NT-proBNP [40,41]. Further, both serum galectin-3 and NT-proBNP well distinguished patients with HFpEF from healthy individuals in ROC analysis [41]. In contrast to NT-proBNP, serum galectin-3 retained its association with ventricular remodeling in HFpEF patients in multivariate analysis, although NT-proBNP was significantly associated with HF symptoms [42]. Regarding to the long-term outcomes, elevated galectin-3 at 6 or 12 months was associated with all-cause death and hospitalization independent of treatment arm and NT-proBNP [43]. We found an increase in serum galectin-3 at both time points, yet no significant correlations with echocardiographic parameters were detected excepting a positive correlation with myocardial performance (Tei) index on the first day after STEMI onset.

MMPs represent a large family of zinc-dependent proteases degrading extracellular matrix and are informative of ventricular remodeling following the first hours after STEMI onset [44]. However, it is unknown whether the initial elevation of serum MMPs and TIMP-1 affects further cardiac remodeling and development of CHF. Concentrations of MMP-9 and TIMP-1 are frequently augmented in patients with CHF, being associated with a number of echocardiographic parameters [45,46]. Notably, NT-proBNP and MMP-9 levels have been found increased at all time points from the acute phase until >4 years after STEMI, and their levels showed a significant correlation [47]. In addition, higher serum MMP-9 correlated with lower LVEF and functional myocardial mass in long-term survivors of complicated STEMI [47] and with increased left ventricular end-diastolic diameter and left ventricular wall thickness in Framingham study participants free of previous MI and CHF [48]. In relation to the HF progression, the predictive value of serum MMP-2 in patients with HFpEF was found to be higher as compared with NT-proBNP [49]. Here, we did not reveal a significant increase in MMPs in the early period upon STEMI, yet MMP-1 and TIMP-1 showed a positive correlation with left ventricular mass to body surface area index at sequential time points. Further, higher MMP-1 on the 10th–12th day after STEMI correlated with left ventricular end-diastolic volume and left ventricular end-systolic volume normalized to the body surface area while MMP-3 at the time of admission inversely correlated with LVEF before hospital discharge. Intriguingly, serum levels of MMP-2 and MMP-3, although being within the reference range, significantly augmented from the admission to the discharge regardless of the ejection fraction, suggesting these molecules are gradually released during ventricular remodeling. Further studies in this direction might address this point.

An important limitation of the study includes differences in risk factors and treatments between the patients resulting in a relatively heterogeneous variable. However, it was expected when considering the patient groups with distinct LVEF (HFpEF and HFrEF). A replication of our study on a larger sample would be beneficial for the field to confirm our results. Another limitation is relatively short observation interval (two weeks), which should possibly be extended in replicating studies.

Notably, patients with HFrEF had multiple correlations of serum markers (NT-proBNP, sST2, galectin-3, MMP-3) with LVEF, as well as left ventricular end-systolic volume and diameter, whereas in those with HFpEF, only NT-proBNP showed significant negative correlations with LVEF. Probably, patients with HFpEF share a number of pathophysiological pathways with those suffering from HFrEF, yet cardiac remodeling in the former patient category is related to the diastolic dysfunction rather than LVEF.

5. Conclusions

In the present study, we found a reduction in NT-proBNP, sST2, galectin-3, and TIMP-1 in patients with HFpEF and HFrEF from hospital admission to the discharge, as well as numerous correlations between the indicated biomarkers and echocardiographic parameters, testifying to the ongoing ventricular remodeling. In patients with HFpEF, studied biomarkers of ventricular remodeling (NT-proBNP, sST2, galectin-3, and MMP-3) correlated with the parameters, reflecting the diastolic dysfunction (myocardial stretch, transmitral flow profile, and myocardial performance (Tei) index). Contrariwise, in patients with HFrEF, these markers are mainly associated with LVEF and left ventricular end-systolic volume/diameter. Therefore, the combination of serum biomarkers and echocardiographic parameters might be useful for the prediction of adverse cardiac remodeling in patients with HFpEF, particularly after STEMI.

Author Contributions: Conceptualization, T.P., A.K., V.K. (Vasiliy Kashtalap) and O.B.; Data curation, T.P. and O.B.; Formal analysis, T.P., A.K., V.K. (Vasiliy Kashtalap) and O.B.; Funding acquisition, O.B.; Investigation, T.P., V.K. (Victoria Karetnikova), O.G. and O.H.; Methodology, T.P., V.K. (Vasiliy Kashtalap), V.K. (Victoria Karetnikova), O.G. and O.H.; Project administration, V.K. (Vasiliy Kashtalap) and O.B.; Resources, V.K. (Vasiliy Kashtalap) and O.G.; Supervision, O.B.; Validation, T.P. and V.K. (Vasiliy Kashtalap); Visualization, T.P.; Writing—original draft, T.P. and A.K.; Writing—review & editing, T.P., A.K. and O.B. All authors have read and agreed to the published version of the manuscript.

Funding: This research was funded by the Complex Program of Basic Research under the Siberian Branch of the Russian Academy of Sciences within the Basic Research Topic of Research Institute for Complex Issues of Cardiovascular Diseases NO. 0546-2019-0003 "Atherosclerosis and its comorbidities. Features of diagnostics and risk management in a large industrial region of Siberia".

Conflicts of Interest: The authors declare no conflict of interest. The funders had no role in the design of the study; in the collection, analyses, or interpretation of data; in the writing of the manuscript, or in the decision to publish the results.

References

1. GBD 2017 Causes of Death Collaborators. Global, regional, and national age-sex-specific mortality for 282 causes of death in 195 countries and territories, 1980–2017: A systematic analysis for the Global Burden of Disease Study 2017. *Lancet* **2018**, *392*, 1736–1788. [CrossRef]
2. Ezzati, M.; Obermeyer, Z.; Tzoulaki, I.; Mayosi, B.M.; Elliott, P.; Leon, D.A. Contributions of risk factors and medical care to cardiovascular mortality trends. *Nat. Rev. Cardiol.* **2015**, *12*, 508–530. [CrossRef] [PubMed]
3. Boytsov, S.A.; Shalnova, S.A.; Deev, A.D. Cardiovascular mortality in the Russian Federation and possible mechanisms of its changes. *Zh. Nevrol. Psikhiatr. Im. S. S. Korsakova* **2018**, *118*, 98–103. [CrossRef]
4. Shah, K.S.; Xu, H.; Matsouaka, R.A.; Bhatt, D.L.; Heidenreich, P.A.; Hernandez, A.F.; Devore, A.D.; Yancy, C.W.; Fonarow, G.C. Heart Failure with Preserved, Borderline, and Reduced Ejection Fraction: 5-Year Outcomes. *J. Am. Coll. Cardiol.* **2017**, *70*, 2476–2486. [CrossRef]

5. González, A.; Schelbert, E.B.; Díez, J.; Butler, J. Myocardial Interstitial Fibrosis in Heart Failure: Biological and Translational Perspectives. *J. Am. Coll. Cardiol.* **2018**, *71*, 1696–1706. [CrossRef] [PubMed]
6. Oatmen, K.E.; Cull, E.; Spinale, F.G. Heart failure as interstitial cancer: Emergence of a malignant fibroblast phenotype. *Nat. Rev. Cardiol.* **2019**, *4*. [CrossRef]
7. Carnes, J.; Gordon, G. Biomarkers in Heart Failure with Preserved Ejection Fraction: An Update on Progress and Future Challenges. *Heart Lung Circ.* **2020**, *29*, 62–68. [CrossRef]
8. Sarhene, M.; Wang, Y.; Wei, J.; Huang, Y.; Li, M.; Li, L.; Acheampong, E.; Zhou, Z.; Qin, X.; Yunsheng, X.; et al. Biomarkers in heart failure: The past, current and future. *Heart Fail. Rev.* **2019**, *24*, 867–903. [CrossRef]
9. Ranjan, P.; Kumari, R.; Verma, S.K. Cardiac Fibroblasts and Cardiac Fibrosis: Precise Role of Exosomes. *Front. Cell Dev. Biol.* **2019**, *7*, 318. [CrossRef]
10. Borlaug, B.A. Evaluation and management of heart failure with preserved ejection fraction. *Nat. Rev. Cardiol.* **2020**, *30*. [CrossRef]
11. Vinereanu, D.; Mărgulescu, A.D. The fallacy of resting echocardiographic parameters of cardiac function in heart failure with preserved ejection fraction: Add global longitudinal strain to the list. *Eur. J. Heart Fail.* **2017**, *19*, 901–903. [CrossRef] [PubMed]
12. Špinarová, M.; Meluzín, J.; Podroužková, H.; Štěpánová, R.; Špinarová, L. New echocardiographic parameters in the diagnosis of heart failure with preserved ejection fraction. *Int. J. Cardiovasc. Imaging* **2018**, *34*, 229–235. [CrossRef] [PubMed]
13. Ibrahim, I.M.; Hafez, H.; Al-Shair, M.H.A.; El Zayat, A. Echocardiographic parameters differentiating heart failure with preserved ejection fraction from asymptomatic left ventricular diastolic dysfunction. *Echocardiography* **2020**, *37*, 247–252. [CrossRef] [PubMed]
14. Iyngkaran, P.; Thomas, M.C.; Neil, C.; Jelinek, M.; Cooper, M.; Horowitz, J.D.; Hare, D.L.; Kaye, D.M. The Heart Failure with Preserved Ejection Fraction Conundrum-Redefining the Problem and Finding Common Ground? *Curr. Heart Fail. Rep.* **2020**, *17*, 34–42. [CrossRef]
15. Task Force on the Management of ST-Segment Elevation Acute Myocardial Infarction of the European Society of Cardiology (ESC); Steg, P.G.; James, S.K.; Atar, D.; Badano, L.P.; Blömstrom-Lundqvist, C.; Borger, M.A.; Di Mario, C.; Dickstein, K.; Ducrocq, G.; et al. ESC Guidelines for the management of acute myocardial infarction in patients presenting with ST-segment elevation. *Eur. Heart J.* **2012**, *33*, 2569–2619. [CrossRef]
16. Montalescot, G.; Sechtem, U.; Achenbach, S.; Andreotti, F.; Arden, C.; Budaj, A.; Bugiardini, R.; Crea, F.; Cuisset, T.; Di Mario, C.; et al. 2013 ESC guidelines on the management of stable coronary artery disease: The Task Force on the management of stable coronary artery disease of the European Society of Cardiology. *Eur. Heart J.* **2013**, *34*, 2949–3003. [CrossRef]
17. McMurray, J.J.; Adamopoulos, S.; Anker, S.D.; Auricchio, A.; Böhm, M.; Dickstein, K.; Falk, V.; Filippatos, G.; Fonseca, C.; Gomez-Sanchez, M.A.; et al. ESC guidelines for the diagnosis and treatment of acute and chronic heart failure 2012: The Task Force for the Diagnosis and Treatment of Acute and Chronic Heart Failure 2012 of the European Society of Cardiology. Developed in collaboration with the Heart Failure Association (HFA) of the ESC. *Eur. J. Heart Fail.* **2012**, *14*, 803–869. [CrossRef]
18. Camm, A.J.; Lip, G.Y.; De Caterina, R.; Savelieva, I.; Atar, D.; Hohnloser, S.H.; Hindricks, G.; Kirchhof, P.; ESC Committee for Practice Guidelines (CPG). 2012 focused update of the ESC Guidelines for the management of atrial fibrillation: An update of the 2010 ESC Guidelines for the management of atrial fibrillation. Developed with the special contribution of the European Heart Rhythm Association. *Eur. Heart J.* **2012**, *33*, 2719–2747. [CrossRef]
19. Tendera, M.; Aboyans, V.; Bartelink, M.L.; Baumgartner, I.; Clément, D.; Collet, J.P.; Cremonesi, A.; De Carlo, M.; Erbel, R.; Fowkes, F.G.; et al. ESC Committee for Practice Guidelines. ESC Guidelines on the diagnosis and treatment of peripheral artery diseases: Document covering atherosclerotic disease of extracranial carotid and vertebral, mesenteric, renal, upper and lower extremity arteries: The Task Force on the Diagnosis and Treatment of Peripheral Artery Diseases of the European Society of Cardiology (ESC). *Eur. Heart J.* **2011**, *32*, 2851–2906. [CrossRef]
20. Mancia, G.; Fagard, R.; Narkiewicz, K.; Redon, J.; Zanchetti, A.; Böhm, M.; Christiaens, T.; Cifkova, R.; De Backer, G.; Dominiczak, A.; et al. 2013 ESH/ESC guidelines for the management of arterial hypertension: The Task Force for the Management of Arterial Hypertension of the European Society of Hypertension (ESH) and of the European Society of Cardiology (ESC). *Eur. Heart J.* **2013**, *34*, 2159–2219. [CrossRef]

21. European Association for Cardiovascular Prevention & Rehabilitation; Reiner, Z.; Catapano, A.L.; De Backer, G.; Graham, I.; Taskinen, M.R.; Wiklund, O.; Agewall, S.; Alegria, E.; Chapman, M.J.; et al. ESC Committee for Practice Guidelines (CPG) 2008–2010 and 2010–2012 Committees. ESC/EAS Guidelines for the management of dyslipidaemias: The Task Force for the management of dyslipidaemias of the European Society of Cardiology (ESC) and the European Atherosclerosis Society (EAS). *Eur. Heart J.* **2011**, *32*, 1769–1818. [CrossRef] [PubMed]
22. Rydén, L.; Grant, P.J.; Anker, S.D.; Berne, C.; Cosentino, F.; Danchin, N.; Deaton, C.; Escaned, J.; Hammes, H.P.; Huikuri, H.; et al. ESC Guidelines on diabetes, pre-diabetes, and cardiovascular diseases developed in collaboration with the EASD: The Task Force on diabetes, pre-diabetes, and cardiovascular diseases of the European Society of Cardiology (ESC) and developed in collaboration with the European Association for the Study of Diabetes (EASD). *Eur. Heart J.* **2013**, *34*, 3035–3087. [CrossRef] [PubMed]
23. Wang, A.Y.; Akizawa, T.; Bavanandan, S.; Hamano, T.; Liew, A.; Lu, K.C.; Lumlertgul, D.; Oh, K.H.; Zhao, M.H.; Ka-Shun Fung, S.; et al. 2017 Kidney Disease: Improving Global Outcomes (KDIGO) Chronic Kidney Disease-Mineral and Bone Disorder (CKD-MBD) Guideline Update Implementation: Asia Summit Conference Report. *Kidney Int. Rep.* **2019**, *4*, 1523–1537. [CrossRef] [PubMed]
24. National Clinical Guideline Centre (UK). *Obesity: Identification, Assessment and Management of Overweight and Obesity in Children, Young People and Adults: Partial Update of CG43*; NICE Clinical Guidelines, No. 189; National Institute for Health and Care Excellence: London, UK, 2014; pp. 1–149.
25. Xu, M.; Yan, L.; Xu, J.; Yang, X.; Jiang, T. Predictors and prognosis for incident in-hospital heart failure in patients with preserved ejection fraction after first acute myocardial infarction: An observational study. *Med. (Baltim.)* **2018**, *97*, e11093. [CrossRef] [PubMed]
26. Bhatia, R.S.; Tu, J.V.; Lee, D.S.; Austin, P.C.; Fang, J.; Haouzi, A.; Gong, Y.; Liu, P.P. Outcome of heart failure with preserved ejection fraction in a population-based study. *N. Engl. J. Med.* **2006**, *355*, 260–269. [CrossRef]
27. Brunner-La Rocca, H.P.; Sanders-van Wijk, S. Natriuretic Peptides in Chronic Heart Failure. *Card. Fail. Rev.* **2019**, *5*, 44–49. [CrossRef]
28. Pagel-Langenickel, I. Evolving Role of Natriuretic Peptides from Diagnostic Tool to Therapeutic Modality. *Adv. Exp. Med. Biol.* **2018**, *1067*, 109–131. [CrossRef]
29. Salah, K.; Stienen, S.; Pinto, Y.M.; Eurlings, L.W.; Metra, M.; Bayes-Genis, A.; Verdiani, V.; Tijssen, J.G.P.; Kok, W.E. Prognosis and NT-proBNP in heart failure patients with preserved versus reduced ejection fraction. *Heart* **2019**, *105*, 1182–1189. [CrossRef]
30. Savarese, G.; Orsini, N.; Hage, C.; Vedin, O.; Cosentino, F.; Rosano, G.M.C.; Dahlström, U.; Lund, L.H. Utilizing NT-proBNP for Eligibility and Enrichment in Trials in HFpEF, HFmrEF, and HFrEF. *JACC Heart Fail.* **2018**, *6*, 246–256. [CrossRef]
31. Magnussen, C.; Blankenberg, S. Biomarkers for heart failure: Small molecules with high clinical relevance. *J. Intern. Med.* **2018**, *283*, 530–543. [CrossRef]
32. Vianello, E.; Dozio, E.; Tacchini, L.; Frati, L.; Corsi Romanelli, M.M. ST2/IL-33 signaling in cardiac fibrosis. *Int. J. Biochem. Cell Biol.* **2019**, *116*, 105619. [CrossRef] [PubMed]
33. Bartunek, J.; Delrue, L.; Van Durme, F.; Muller, O.; Casselman, F.; De Wiest, B.; Croes, R.; Verstreken, S.; Goethals, M.; de Raedt, H.; et al. Nonmyocardial production of ST2 protein in human hypertrophy and failure is related to diastolic load. *J. Am. Coll. Cardiol.* **2008**, *52*, 2166–2174. [CrossRef] [PubMed]
34. Wang, Y.C.; Yu, C.C.; Chiu, F.C.; Tsai, C.T.; Lai, L.P.; Hwang, J.J.; Lin, J.L. Soluble ST2 as a biomarker for detecting stable heart failure with a normal ejection fraction in hypertensive patients. *J. Card. Fail.* **2013**, *19*, 163–168. [CrossRef]
35. Song, Y.; Li, F.; Xu, Y.; Liu, Y.; Wang, Y.; Han, X.; Fan, Y.; Cao, J.; Luo, J.; Sun, A.; et al. Prognostic value of sST2 in patients with heart failure with reduced, mid-range and preserved ejection fraction. *Int. J. Cardiol.* **2020**, *304*, 95–100. [CrossRef] [PubMed]
36. Hara, A.; Niwa, M.; Noguchi, K.; Kanayama, T.; Niwa, A.; Matsuo, M.; Hatano, Y.; Tomita, H. Galectin-3 as a Next-Generation Biomarker for Detecting Early Stage of Various Diseases. *Biomolecules* **2020**, *10*, 389. [CrossRef] [PubMed]
37. Felker, G.M.; Fiuzat, M.; Shaw, L.K.; Clare, R.; Whellan, D.J.; Bettari, L.; Shirolkar, S.C.; Donahue, M.; Kitzman, D.W.; Zannad, F.; et al. Galectin-3 in ambulatory patients with heart failure: Results from the HF-ACTION study. *Circ. Heart Fail.* **2012**, *5*, 72–78. [CrossRef]

38. Di Tano, G.; Caretta, G.; De Maria, R. Galectin-3 predicts left ventricular remodelling after anterior-wall myocardial infarction treated by primary percutaneous coronary intervention. *Heart* **2017**, *103*, 71–77. [CrossRef]
39. Ho, J.E.; Liu, C.; Lyass, A. Galectin-3, a marker of cardiac fibrosis, predicts incident heart failure in the community. *J. Am. Coll. Cardiol.* **2012**, *60*, 1249–1256. [CrossRef]
40. Polat, V.; Bozcali, E.; Uygun, T.; Opan, S.; Karakaya, O. Diagnostic significance of serum galectin-3 levels in heart failure with preserved ejection fraction. *Acta Cardiol.* **2016**, *71*, 191–197. [CrossRef]
41. Cui, Y.; Qi, X.; Huang, A.; Li, J.; Hou, W.; Liu, K. Differential and Predictive Value of Galectin-3 and Soluble Suppression of Tumorigenicity-2 (sST2) in Heart Failure with Preserved Ejection Fraction. *Med. Sci. Monit.* **2018**, *24*, 5139–5146. [CrossRef]
42. Wu, C.K.; Su, M.M.; Wu, Y.F.; Hwang, J.J.; Lin, L.Y. Combination of Plasma Biomarkers and Clinical Data for the Detection of Myocardial Fibrosis or Aggravation of Heart Failure Symptoms in Heart Failure with Preserved Ejection Fraction Patients. *J. Clin. Med.* **2018**, *7*, 427. [CrossRef] [PubMed]
43. Edelmann, F.; Holzendorf, V.; Wachter, R.; Nolte, K.; Schmidt, A.G.; Kraigher-Krainer, E.; Duvinage, A.; Unkelbach, I.; Düngen, H.D.; Tschöpe, C.; et al. Galectin-3 in patients with heart failure with preserved ejection fraction: Results from the Aldo-DHF trial. *Eur. J. Heart Fail.* **2015**, *17*, 214–223. [CrossRef] [PubMed]
44. Lindsey, M.L. Assigning matrix metalloproteinase roles in ischaemic cardiac remodelling. *Nat. Rev. Cardiol.* **2018**, *15*, 471–479. [CrossRef]
45. Kelly, D.; Khan, S.Q.; Thompson, M.; Cockerill, G.; Ng, L.L.; Samani, N.; Squire, I.B. Plasma tissue inhibitor of metalloproteinase-1 and matrix metalloproteinase-9: Novel indicators of left ventricular remodelling and prognosis after acute myocardial infarction. *Eur. Heart J.* **2008**, *29*, 2116–2124. [CrossRef]
46. Jordán, A.; Roldán, V.; García, M.; Monmeneu, J.; de Burgos, F.G.; Lip, G.Y.; Marín, F. Matrix metalloproteinase-1 and its inhibitor, TIMP-1, in systolic heart failure: Relation to functional data and prognosis. *J. Intern. Med.* **2007**, *262*, 385–392. [CrossRef]
47. Orn, S.; Manhenke, C.; Squire, I.B.; Ng, L.; Anand, I.; Dickstein, K. Plasma MMP-2, MMP-9 and N-BNP in long-term survivors following complicated myocardial infarction: Relation to cardiac magnetic resonance imaging measures of left ventricular structure and function. *J. Card. Fail.* **2007**, *13*, 843–849. [CrossRef] [PubMed]
48. Sundström, J.; Evans, J.C.; Benjamin, E.J.; Levy, D.; Larson, M.G.; Sawyer, D.B.; Siwik, D.A.; Colucci, W.S.; Sutherland, P.; Wilson, P.W.; et al. Relations of plasma matrix metalloproteinase-9 to clinical cardiovascular risk factors and echocardiographic left ventricular measures: The Framingham Heart Study. *Circulation* **2004**, *109*, 2850–2856. [CrossRef] [PubMed]
49. Martos, R.; Baugh, J.; Ledwidge, M.; O'Loughlin, C.; Murphy, N.F.; Conlon, C.; Patle, A.; Donnelly, S.C.; McDonald, K. Diagnosis of heart failure with preserved ejection fraction: Improved accuracy with the use of markers of collagen turnover. *Eur. J. Heart Fail.* **2009**, *11*, 191–197. [CrossRef]

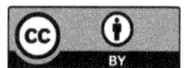

© 2020 by the authors. Licensee MDPI, Basel, Switzerland. This article is an open access article distributed under the terms and conditions of the Creative Commons Attribution (CC BY) license (http://creativecommons.org/licenses/by/4.0/).

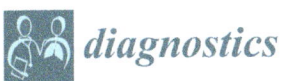

Article

Prediction of Adverse Post-Infarction Left Ventricular Remodeling Using a Multivariate Regression Model

Valentin Oleynikov, Lyudmila Salyamova, Olga Kvasova and Nadezhda Burko *

Department of Therapy, Medical Institute, Penza State University, 440026 Penza, Russia;
v.oleynikof@gmail.com (V.O.); l.salyamova@yandex.ru (L.S.); olgkvasova@rambler.ru (O.K.)
* Correspondence: hopeful.n@mail.ru; Tel.: +7-986-936-6220

Abstract: Background. In order to provide personalized medicine and improve cardiovascular outcomes, a method for predicting adverse left ventricular remodeling (ALVR) after ST-segment elevation myocardial infarction (STEMI) is needed. Methods. A total of 125 STEMI patients, mean age 51.2 (95% CI 49.6; 52.7) years were prospectively enrolled. The clinical, laboratory, and instrumental examinations were performed between the 7th and 9th day, and after 24 and 48 weeks, including plasma analysis of brain natriuretic peptide (BNP), transthoracic echocardiography, analysis of left ventricular-arterial coupling, applanation tonometry, ultrasound examination of the common carotid arteries with RF signal amplification. Results. Patients were divided into 2 groups according to echocardiography: "ALVR" (n = 63)—end-diastolic volume index (EDVI) >20% and/or end-systolic volume index (ESVI) >15% after 24 weeks compared with initial values; "non-ALVR" (n = 62)—EDVI <20% and ESVI <15%. In the ALVR group, hard endpoints (recurrent myocardial infarction, unstable angina, hospitalization for decompensated heart failure, ventricular arrhythmias, cardiac surgery, cardiovascular death) were detected in 19 people (30%). In the non-ALVR group, hard endpoints were noted in 3 patients (5%). The odds ratio of developing an adverse outcome in ALVR vs. non-ALVR group was 8.5 (95% CI 2.4–30.5) (p = 0.0004). According to the multivariate analysis, the contribution of each of the indicators to the relative risk (RR) of adverse cardiac remodeling: waist circumference, RR = 1.02 (95% CI 1.001–1.05) (p = 0.042), plasma BNP—RR = 1.81 (95% CI 1.05–3.13) (p = 0.033), arterial elastance to left ventricular end-systolic elastance (Ea/Ees)—RR = 1.96 (95% CI 1.11–3.46) (p = 0.020). Conclusion. Determining ALVR status in early stages of the disease can accurately predict and stratify the risk of adverse outcomes in STEMI patients.

Keywords: myocardial infarction; adverse left ventricular remodeling; echocardiography; left ventricular-arterial coupling

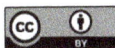

1. Introduction

Chronic heart failure (CHF) is one of the main causes of hospitalization and mortality in the world, including the Russian Federation [1,2]. The progressive nature of the course, early disability, the need for long-term pharmacotherapy and cardiac surgery are associated with significant economic costs for the healthcare system.

The results of a meta-analysis conducted by N.R. Jones et al. showed a significant improvement in the survival rates of patients with CHF from the 1970s to the 1990s. However, mortality has declined slightly over the past two decades. In 2010–2019, one-year and five- year survival amounted to 89.3% (84.3–93.4%) and 59.7% (54.7–64.6%), respectively [3]. Another study showed five times increase in the risk of a fatal outcome in the development of CHF [4].

According to the American Heart Association report, CHF prevalence is predicted to increase by 46% in the USA by 2030 [5]. CHF often complicates the postinfarction period. According to the results of the Russian EPOCHA-CHF study, along with arterial hypertension and chronic ischemic heart disease, myocardial infarction (MI) has become a competing cause of CHF, accounting for 15.8% in 2017 vs. 5.8% in 1998 [6]. The results of the European Society of Cardiology Heart Failure Long-Term Registry (ESC-HF-LT-R) also demonstrate the prevailing role of coronary heart disease in the development of CHF [7].

The widespread introduction of high-tech methods for the treatment of acute MI has led to a decrease in hospital mortality; this has been accompanied, however, by an increase in the number of patients with CHF [1,6]. Due to the very typical prolongation of myocardial revascularization terms, adverse postinfarction remodeling often develops being a key pathogenetic element of CHF and a significant predictor of mortality.

Adverse postinfarction left ventricular remodeling (ALVR) is characterized by an increase in the end-diastolic volume (EDV) >20% or the end-systolic volume (ESV) >15% compared with baseline values [8]. Ventricular remodeling already occurs within the first hours after cardiomyocyte necrosis and proceeds for several months. This process is characterized by a change in the left ventricular (LV) shape and size, and its dysfunction [8,9]. Early remodeling develops within three months after acute MI; mid-term and late remodeling develop within six and twelve months, respectively [10].

Identification of patients with a high probability of ALVR development in the early stages of the disease is important for the stratification of cardiovascular risk, the choice of personalized anti-remodeling therapy and rehabilitation.

The aim of this study was to search for early predictors and develop a model for predicting adverse remodeling in patients who had ST-segment elevation myocardial infarction (STEMI).

2. Materials and Methods

An open prospective single-center study involving 141 STEMI patients was conducted at the Department of Therapy of Penza State University (Penza, Russia). The study protocol and informed consent were approved by the Local Ethics Committee at Penza State University (approval code 317, on 15 May 2020).

The study included patients which met the following criteria: aged 35–65 years; acute STEMI, confirmed by an electrocardiogram, a diagnostically significant increase in specific cardiac enzymes (troponin I, CPK-MB); the presence of hemodynamically significant stenosis of the infarct-related artery according to coronary angiography with occlusion of other coronary arteries less than 50%, including the trunk of the left coronary artery less than 30%. The main exclusion criteria included: repeated or recurrent MI; type 1 or type 2 diabetes (requiring insulin therapy); NYHA class II-IV of CHF, severe concomitant diseases.

The treatment of STEMI patients has been carried out in full accordance with the guidelines [11] over the entire follow-up period.

A comprehensive clinical, laboratory and instrumental examination has been conducted with preserved pharmacotherapy initially in the period from the 7th to the 9th day of the STEMI, and after 24- and 48-week follow up (Figure 1).

Plasma brain natriuretic peptide (BNP) (with EDTA-ethylenediaminetetraacetic acid) has been measured using the OLYMPUS AU400 chemistry analyzer (Olympus Corporation, Tokyo, Japan).

Transthoracic echocardiography (EchoCG) has been performed using the MyLab90 ultrasound scanner (Esaote, Genoa, Italy) for determination of standard parameters and subsequent calculation of indexed values for the end-diastolic volume (EDVI) and the end-systolic volume (ESVI). An increase in EDVI >20% and/or ESVI >15% has been taken as ALVR after 24 weeks compared with the initial values (7–9th day). The interaction of the left ventricle and the arterial bed has been analyzed according to the following parameters: LV end-systolic elastance, which is the ratio of the end-systolic pressure to the end-systolic volume and reduced to body surface area (Ees/BSA); the arterial elastance calculated as the ratio of the end-systolic pressure over stroke volume divided by body surface area (Ea/BSA); LV-arterial coupling (LVAC) index, defined as the ratio of arterial elastance to left ventricular end-systolic elastance (Ea/Ees) [12].

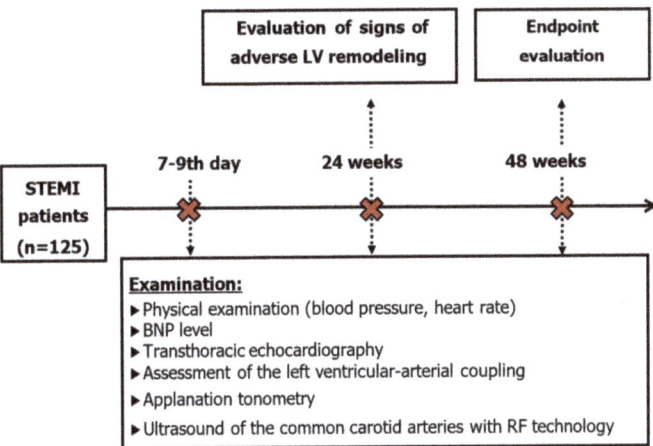

Figure 1. Flowchart of the study.

The structural and functional state of the common carotid arteries (CCA) has been assessed with the MyLab ultrasound machine (Esaote, Genoa, Italy) using radiofrequency (RF)- based technology. The following indicators were recorded: quality intima-media thickness (QIMT); stiffness index β; local systolic arterial pressure in CCA (loc Psys); local diastolic arterial pressure in CCA (loc Pdia). The above indicators of local pressure and stiffness are calculated using special software based on the level of blood pressure in the brachial artery, changes in the diameter and volume of the CCA in systole and diastole [13].

Applanation tonometry has been used to determine systolic aortic pressure (SBPao) and diastolic (DBPao) aortic pressure, and carotid-femoral pulse wave velocity (cfPWV) using the SphygmoCor device (AtCor Medical, Sydney, Australia) [14].

Statistical Analysis

Statistical data processing was performed using the licensed version of STATISTICA 13.0 program (StatSoft, Inc., Tulsa, OK, USA). All indicator values were given with the 95% confidence interval (CI). The dynamics of indicators was analyzed by the method of one-way analysis of variance (ANOVA) using the Newman-Keuls test. The Cox multiple linear regression was used when constructing a multivariate model. The frequency of the endpoint development was determined by the Kaplan-Meier method. The level of statistical significance was $p < 0.05$.

3. Results

We have summed up a 48-week follow-up for 125 patients (88.7%). There were some reasons for early termination of study participation: 1 patient died due to myocardial rupture on the 16th day; 1 patient died from pulmonary edema (according to the autopsy report) at the 10th month; 3 patients moved to another city; 11 patients discontinued the follow-up due to low adherence.

The age of the patients included in the study was 51.2 (49.6; 52.7) years, men prevailed—109 patients (87.2%). The body mass index was 27.4 (26.7; 28.0) kg/m^2. Symptoms of abdominal obesity were diagnosed in 74 patients (59.2%) [14]. Coronary heart disease was noted in 21 patients in the history (16.8%). Heredity cardiovascular diseases burdened 51 patients (40.8%) and 80 patients were smokers (64%). Arterial hypertension was observed in 61.6% (n = 77) with a disease duration of 6.5 (5.2; 7.8) years. The mean level of systolic blood pressure (SBP) was 118.8 (116.3; 121.3) mmHg and that of diastolic blood pressure (DBP)—76.2 (74.6; 77.9) mmHg. Prior to the STEMI, antihypertensive therapy was received regularly by 16 patients (20.8%), and irregularly by 24 patients (31.2%); 37 patients (48%) were not treated.

Primary percutaneous coronary intervention has been performed in 56 patients (44.8%); pharmacoinvasive strategy has been performed in 68 cases (54.4%). One patient only received thrombolytic therapy at the pre-hospital stage.

The analysis of EDVI and ESVI dynamics within 24 weeks after acute myocardial infarction has made it possible to divide the patients into 2 groups. The first group included 63 patients with ALVR revealed after 24 weeks according to the echocardiography. The second group included 62 patients without ALVR (non-ALVR group). A comparative analysis of patients by age, some anthropometric and anamnestic indicators and therapy is presented in Table 1.

Table 1. A comparative analysis of ALVR and non-ALVR groups (n = 125).

Indicators	ALVR Group (n = 63)	non-ALVR Group (n = 62)	p
Age, years	51.4 (49.2; 53.6)	50.9 (48.7; 53.1)	0.724
Female, n (%)	9 (14.3%)	6 (9.7%)	0.246
Male, n (%)	54 (85.7%)	56 (90.3%)	0.246
Abdominal obesity, n (%)	41 (65%)	33 (53.2%)	0.086
Waist circumference (WC), cm	99.1 (96.4; 101.9)	92.9 (90.1; 95.6)	**0.002**
BMI, kg/m^2	28 (27.1; 28.9)	26.7 (25.8; 27.6)	0.056
Tobacco smoking, n (%)	38 (60.3%)	42 (67.7%)	0.176
Smoking history, years	26.4 (23.4; 29.4)	27.4 (24.6; 30.3)	0.619
Burdened heredity, n (%)	27 (42.8%)	24 (38.7%)	0.325
History of CHD, n (%)	11 (17.5%)	10 (16.1%)	0.383
CHD duration, years	2.4 (0; 4.9)	2.8 (0.2; 5.5)	0.798
AH, n (%)	37 (58.7%)	40 (64.5%)	0.245
AH duration, years	7.6 (5.8; 9.5)	5.4 (3.7; 7.2)	0.090
SBP, mmHg	118.1 (114.5; 121.6)	119.4 (115.9; 122.9)	0.586
DBP, mmHg	76.6 (74.2; 78.9)	75.9 (73.6; 78.2)	0.696
HR, bpm	71.1 (69.4; 72.8)	69.9 (68.2; 71.5)	0.305
Drug therapy			
Dual antiplatelet therapy, n (%)	63 (100%)	62 (100%)	0.500
Statins, n (%)	63 (100%)	62 (100%)	0.500
Beta blockers, n (%)	56 (89%)	51 (82%)	0.133
ACE (angiotensin converting enzyme) inhibitors/sartans, n (%)	49 (78%)	53 (86%)	0.122
Calcium channel block-ers, n (%)	5 (8%)	5 (8%)	0.500
Diuretics, n (%)	12 (19%)	10 (16%)	0.329

Note: the data are presented as M ± SD with a normal distribution, and as Me (Q25%; Q75%) with an incorrect distribution; n is the number of patients; BMI is body mass index; CHD is coronary heart disease; AH is arterial hypertension; SBP is systolic blood pressure; DBP is diastolic blood pressure; HR is heart rate.

The study of echocardiographic parameters in patients with ALVR revealed a progressive increase in EDVI and ESVI during the entire follow-up period. Thus, within 24–48 weeks, EDVI increased by 22.3–21.1%, and ESVI by 26.9–25.7%, respectively (Figure 2, Supplementary Materials). Besides, negative dynamics of ejection fraction (EF) has been noted during the repeated studies. At the same time, some negative dynamics of ESVI were accompanied by an increase in EF by 3.4% in patients without ALVR by the end of the follow-up. Differences in the presented echocardiographic parameters of the compared groups were noted for 48 weeks (Figure 1).

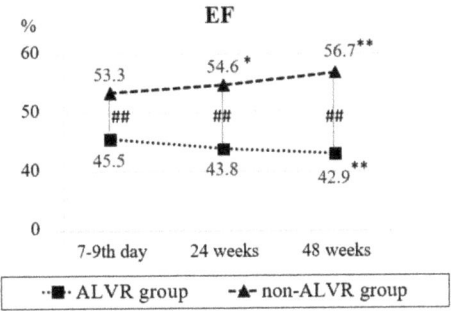

Figure 2. Dynamics of EF values in the comparison groups. Note: * $p < 0.05$, ** $p < 0.01$ are significant differences between the initial values and subsequent visits; ## $p < 0.01$ are significant intergroup differences. EF—ejection fraction.

Patients with adverse LV remodeling and without it initially varied by BNP level: 231.9 (95% CI 122.9; 340.9) vs. 72.1 (95% CI 51.0; 93.2) ($p = 0.003$). Despite the improvement in laboratory values for each group, the differences persisted at subsequent visits (Figure 3).

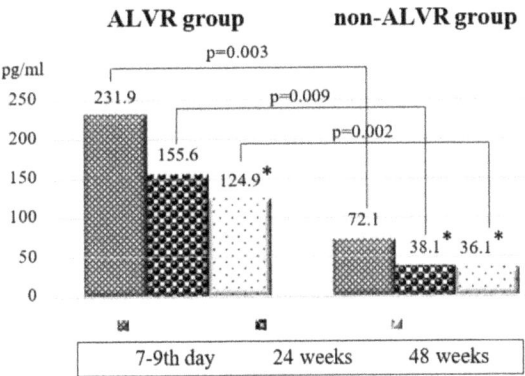

Figure 3. Dynamics of BNP in the comparison groups. Note: * $p < 0.05$ are significant differences between the initial values and subsequent visits. BNP –brain natriuretic peptide.

In the analyzed groups, the inverse dynamics of LVAC indicators were revealed. Initially, the patients of two groups had comparable values of arterial elastance. Ea/BSA indicator in ALVR group decreased after 24 weeks and returned to the baseline after 48 weeks; in non-ALVR group, it decreased by the end of the follow-up (Table 2).

Table 2. Comparative characteristics of LVAC indicators, and structural and functional features of arteries in the comparison groups.

Indicator	7th–9th Day		24 Weeks		48 Weeks	
	ALVR	non-ALVR	ALVR	non-ALVR	ALVR	non-ALVR
Ea/BSA, mmHg/mL	0.97 (0.89; 1.05)	1.01 (0.92; 1.09)	0.86 (0.78; 0.94) ##	0.98 (0.92; 1.05) *	0.93 (0.84; 1.02)	0.92 (0.86; 0.99) #
Ees/BSA, mmHg/mL	0.86 (0.77; 0.96)	1.13 (1.04; 1.23) **	0.70 (0.62; 0.78) ##	1.19 (1.10; 1.28) **	0.74 (0.65; 0.84) ##	1.20 (1.12; 1.28) **
Ea/Ees	1.27 (1.14; 1.39)	0.94 (0.85; 1.02) **	1.36 (1.23; 1.49)	0.84 (0.80; 0.88) **#	1.41 (1.25; 1.56) #	0.79 (0.74; 0.83) **##
SBPao, mmHg	98.9 (96.4; 101.5)	102.8 (100.2; 105.4) *	107.5 (104.3; 110.7) ##	109.7 (106.2; 113.1) ##	108.6 (105.7; 111.4) ##	112.4 (108.4; 116.3) ##
DBPao, mmHg	71.8 (69.6; 74.0)	72.7 (70.2; 75.2)	74.8 (72.0; 77.7) #	76.3 (73.8; 78.8) #	77.4 (75.3; 79.4) ##	77.1 (74.9; 79.3) #
cfPWV, m/s	7.8 (7.4; 8.3)	8.1 (7.6; 8.7)	7.7 (7.3; 8.2)	8.0 (7.5; 8.5)	7.6 (7.1; 8.0)	7.8 (7.3; 8.3)
QIMT, μm	798.2 (750.8; 845.6)	762.9 (722.9; 802.8)	758.2 (714.8; 801.6) ##	725.7 (692.0; 759.4) ##	735.7 (702.1; 769.2) ##	705.3 (669.7; 740.9) ##
β index	10.7 (9.5; 11.9)	9.3 (8.3; 10.2)	8.9 (8.2; 9.7) ##	8.2 (7.5; 8.9)	9.7 (8.5; 10.8) ##	8.5 (7.7; 9.2)
loc Psys, mmHg	101.8 (98.5; 105.1)	108.7 (105.8; 111.5) **	107.6 (105.3; 109.9) ##	113.1 (109.3; 116.8) *	111.2 (108.5; 113.8) ##	111.8 (108.7; 114.9)
loc Pdia, mmHg	68.7 (66.2; 71.2)	72.2 (70.2; 74.3) *	73.2 (71.1; 75.2) ##	75.3 (72.9; 77.7) #	75.9 (73.9; 77.8) ##	75.6 (73.8; 77.4) #

Note: the data are presented with 95% confidence interval; * $p < 0.05$, ** $p < 0.01$ is significance for intergroup differences; # $p < 0.05$, ## $p < 0.01$ is significance for intragroup differences on the baseline with subsequent visits; Ea/BSA is arterial elastance normalized to body surface area; Ees/BSA is end-systolic left ventricular elastance normalized to body surface area; Ea/Ees is left ventricular-arterial coupling index; SBPao is aortic systolic pressure; DBPao is aortic diastolic pressure; cfPWV is carotid-femoral pulse wave velocity; QIMT is quality intima-media thickness; loc Psys is local systolic blood pressure; loc Pdia is local diastolic blood pressure.

Initially, in patients with ALVR, the level of LV elastance was significantly reduced, and LVAC index predominated compared to non-ALVR group. After 24 and 48 weeks, a decrease in Ees/BSA by 18.6–14%, and an increase in Ea/Ees were denoted by the end of the follow-up in ALVR group. At the same time in the comparison group the LV elastance has not changed, and LVAC index decreased by 10.6% after 24 weeks and by 16% after 48 weeks. Intergroup differences in Ees/BSA and Ea/Ees values persisted over the entire follow-up period.

A detailed analysis of LVAC index has elicited abnormal values in ALVR group: initially in 29 patients (46%), then in 36 patients (57%; unreliable) after 24 weeks, and finally in 33 patients (52.4%; unreliable) after 48 weeks. As for non-ALVR group, there were initially 7 patients (11.3%), and 2 patients (3%; $p = 0.08$) at the interval visit with abnormal LVAC values. By the end of the follow-up, all of the patients of the comparison group demonstrated a normal level of LVAC index (0%; $p = 0.008$).

An analysis of applanation tonometry indicators has shown low SBPao values in ALVR group. Within 48 weeks, a comparable increase in central pressure parameters in the comparison groups has been found. In patients with ALVR and without it cfPWV has not shown differences and was stable over the entire follow-up period.

According to the ultrasound of CCA using the RF-technology, the groups had a comparable QIMT level and β index in the period from the 7th to the 9th day of the STEMI. In ALVR group, indicators have decreased after 24 and 48 weeks; in non-ALVR group, QIMT values have also improved during therapy.

A comparative analysis of the dynamics of local pressure in CCA is essential. The level of loc Psys and loc Pdia has been initially reduced in patients with ALVR compared with non-ALVR group. Subsequently, the pressure values in CCA in ALVR group were restored after 24–48 weeks.

One of the important results of this study is the relationship between ALVR and cardiovascular events. In the comparison groups, the frequency of hard endpoints, such as recurrent MI, unstable angina, hospitalization for decompensated heart failure, ventricular arrhythmias, cardiac surgery, and death from cardiac causes has been analyzed (Figure 4). In ALVR group, the above endpoints were detected in 19 patients (30%): 7 patients were hospitalized for unstable angina (11.1%); 1 patient (1.6%) was diagnosed with recurrent acute MI and 2 patients (3.2%) due to decompensated CHF. Cardiac surgery was performed in 7 patients (11.1%). Moreover, 2 patients were diagnosed with life-threatening arrhythmias (3.2%). In non-ALVR group, hard endpoints were noted in 3 patients (5%); 1 patient underwent cardiac surgery (1.6%), 2 patients (3.2%) were hospitalized for unstable angina. The odds ratio of developing an adverse outcome in group 1 compared with group 2 was 8.5 [95% CI 2.4–30.5] ($p = 0.0004$).

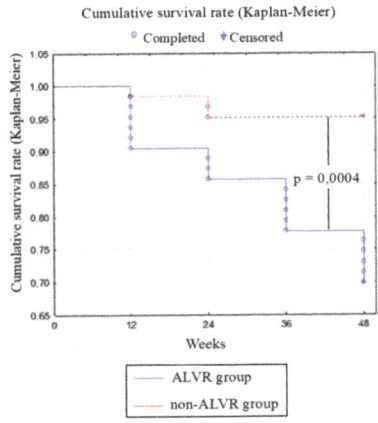

Figure 4. The incidence of hard endpoints in the comparison groups.

The predictors of adverse postinfarction remodeling were identified according to the univariate and multivariate logistic regression analysis of clinical, laboratory and instrumental parameters recorded in the period of the 7th-9th days from the index event. Since the determination of postinfarction remodeling is based on echocardiographic parameters, the latter were excluded from the analysis [8]. According to the univariate analysis, the independent variables of ALVR were waist circumference (WC), determination of BNP in a bimodal distribution ("0"—with BNP <100 pg/mL; "1"—BNP ≥100 pg/mL), EF, Ees/BSA, Ea/Ees, Ea/Ees in bimodal distribution ("0"—at Ea/Ees 0.6–1.2; "1"—at Ea/Ees <0.6 or >1.2), Loc Psys (Table 3).

Table 3. Predictors of adverse left ventricular remodeling in patients after STEMI according to univariate analysis.

Indicator	β	Chi-Squared	p	RR (95% CI)
WC, cm	0.025	4.69	0.030	1.03 (1.002–1.05)
BNP, pg/mL	0.0009	6.50	0.011	1.001 (1.0002–1.002)
Abnormal BNP	0.88	10.11	0.001	2.41 (1.402–4.15)
EF, %	−0.057	14.57	0.0001	0.94 (0.92–0.97)
Ees/BSA, mmHg/mL/m²	−1.07	7.39	0.007	0.34 (0.16–0.74)
Ea/Ees	0.66	7.85	0.005	1.94 (1.22–3.08)
Abnormal Ea/Ees	0.82	10.42	0.001	2.27 (1.38–3.74)
loc Psys, mmHg	−0.020	4.07	0.044	0.98 (0.96–0.999)

Note: β is regression coefficient; p is significance; RR is relative risk; CI is confidence interval; WC is waist circumference; BNP is brain natriuretic peptide; EF is ejection fraction; Ees/BSA is end-systolic left ventricular elastance normalized to body surface area; Ea/Ees is Ea/Ees is left ventricular-arterial coupling index; loc Psys is local carotid systolic blood pressure.

A multivariate model for the development of various types of postinfarction remodeling including WC, abnormal values of BNP and Ea/Ees was created based on the results of the univariate analysis and considering the correlations between the indicators (Table 4).

Table 4. A multivariate model for the development of ALVR in STEMI patients.

Indicator	β	Chi-Squared	p	RR (95% CI)
WC, cm	0.024	4.11	0.042	1.02 (1.001–1.05)
Abnormal BNP	0.59	4.50	0.033	1.81 (1.05–3.13)
Abnormal Ea/Ees	0.68	5.45	0.020	1.96 (1.11–3.46)

Note: β—regression coefficient, p—significance, RR—relative risk, CI—confidence interval. WC, waist circumference; BNP, brain natriuretic peptide; Ea/Ees, left ventricular-arterial coupling index.

The multivariate regression model presented in Table 4 uses the Formula (1):

$$h = h_0 \cdot \exp(0.024 \cdot X_1 + 0.59 \cdot X_2 + 0.68 \cdot X_3) \tag{1}$$

where: X_1 is WC, cm; X_2 is equal to 1.0 with BNP $\geq$100 pg/mL, and it is equal to 0 with BNP <100 pg/mL; X_3 is equal to 1.0 with Ea/Ees ranging between 0.6 and 1.2, and it is equal to 0 with a normal value of Ea/Ees; $h_0(t)$ is baseline risk of 0.024329 at the 24th week after STEMI. If the value of h is higher than 1.0, the development of ALVR is predicted; if the value of h is less than 1.0, a conclusion is made about the absence of ALVR.

The created model for determining the risk of developing the postinfarction remodeling has shown good informative results: the Wilks' lambda = 0.65256; $F_{(3,105)}$ = 18.63467 ($p < 0.00001$).

4. Discussion

The development of CHF post-MI is driven by the complex pathophysiological mechanisms underlying cardiac remodeling: an inflammatory reaction in the area of myocardial necrosis, isolation of intracellular signaling proteins, activation of neurohumoral systems, followed by the development of hypertrophy and cardiac dilatation, and the formation of a connective tissue scar.

The structural and functional remodeling of LV was followed by a decrease in its contractile function leading to impairment of hemodynamics in organs and tissues [15,16]. The adverse cardiac remodeling post-MI leads to CHF development, associated with increased re-hospitalization rate, disability, and mortality of patients [10,17]. The present study demonstrates that adverse postinfarction remodeling is associated with a high risk of cardiovascular events, being 8.5 times higher than that compared with non-ALVR group during the 48-week follow-up. Thus, the authors have developed a model for predicting various forms of cardiac remodeling to timely prescribe medication and conduct dynamic monitoring for patients with a high risk of an adverse outcome.

Traditional factors have little effect on prognosis after STEMI [18]. In our study, the patients who subsequently developed different types of postinfarction remodeling did not experience differences in most risk factors, except for WC. In this connection, a search for new predictors of unfavorable structural and functional cardiac remodeling seems to be highly relevant.

The high frequency of thrombolytic therapy as part of the pharma-coinvasive treatment strategy should be noted; this was present in 54.4% of cases, which is due to the late presentation of the patients and the territorial remoteness of the place of residence of the patients from the hospital.

In accordance with the clinical practice guidelines for CHF, the determination of natriuretic peptides is used in diagnosing this complication and in assessing the prognosis [2,19]. A high level of N-terminal pro-brain natriuretic peptide (NT-proBNP) indicates an increasing risk of sudden death, recurrent MI, and CHF in patients with MI and unstable angina [20]. The level of BNP was significantly higher in patients with ALVR as compared to non-ALVR group over the entire follow-up period. As a result, the indicator was included in both univariate and multivariate models for predicting adverse postinfarction cardiac remodeling.

The development and progression of cardiovascular diseases are associated with deterioration in the structural and functional properties of the vascular wall, being an important predictor of an adverse outcome, regardless of traditional factors [21]. According to Lechner I. et al., an enhanced level of pulse wave velocity (PWV) in STEMI patients predicted the development of cardiac and cerebrovascular adverse events 13 months after the index event. In another study, cfPWV appeared to be an important predictor of recovery of LV contractile function three and six months after STEMI [22].

An increased aortic stiffness causes impairment of the coronary blood flow and the development of ischemia of the subendocardial layer even without the coronary artery stenosis. Early return of the reflected pulse wave is accompanied by an increase in SBP and decrease in DBP. The LV load and myocardial oxygen demand increase, but perfusion pressure deteriorates, and myocardial ischemia develops due to lower DBP [23]. Besides, a decrease in the damping function of the aorta, combined with an increase in total peripheral vascular resistance, significantly reduces the efficiency of LV contraction [24].

In this study, the compared groups initially differed in the level of SBPao, and SBP and DBP in CCA. Loc Psys has only shown predictive value in the development of ALVR in univariate logistic regression analysis. However, the indicators of the structural and functional state of the aorta and CCA have not been included in the multivariate model.

The functioning of the cardiovascular system as a whole is determined by the adequacy of the interaction between the heart and the arterial system during the ejection of blood from the LV and is called LVAC [25]. The predictive significance of this parameter has been demonstrated in a number of studies. In particular, in patients with ischemic cardiomyopathy, the ratio Ea/Ees < 1.47 was characterized by better survival rate compared to those whose indicator exceeded the specified threshold value [12]. LVAC can be used both to clarify cardiovascular risk and to study the efficiency of treatment.

LVAC indicator is calculated as the ratio of arterial elastance (Ea) to LV end-systolic elastance (Ees). The Ea parameter indicates the arterial load exerted on LV during the blood ejection, regardless of its functional ability. Arterial afterload includes aortic valve resistance, systemic vascular resistance (SVR), arterial capacitance and stiffness, and duration of systole and diastole. The Ees parameter indicates LV contractility and systolic stiffness. In our study, a low level of Ees/BSA and higher LVAC values were initially diagnosed in the ALVR group. These differences have remained over the entire follow-up period. Besides, these indicators of LV-arterial interaction have evidenced predictive significance according to univariate regression analysis. The determination of the normal/abnormal LVAC level was adequate for inclusion in the mul tivariate model based on the studied parameters.

With the results obtained, a complex model for predicting ALVR in the period from the 7th to the 9th day of the STEMI was developed based on the analysis of WC, BNP, and LVAC.

5. Conclusions

In the present study, the development of adverse postinfarction LV remodeling is associated with an 8.5-fold increase in the risk of cardiovascular events. The following independent factors of adverse cardiac remodeling were determined 24 weeks after STEMI: waist circumference; abnormal values of brain natriuretic peptide; end-systolic left ventricular elastance normalized to body sur- face area; abnormal level of Ea/Ees index; local systolic pres sure in the common carotid arteries.

Based on the results of multivariate regression analysis, a model for predicting various types of postinfarction remodeling based on waist circumference, abnormal values of brain natriuretic peptide, and the LV arterial coupling index has been developed.

6. Study limitations

The study was conducted in patients with single-vessel lesion of the coronary bed according to coronary angiography: the presence of hemodynamically significant stenosis of only the infarct-related artery with occlusion of other coronary arteries less than 50%, including the trunk of the left coronary artery—less than 30%. Moreover, the proposed multivariate model was developed for patients with primary STEMI aged 35 to 65 years and is not applicable to patients with recurrent MI, as well as MI without ST segment elevation, younger or older than this age.

Supplementary Materials: The following supporting information can be downloaded at: https://www.mdpi.com/article/10.3390/diagnostics12030770/s1, Figure S1: Dynamics of indexed values of EDV and ESV in the comparison groups.

Author Contributions: Conceptualization, V.O. and L.S.; methodology, software O.K.; validation, V.O., L.S., O.K.; formal analysis, investigation, L.S., O.K.; resources, V.O.; data curation, L.S.; writing—original draft preparation, O.K.; writing—review and editing, L.S., N.B.; project administration, V.O.; funding acquisition, V.O. All authors have read and agreed to the published version of the manuscript.

Funding: The work was carried out with financial support: a grant from the President of the Russian Federation for the government support of the young Russian scientists—Candidates and Doctors of sciences.

Institutional Review Board Statement: The study was conducted according to the guidelines of the Declaration of Helsinki, and approved by the Local Ethics Committee of the Penza State University (protocol code 317 and date of approval—15 May 2020).

Informed Consent Statement: Informed consent was obtained from all subjects involved in the study.

Data Availability Statement: The data presented in this study are available on request from the corresponding author. The data are not publicly available due to ethical reasons.

Conflicts of Interest: The authors declare no conflict of interest.

References

1. Shlyakhto, E.V.; Zvartau, N.E.; Villevalde, S.V.; Yakovlev, A.N.; Solovyeva, A.E.; Fedorenko, A.A.; Karlina, V.A.; Avdonina, N.G.; Endubaeva, G.V.; Zaitsev, V.V.; et al. Assessment of prevalence and monitoring of outcomes in patients with heart failure in Russia. *Russ. J. Cardiol.* **2020**, *25*, 4204. [CrossRef]
2. McDonagh, T.A.; Metra, M.; Adamo, M.; Gardner, R.S.; Baumbach, A.; Böhm, M.; Burri, H.; Butler, J.; Čelutkienė, J.; Chioncel, O.; et al. 2021 ESC Guidelines for the diagnosis and treatment of acute and chronic heart failure. *Eur. Heart J.* **2021**, *42*, 3599–3726. [CrossRef] [PubMed]
3. Jones, N.R.; Roalfe, A.K.; Adoki, I.; Hobbs, F.D.R.; Taylor, C.J. Survival of patients with chronic heart failure in the community: A systematic review and meta-analysis. *Eur. J. Heart Fail.* **2019**, *21*, 1306–1325. [CrossRef] [PubMed]
4. Magnussen, C.; Niiranen, T.J.; Ojeda, F.M.; Gianfagna, F.; Blankenberg, S.; Vartiainen, E.; Sans, S.; Pasterkamp, G.; Hughes, M.; Costanzo, S.; et al. Sex-Specific Epidemiology of Heart Failure Risk and Mortality in Europe: Results from the BiomarCaRE Consortium. *JACC Heart Fail.* **2019**, *7*, 204–213. [CrossRef] [PubMed]
5. Savarese, G.; Lund, L.H. Global Public Health Burden of Heart Failure. *Card. Fail. Rev.* **2017**, *3*, 7–11. [CrossRef]
6. Polyakov, D.S.; Fomin, I.V.; Belenkov, Y.N.; Mareev, V.Y.; Ageev, F.T.; Artemjeva, E.G.; Badin, Y.V.; Bakulina, E.V.; Vinogradova, N.G.; Galyavich, A.S.; et al. Chronic heart failure in the Russian Federation: What has changed over 20 years of follow-up? Results of the EPOCH-CHF study. *Kardiologiia* **2021**, *61*, 4–14. [CrossRef]
7. Crespo-Leiro, M.G.; Anker, S.D.; Maggioni, A.P.; Coats, A.J.; Filippatos, G.; Ruschitzka, F.; Ferrari, R.; Piepoli, M.F.; Jimenez, J.F.D.; Metra, M.; et al. European Society of Cardiology Heart Failure Long-Term Registry (ESC-HF-LT): 1-year follow-up outcomes and differences across regions. *Eur. J. Heart Fail.* **2016**, *18*, 613–625. [CrossRef]
8. Shetye, A.; Nazir, S.A.; Squire, I.B.; McCann, G.P. Global myocardial strain assessment by different imaging modalities to predict outcomes after ST-elevation myocardial infarction: A systematic review. *World J. Cardiol.* **2015**, *7*, 948–960. [CrossRef]
9. Galli, A.; Lombardi, F. Postinfarct Left Ventricular Remodelling: A Prevailing Cause of Heart Failure. *Cardiol. Res. Pract.* **2016**, *2016*, 1–12. [CrossRef]
10. Van der Bijl, P.; Abou, R.; Goedemans, L.; Gersh, B.J.; Holmes, D.R.; Marsan, N.A.; Delgado, V.; Bax, J.J. Left Ventricular Post-Infarct Remodeling: Implications for Systolic Function Im-provement and Outcomes in the Modern Era. *JACC Heart Fail.* **2020**, *8*, 131–140. [CrossRef]

11. Ibanez, B.; James, S.; Agewall, S.; Antunes, M.J.; Bucciarelli-Ducci, C.; Bueno, H.; Caforio, A.L.P.; Crea, F.; Goudevenos, J.A.; Halvorsen, S.; et al. 2017 ESC Guidelines for the management of acute myocardial infarction in patients presenting with ST-segment elevation: The Task Force for the management of acute myocardial infarction in patients presenting with ST-segment elevation of the European Society of Cardiology (ESC). *Eur. Heart J.* **2018**, *39*, 119–177. [CrossRef] [PubMed]
12. Ikonomidis, I.; Aboyans, V.; Blacher, J.; Brodmann, M.; Brutsaert, D.L.; Chirinos, J.A.; De Carlo, M.; Delgado, V.; Lancellotti, P.; Lekakis, J.; et al. The role of ventricular–arterial coupling in cardiac disease and heart failure: Assessment, clinical implications and therapeutic interventions. A consensus document of the European Society of Cardiology Working Group on Aorta & Peripheral Vascular Diseases, European Association of Cardiovascular Imaging, and Heart Failure Association. *Eur. J. Heart Fail.* **2019**, *21*, 402–424. [CrossRef] [PubMed]
13. Oleynikov, V.E.; Salyamova, L.I.; Burko, N.V.; Khromova, A.A.; Krivonogov, L.Y.; Melnikova, E.A. Ultrasound Evaluation of the Great Arteries Based on the Analysis of Radio-Frequency Signal. *Biomed. Eng.* **2017**, *50*, 352–356. [CrossRef]
14. Kobalava, Z.D.; Konradi, A.O.; Nedogoda, S.V.; Shlyakhto, E.V.; Arutyunov, G.P.; Baranova, E.I.; Barbarash, O.L.; Boitsov, S.A.; Vavilova, T.V.; Villevalde, S.; et al. Arterial hypertension in adults. Clinical guidelines 2020. *Russ. J. Cardiol.* **2020**, *25*, 149–218. [CrossRef]
15. Bhatt, A.S.; Ambrosy, A.P.; Velazquez, E.J. Adverse Remodeling and Reverse Remodeling After Myocardial Infarction. *Curr. Cardiol. Rep.* **2017**, *19*, 71. [CrossRef] [PubMed]
16. Ferrari, R.; Malagù, M.; Biscaglia, S.; Fucili, A.; Rizzo, P. Remodelling after an Infarct: Crosstalk between Life and Death. *Cardiology* **2016**, *135*, 68–76. [CrossRef]
17. Roger, V.L. Epidemiology of Heart Failure: A Contemporary Perspective. *Circ. Res.* **2021**, *128*, 1421–1434. [CrossRef]
18. Lustosa, R.P.; van der Bijl, P.; El Mahdiui, M.; Montero-Cabezas, J.M.; Kostyukevich, M.V.; Marsan, N.A.; Bax, J.J.; Delgado, V. Noninvasive Myocardial Work Indices 3 Months after ST-Segment Elevation Myocardial Infarction: Prevalence and Characteristics of Patients with Postinfarction Cardiac Remodeling. *J. Am. Soc. Echocardiogr.* **2020**, *33*, 1172–1179. [CrossRef]
19. Russian Society of Cardiology (RSC). 2020 Clinical practice guidelines for Chronic heart failure. *Russ. J. Cardiol.* **2020**, *25*, 4083. [CrossRef]
20. Zagidullin, N.; Motloch, L.J.; Gareeva, D.; Hamitova, A.; Lakman, I.; Krioni, I.; Popov, D.; Zulkarneev, R.; Paar, V.; Kopp, K.; et al. Combining Novel Biomarkers for Risk Stratification of Two-Year Cardiovascular Mortality in Patients with ST-Elevation Myocardial Infarction. *J. Clin. Med.* **2020**, *9*, 550. [CrossRef]
21. Bonarjee, V.V.S. Arterial Stiffness: A Prognostic Marker in Coronary Heart Disease. Available Methods and Clinical Application. *Front. Cardiovasc. Med.* **2018**, *5*, 64. [CrossRef] [PubMed]
22. Imbalzano, E.; Vatrano, M.; Mandraffino, G.; Ghiadoni, L.; Gangemi, S.; Bruno, R.M.; Ciconte, V.A.; Paunovic, N.; Costantino, R.; Mormina, E.; et al. Arterial stiffness as a predictor of recovery of left ventricular systolic function after acute myocardial infarction treated with primary percutaneous coronary intervention. *Int. J. Cardiovasc. Imaging* **2015**, *31*, 1545–1551. [CrossRef] [PubMed]
23. Lønnebakken, M.T.; Eskerud, I.; Larsen, T.H.; Midtbø, H.B.; Kokorina, M.V.; Gerdts, E. Impact of aortic stiffness on myocardial ischaemia in non-obstructive coronary artery disease. *Open Heart* **2019**, *6*, e000981. [CrossRef] [PubMed]
24. Bell, V.; McCabe, E.L.; Larson, M.G.; Rong, J.; Merz, A.; Osypiuk, E.; Lehman, B.T.; Stantchev, P.; Aragam, J.; Benjamin, E.J.; et al. Relations Between Aortic Stiffness and Left Ventricular Mechanical Function in the Community. *J. Am. Heart Assoc.* **2017**, *6*, 004903. [CrossRef] [PubMed]
25. Chirinos, J.A. Ventricular–arterial coupling: Invasive and non-invasive assessment. *Artery Res.* **2013**, *7*, 2–14. [CrossRef]

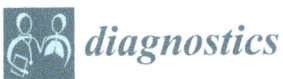

Article

Association of Non-Alcoholic Fatty Liver Disease and Hepatic Fibrosis with Epicardial Adipose Tissue Volume and Atrial Deformation Mechanics in a Large Asian Population Free from Clinical Heart Failure

Yau-Huei Lai [1,2,3], Cheng-Huang Su [1,3,4], Ta-Chuan Hung [1,3,4], Chun-Ho Yun [1,3,5,*,†], Cheng-Ting Tsai [1,3,4,*,†], Hung-I Yeh [1,3,4] and Chung-Lieh Hung [1,3,4]

1. Department of Medicine, Mackay Medical College, New Taipei City 25245, Taiwan; garak1109@mmh.org.tw (Y.-H.L.); chsu007@gmail.com (C.-H.S.); hung0787@ms67.hinet.net (T.-C.H.); hiyeh@mmh.org.tw (H.-I.Y.); jotaro3791@gmail.com (C.-L.H.)
2. Division of Cardiology, Department of Internal Medicine, Hsinchu MacKay Memorial Hospital, Hsinchu City 30071, Taiwan
3. MacKay Junior College of Medicine, Nursing, and Management, Taipei City 11260, Taiwan
4. Division of Cardiology, Department of Internal Medicine, MacKay Memorial Hospital, Zhongshan North Road, Taipei City 10449, Taiwan
5. Department of Radiology, MacKay Memorial Hospital, Zhongshan North Road, Taipei City 10449, Taiwan
* Correspondence: med202657@gmail.com (C.-H.Y.); chengtingtsai@gmail.com (C.-T.T.); Tel.: +886-2-2543-3535 (C.-H.Y. & C.-T.T.); Fax: +886-2-2543-3642 (C.-H.Y. & C.-T.T.)
† These authors contribute equally to this work.

Abstract: Non-alcoholic fatty liver disease (NAFLD) and cardiovascular disease share several cardiometabolic risk factors. Excessive visceral fat can manifest as ectopic fat depots over vital organs, such as the heart and liver. This study assessed the associations of NAFLD and liver fibrosis with cardiac structural and functional disturbances. We assessed 2161 participants using ultrasound, and categorized them as per the NAFLD Fibrosis Score into three groups: (1) non-fatty liver; (2) fatty liver with low fibrosis score; and (3) fatty liver with high fibrosis score. Epicardial fat volume (EFV) was measured through multidetector computed tomography. All participants underwent echocardiographic study, including tissue Doppler-based E/e' ratio and speckle tracking-based left ventricular global longitudinal strain, peak atrial longitudinal strain (PALS), and atrial longitudinal strain rates during systolic, early and late-diastolic phases ($ALSR_{syst}$, $ALSR_{early}$. $ALSR_{late}$). Larger EFV, decreased e' velocity, PALS, $ALSR_{syst}$, and $ALSR_{early}$, along with elevated E/e' ratio, were seen in all groups, especially in those with high fibrosis scores. After multivariate adjustment for traditional risk factors and EFV, fibrosis scores remained significantly associated with elevated E/e' ratio, LA stiffness, and decreased PALS (β: 0.06, 1.4, −0.01, all $p < 0.05$). Thus, NAFLD is associated with LV diastolic dysfunction and subclinical changes in LA contractile mechanics.

Keywords: fatty liver; cardiovascular disease; fibrosis; epicardial fat; left atrial strain

1. Introduction

Obesity and metabolic disorders have long been recognized as global health issues. Non-alcoholic fatty liver disease (NAFLD), also known as metabolic-associated fatty liver disease (MAFLD) [1,2], is one of the most widespread forms of chronic liver disease. It represents a spectrum of conditions ranging from simple steatosis to non-alcoholic steatohepatitis, which can progress to various grades of fibrosis, cirrhosis, and hepatocellular carcinoma [3,4]. NAFLD has also been identified as a precipitating factor for early subclinical cardiac disorders since it shares several cardiometabolic risk factors with cardiovascular disease (CVD) [5]. Numerous studies have evaluated the pathological mechanisms connecting these two entities [6,7]. For example, NAFLD has been shown to induce hepatic insulin resistance and atherogenic dyslipidemia [8], which makes the affected individuals susceptible to premature atherosclerosis.

Excessive visceral fat can accumulate at various body sites besides the liver, most notably presenting as epicardial fat. As a biologically active source of pro-atherogenic cytokines that mediate systemic vascular inflammation and metabolic derangements [9], epicardial fat has been shown to influence left ventricular (LV) structure and function through mechanical or paracrine effects [10]. The term "cardiac steatosis" has been used to describe the exaggerated lipid deposition and elevated oxidative stress that up-regulates myocardial fibrosis and cellular apoptosis, leading to cardiomyopathy [11,12]. The release of a variety of pro-inflammatory and pro-fibrogenic mediators in this condition may play important roles in the pathophysiology of cardiac and arrhythmic complications. Furthermore, the surrounding ectopic fat depots may mechanistically impede diastolic filling due to the physical constraints on the epicardium [13].

Previous studies utilizing strain imaging have shown both cross-sectional and longitudinal association of NAFLD with subclinical myocardial remodeling and diastolic dysfunction [14,15]. It has been hypothesized that these changes may be mediated by the interaction between epicardial fat and cardiac structures. A few small histological studies have demonstrated a graded relationship between LV systolic dysfunction, epicardial fat thickness, and liver fibrosis severity in NAFLD, suggesting that systemic inflammation may also contribute to the development and progression of myocardial dysfunction [16,17]. Due to the cost of biopsy and procedural risks, alternative noninvasive tools have been developed to predict the fibrosis stage, including the NAFLD Fibrosis Score [18], which we employed in this study.

Whether or not NAFLD is an independent risk factor for cardiovascular mortality and other cardiovascular events has been studied, but remains controversial [19,20]. Relatively little is known about the underlying pathophysiological mechanisms behind the cardiac remodeling process in Asians with NAFLD. Therefore, we aim to investigate the potential impact of fatty liver and epicardial fat on various aspects of diastolic function and myocardial deformation mechanics in a large Asian population with normal LV ejection fraction, and who free from clinical heart failure (HF).

2. Materials and Methods

2.1. Study Population

We retrospectively examined individuals who participated in an ongoing cardiovascular health screening program between June 2009 and January 2013 at a tertiary medical center in Taipei, Taiwan. The original study setting and design have been published previously [21]. The baseline clinical information, medical history, symptoms/signs, and lifestyle patterns were obtained. Informed consent was waived for each participant owing to the retrospective study design. This study conformed to the principles outlined in the Declaration of Helsinki, and was approved by the local ethical board committee (18MMHIS180e, 8 January 2019). Subjects with a history of chronic viral hepatitis, liver cirrhosis, heavy alcohol consumption, any prevalent clinical HF, CVD (defined as a history of previous myocardial infarction, symptom-driven angioplasty, peripheral arterial disease, or cerebrovascular disease), and significant valvular diseases or cardiac arrhythmias were excluded from the analysis. Those with a high fibrosis risk score but diagnosed as non-fatty liver by abdominal ultrasound were also excluded, since it is unlikely for them to have liver fibrosis. (Figure 1).

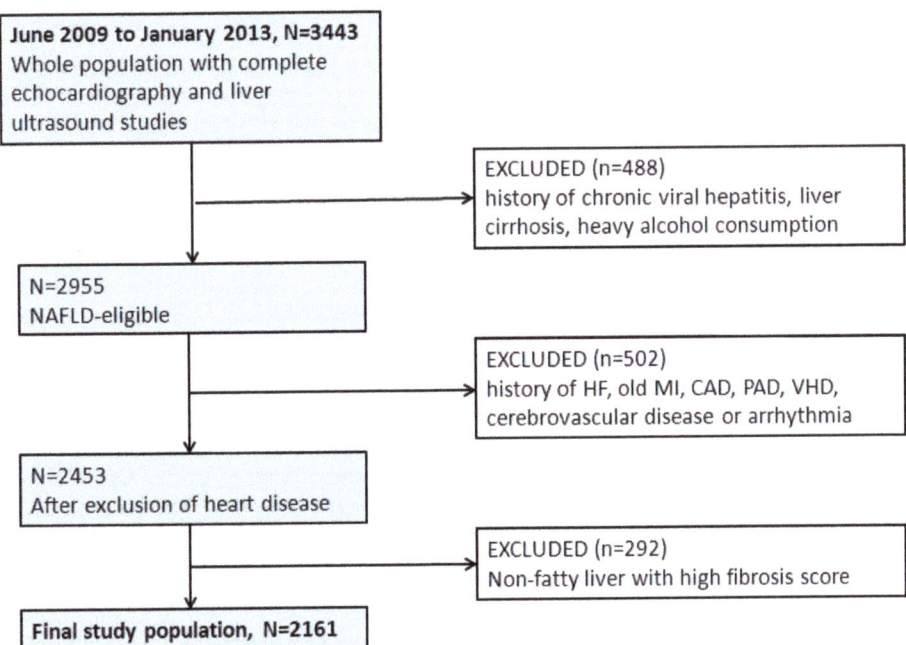

Figure 1. Study design and exclusion flowchart. Abbreviations: HF = heart failure, MI = myocardial infarction, CAD = coronary artery disease, PAD = peripheral artery disease, VHD = valvular heart disease.

2.2. Laboratory Data and Body Fat Assessment

All biochemical and laboratory parameters, including homeostatic model assessment for insulin resistance (HOMA-IR) and high-sensitivity C-reactive protein (Hs-CRP), were measured at a standardized central laboratory using a Hitachi 7170 Automatic Analyzer (Hitachi Corp., Hitachinaka, Ibaraki, Japan). Body fat composition was calculated by foot-to-foot bioelectrical impedance-based analysis (Tanita-305 Body-Fat Analyzer; Tanita Corp, Tokyo, Japan), which estimated the total body fat percentage.

2.3. Assessment of Fatty Liver and Fibrosis Score

Abdominal sonography was performed with a Toshiba Nemio SSA-550A instrument (Toshiba, Tochigi-ken, Japan) by hepatology specialists who were completely blinded to other laboratory results. The degree of fatty liver was graded semi-quantitatively according to the level of echoes arising from the hepatic parenchyma [22]. Since interpretation of fatty liver by abdominal ultrasound can be subjective, we defined subjects with at least moderate-degree fatty liver disease as significant NAFLD. By applying the low cut-off value (−1.455) of the NAFLD Fibrosis Score [18] (calculated as [−1.675 + 0.037 × age (years) + 0.094 × BMI (kg/m^2) + 1.13 × hyperglycemia/diabetes mellitus (yes = 1, no = 0) + 0.95 × AST (U/L) to ALT (U/L) ratio − 0.013 × platelet count (10^{-9}/L) − 0.66 × albumin (g/dL)]), the study population was categorized into three groups: (1) non-fatty liver; (2) NAFLD with low fibrosis score; and (3) NAFLD with high fibrosis score. APRI and FIB-4 scores were also calculated for comparison [23].

2.4. Assessment of Epicardial Fat

Multidetector computed tomography study was performed using a 16-slice scanner (Sensation 16, Siemens Medical Solutions, Forchheim, Germany) with 16 mm × 0.75 mm collimation, rotation time of 420 ms, and tube voltage of 120 kV. In one breath-hold, images were acquired from a level above the tracheal bifurcation to below the base of the heart, using prospective ECG-triggering at 70% of the R-R interval. From the raw data, the images were reconstructed with a standard kernel in 3-mm thick axial, non-overlapping slices, and a 25-cm field of view. Epicardial fat volume (EFV) was measured offline on a single workstation (Aquarius iNtuition Cloud, TeraRecon, SanMateo, CA, USA), using methods validated in previous studies [24].

2.5. Conventional Echocardiography and Diastolic Function Indices

Each participant underwent an extensive two-dimensional (2D) and tissue Doppler echocardiography with strain analysis. All assessments were performed by a single experienced sonographer blinded to the participants' clinical information, using a commercially available ultrasound system equipped with a 2–4 MHz multifrequency transducer (Vivid 7; GE Medical System, Vingmed, Norway), in adherence with the American Society of Echocardiography guidelines [25]. Using the modified biplane Simpson's method, the maximum values of left atrial volume (LAV) were presented in this study. All measurements were the average value derived from three consecutive cardiac cycles. Diastolic functional indices were assessed using transmitral pulsed-wave Doppler and tissue Doppler-derived mitral annular velocities. Systolic and early diastolic velocities (LV s' and LV e') were averaged from the basal septal and lateral LV segments at the mitral annulus level.

2.6. Two-Dimensional Speckle-Tracking Analysis Protocol

Speckle-tracking analysis was performed offline using 2D cardiac performance software (EchoPAC version 10.8; GE Vingmed Ultrasound, Norway). Semi-automated tracing of endocardial borders was performed at the end-diastolic frame, with minor manual adjustments to ensure optimal delineation. The LV global longitudinal strain (GLS) was calculated as the average peak global values derived from three LV apical planes of the 4-chamber, the 2-chamber, and long-axis views, as described in our previous published work [25]. Peak atrial longitudinal strain (PALS) and triphasic LA strain rates [systolic, early, and late diastolic atrial longitudinal strain rate ($ALSR_{syst}$, $ALSR_{early}$, and $ALSR_{late}$, respectively)] were determined as the average values obtained from both apical 2- and 4-chamber views. The endocardial border of the LA was traced manually so that the LA appendage and pulmonary veins were excluded. LA stiffness (LA_{stiff}) was derived from dividing E/e' by PALS. To avoid confusion regarding the directionality of strain changes, the absolute values of GLS, $ALSR_{early}$, and $ALSR_{late}$ were reported. The inter-and intra-observer analysis of the LA and LV strain/strain rate components in our lab was reported in our previous work [21].

2.7. Statistical Analysis

Data were presented as mean (standard deviation) for continuous variables, and as proportions for categorical variables. One-way ANOVA was used to assess differences of anthropometric, metabolic, and echocardiography parameters between groups with post hoc paired comparisons using the Bonferroni correction. Fisher's exact test was used to test differences between categorical data. Multiple linear regression models were used to assess the independent association of EFV and NAFLD Fibrosis Score with diastolic function and deformation parameters. For EFV, clinical covariates (age, sex, BMI, blood pressure, and clinical risk factors) were sequentially entered into the models. Since age and BMI are components of the NAFLD Fibrosis Score, they were omitted from the multivariate models for its analysis, while ALT was added into them. Statistical analyses were performed using the STATA statistical software package (Version 14. Stata Corp. College Station, Texas). A two-sided *p*-value of less than 0.05 was considered statistically significant.

3. Results

3.1. Baseline Demographics, Adiposity Measures, and Metabolic Profiles

Among the 2161 eligible study participants (mean age: 48.3 ± 9.9 years, 36.5% female), progressive epicardial fat burden, central obesity, stepwise increases in HbA1c, HOMA-IR, GOT, and decreases in platelet count were observed across all three groups (all $p < 0.05$). Both fatty liver groups shared similarly unfavorable lipid profiles and elevated Hs-CRP compared to the normal group. Patients with high fibrosis scores were also older and more likely to have hypertension, diabetes, and hyperlipidemia (Table 1). After excluding the youngest quartile from the normal group, differences in adiposity measures and biomarkers remained mostly unchanged (Supplementary Table S1).

Table 1. Baseline demographics, adiposity measures and biomarkers.

	Non-Fatty Liver	NAFLD, Low Fibrosis Score (<−1.455)	NAFLD, High Fibrosis Score (≥−1.455)	P_{trend}
	N = 1019	N = 840	N = 302	
Age, years	46.32(9.96)	47.69(9.1) *	56.37(8.34) *†	<0.001
Female sex, %	502 (49.3%)	211 (25.1%) *	76 (25.2%) *	<0.001
NAFLD Fibrosis score	−2.76(0.79)	−2.67(0.79) *	−0.82(0.54) *†	<0.001
FIB-4 score	0.86(0.34)	0.93(0.29) *	1.35(0.48) *†	<0.001
APRI score	0.23(0.15)	0.37(0.26) *	0.42(0.28) *†	<0.001
SBP, mmHg	116.93(15.14)	123.86(16.42) *	129.21(16.03) *†	<0.001
DBP, mmHg	72.76(10.22)	78.04(10.21) *	80.45(10.06) *†	<0.001
Adiposity measures				
EFV, ml	65.02(25.5)	79.73(26.25) *	95.13(31.67) *†	<0.001
BMI, kg/m^2	22.26(2.58)	25.69(3.17) *	27.21(3.53) *†	<0.001
WC, cm	77.86(7.9)	87.29(8.24) *	91.06(9.46) *†	<0.001
Body fat, %	23.84(6.26)	27.42(7.38) *	28.9(7.61) *†	<0.001
Biomarkers				
Fasting glucose, mg/dl	93.53(10.59)	100.15(18.17) *	118.17(32.1) *†	<0.001
HbA1c, %	5.54(0.44)	5.74(0.66) *	6.32(1.18) *†	<0.001
Fasting insulin, U/L	6.62(3.61)	10.01(6.16) *	10.86(5.81) *	<0.001
HOMA-IR	1.53(0.94)	2.5(1.78) *	3.23(2.05) *†	<0.001
Hs-CRP, mg/L	1.61(4.36)	2.42(4.16) *	2.67(3.73) *	0.001
Platelet, 10^9/L	257.15(46.67)	243.96(48.03) *	207.87(32.99) *†	<0.001
PT-INR	1.04(0.04)	1.03(0.05) *	1.04(0.05)	0.03
GOT, IU/L	21.21(7.46)	26.11(11.3) *	28.1(14.57) *†	<0.001
GPT, IU/L	21.41(12.29)	36.42(24.24) *	34.44(21.94) *	<0.001
GGT, IU/L	20.55(18.49)	34.28(40.76) *	35.79(48.43) *	<0.001
Bil(d), mg/dL	0.21(0.07)	0.2(0.07)	0.22(0.08)	0.06
Bil(t), mg/dL	0.78(0.34)	0.81(0.36)	0.83(0.37)	0.06
Albumin, g/dL	4.52(0.25)	4.59(0.24) *	4.46(0.24) *†	<0.001
TC, mg/dL	200.91(36.12)	211.29(36.5) *	207.02(35.7) *	<0.001
TG, mg/dL	106.33(78.63)	167.19(95.16) *	170.79(111.15) *	<0.001

Table 1. Cont.

	Non-Fatty Liver	NAFLD, Low Fibrosis Score (<−1.455)	NAFLD, High Fibrosis Score (≥−1.455)	P_{trend}
	N = 1019	N = 840	N = 302	
LDL-C, mg/dL	127.15(33.83)	140.58(33.38) *	136.89(31.84) *	<0.001
HDL-C, mg/dL	60.64(15.49)	48.77(12.45) *	47.96(11.41) *	<0.001
eGFR, mL/min/m^2	91.78(16.6)	89.3(15.2) *	85.39(16.84) *†	0.001
Comorbidities				
Hypertension, %	82 (8%)	149 (17.7%) *	93 (30.8%) *†	<0.001
Diabetes, %	17 (1.7%)	65 (7.7%)	77 (25.5%) *†	<0.001
Hyperlipidemia, %	43 (4.2%)	64 (7.6%)	36 (11.9%) *	<0.001

Data presented as mean (SD). *p*-value < 0.05 for comparisons against * Non-fatty liver, † Fatty liver with low fibrosis score, Abbreviations: SBP = systolic blood pressure, DBP = diastolic blood pressure, EFV = epicardial fat volume, BMI = body mass index, WC = waist circumference, HOMA-IR = homeostasis model assessment-insulin resistance, Hs-CRP = high-sensitivity C-reactive protein, PT-INR = prothrombin time-international normalized ratio, GOT = glutamic oxaloacetic transaminase, GPT = glutamate pyruvate transaminase, GGT = gamma-glutamyl transferase, Bil (d) = direct bilirubin, Bil (t) = total bilirubin, TC = total cholesterol, TG = triglyceride, LDL-C = low-density lipoprotein cholesterol, HDL-C = high-density lipoprotein cholesterol, eGFR = estimated glomerular filtration rate.

3.2. Cardiac Structures, Diastolic Function and Strain Indices

Increasing LV wall thickness, LA and LV volumes, and LV mass (with and without indexation) was observed across all three groups (all $p < 0.05$). Progressive worsening diastolic function with graded reductions in LV e' and elevated E/e' ratio was also present (all $p < 0.05$). Most notably, stepwise reductions in PALS, ALSR$_{syst}$, and ALSR$_{early}$ across all three groups were observed (all $p < 0.05$). Compared to the normal group, both fatty liver groups had similar decreases in LV GLS (Table 2). After excluding the youngest quartile from the normal group, differences in LV geometry, LV e', PALS, ALSR$_{syst}$, ALSR$_{early}$, and LA stiffness remained significant (Supplementary Table S2).

Table 2. Echocardiographic parameters.

	Non-Fatty Liver	NAFLD, Low Fibrosis Score (<−1.455)	NAFLD, High Fibrosis Score (≥−1.455)	P_{trend}
	N = 1019	N = 840	N = 302	
LVST, mm	8.6(1.03)	9.14(0.96) *	9.54(1.02) *†	<0.001
LVPT, mm	8.6(0.94)	9.13(0.88) *	9.48(0.95) *†	<0.001
RWT	0.38(0.04)	0.39(0.04) *	0.4(0.04) *†	<0.001
LVEDV, mL	72.44(13.36)	77.26(12.48) *	80.75(11.04) *†	<0.001
LVEF, %	62.79(5.05)	62.16(5.2) *	62.34(5.08)	0.03
LVM, gm	129.66(29.83)	146.4(27.82) *	159.65(30.33) *†	<0.001
LVMi(BSA), gm/m^2	72.32(13.73)	74.89(12.56) *	80.42(13.79) *†	<0.001
LVMi, gm/m$^{2.7}$	33.66(7.13)	36.86(7.11) *	41.08(7.94) *†	<0.001
LAV, mL	26.69(8.92)	31.44(11.22) *	35.63(12.48) *†	<0.001
LAEF, %	58.9(10.59)	57.72(10.73)	56.94(10.48) *	0.006
Diastolic function				
DT, ms	196.21(37.2)	201.19(35.32) *	214.5(40.65) *†	0.001
IVRT, ms	87.76(13.49)	89.87(13.64) *	94.03(18.93) *†	<0.001

Table 2. Cont.

	Non-Fatty Liver	NAFLD, Low Fibrosis Score (<−1.455)	NAFLD, High Fibrosis Score (≥−1.455)	P$_{trend}$
	N = 1019	N = 840	N = 302	
E/A	1.4(0.49)	1.19(0.37) *	1.04(0.36) *†	<0.001
LV e′, cm/sec	10.27(2.39)	9.11(2.04) *	7.85(1.88) *†	<0.001
LV s′, cm/sec	8.49(1.52)	8.32(2.07)	7.98(1.45) *†	<0.001
E/e′	6.71(2.21)	7.11(2.43) *	8.08(3.05) *†	<0.001
	Strain indices			
LV GLS, %	20.85(1.91)	19.78(1.6) *	19.53(1.71) *	<0.001
PALS, %	40.23(7.39)	36.96(7.77) *	34.05(8.01) *†	<0.001
ALSR$_{syst}$	1.78(0.38)	1.66(0.36) *	1.52(0.35) *†	<0.001
ALSR$_{early}$	2(0.54)	1.66(0.49) *	1.35(0.45) *†	<0.001
ALSR$_{late}$	2(0.49)	2.07(0.5) *	2.05(0.49)	0.006
LA$_{stiff}$	0.17(0.08)	0.2(0.09) *	0.26(0.15) *†	<0.001

Data presented as mean (SD). *p*-value < 0.05 for comparisons against * Non-fatty liver, † Fatty liver with low fibrosis score. Abbreviations: LVST = left ventricular septal wall thickness, LVPT = left ventricular posterior wall thickness, RWT = relative wall thickness, LVEDV = left ventricular end-diastolic volume, LVM = left ventricular mass, LVMi = left ventricular mass index, LAV = left atrial volume, LAEF = left atrial emptying fraction, DT = deceleration time, IVRT = isovolumetric relaxation time, E/A = early-to-late diastolic mitral inflow velocity ratio, e′ = early-diastolic tissue Doppler velocity, s′ = systolic tissue Doppler velocity, GLS= global longitudinal strain, PALS = peak atrial longitudinal strain, ALSRsyst = atrial longitudinal strain rate-systolic phase, ALSRearly = atrial longitudinal strain rate-early diastolic phase, ALSRlate = atrial longitudinal strain rate-late diastolic phase, LAstiff = LA stiffness.

Box plots of EFV, PALS and LV GLS are further illustrated in Figures 2 and 3.

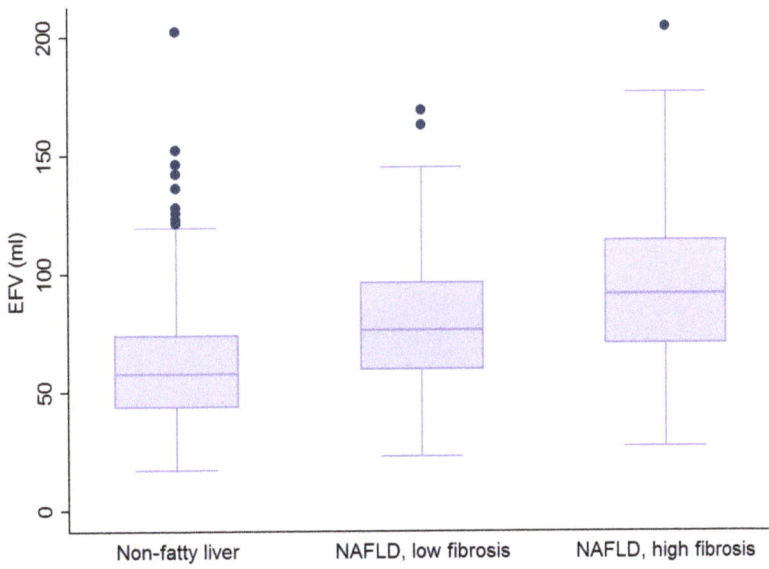

Figure 2. Box plots of epicardial fat volume (EFV). Graded increases in EFV were observed across all three groups (all *p* < 0.05).

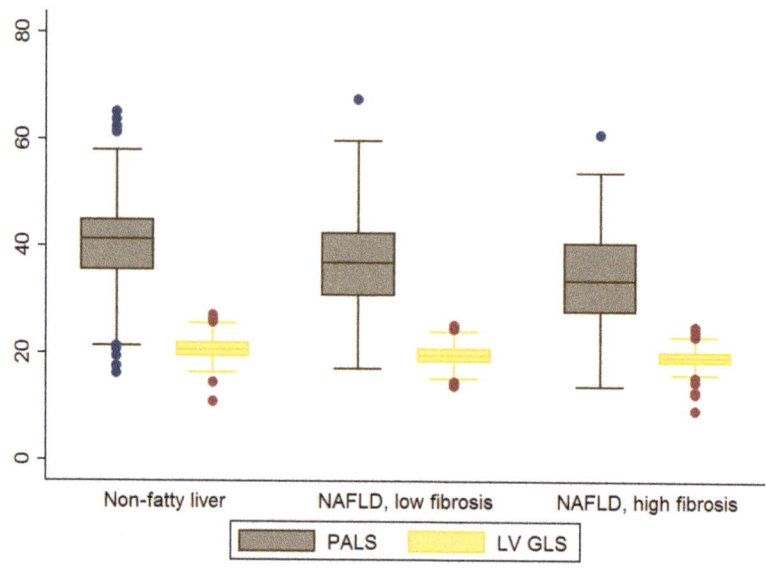

Figure 3. Box plots of LA and LV strain. Graded decreases in LA strain were observed across all three groups (all $p < 0.05$). Abbreviations: GLS= global longitudinal strain, PALS = peak atrial longitudinal strain.

Following multivariate adjustment, EFV remained strongly associated with elevated E/e' ratio, and LA$_{stiff}$ (β: 4.06, 41,14, both $p < 0.05$) and decreased LV e', PALS, ALSR$_{syst}$, and ALSR$_{early}$ (β: −7.62, −2.48, −42.14, −31.94, all $p < 0.05$) (Table 3).

Table 3. Multiple linear regression analysis for association of EFV with diastolic function and deformation parameters.

	Pearson r	Univariate Model β [95% CI]	p	Multivariate Model 1 β [95% CI]	p	Multivariate Model 2 β [95% CI]	p
LAV	0.22	0.76 [0.57, 0.95]	<0.001	0.18 [0.01, 0.36]	0.04	0.7 [−0.67, 2.07]	0.3
LVM	0.33	0.32 [0.25, 0.38]	<0.001	0.06 [−0.01, 0.14]	0.08	0.11 [−0.32, 0.55]	0.59
LV e'	−0.35	−4.75 [−5.66, −3.83]	<0.001	−1.33 [−2.36, −0.29]	0.01	−7.62 [−14.91, −0.32]	0.04
E/e'	0.19	2.23 [1.38, 3.07]	<0.001	0.71 [−0.07, 1.48]	0.08	4.06 [0.17, 7.95]	0.04
LV GLS	−0.27	−4.2 [−5.28, −3.12]	<0.001	−1.14 [−2.15, −0.13]	0.03	0.8 [−6.87, 8.48]	0.83
PALS	−0.34	−1.26 [−1.52, −1.01]	<0.001	−0.54 [−0.78, −0.3]	<0.001	−2.48 [−4.41, −0.55]	0.01
ALSR$_{syst}$	−0.26	−19.51 [−24.8, −14.22]	<0.001	−8.57 [−13.31, −3.84]	<0.001	−42.14 [−68, −16.28]	0.002
ALSR$_{early}$	−0.42	−23.37 [−26.97, −19.78]	<0.001	−8.05 [−12.38, −3.72]	<0.001	−31.94 [−58.13, −5.75]	0.02
LA$_{stiff}$	0.33	102.47 [79.11, 125.83]	<0.001	41.51 [18.99, 64.04]	<0.001	41.14 [18.24, 64.05]	<0.001

Multivariate model 1: adjusted by age, sex, BMI; Multivariate Model 2: Model 1 + systolic blood pressure, total cholesterol, high-density lipoprotein, glomerular filtration rate, history of hypertension, diabetes, hyperlipidemia, and smoking.

After similar adjustments, NAFLD Fibrosis Scores were weakly associated with EFV, yet still statistically significant (β: 0.01, $p < 0.001$). After further correction for EFV, the fibrosis score remained significantly associated with elevated E/e' ratio, LA$_{stiff}$ (β: 0.06, 1.4, both $p < 0.001$) and decreased LV e', PALS, ALSR$_{syst}$, and ALSR$_{early}$ (β: −0.1, −0.01, −0.26, −0.4, all $p < 0.05$) (Table 4).

Table 4. Multiple linear regression analysis for association of NAFLD Fibrosis Score with EFV, diastolic function, and deformation parameters *.

	Pearson r	Univariate Model		Multivariate Model 1		Multivariate Model 2	
		β [95% CI]	p	β [95% CI]	p	β [95% CI]	p
EFV	0.31	0.012 [0.01, 0.014]	<0.001	0.01 [0.007, 0.011]	<0.001	-	-
LAV	0.22	0.02 [0.017, 0.025]	<0.001	0.013 [0.01, 0.017]	<0.001	0.002 [−0.005, 0.01]	0.57
LVM	0.26	0.009 [0.007, 0.01]	<0.001	0.006 [0.004, 0.01]	<0.001	0.004 [0.001, 0.006]	0.002
LV e'	−0.42	−0.18 [−0.19, −0.16]	<0.001	−0.14 [−0.15, −0.12]	<0.001	−0.1 [−0.13, −0.06]	<0.001
E/e'	0.24	0.11 [0.1, 0.13]	<0.001	0.08 [0.06, 0.1]	<0.001	0.06 [0.02, 0.09]	<0.001
LV GLS	−0.14	−0.08 [−0.1, −0.05]	<0.001	−0.02 [−0.04, 0.003]	0.095	−0.01 [−0.05, 0.03]	0.64
PALS	−0.29	−0.036 [−0.03, −0.04]	<0.001	−0.025 [−0.03, −0.02]	<0.001	−0.01 [−0.02, −0.001]	0.02
ALSR$_{syst}$	−0.25	−0.65 [−0.76, −0.55]	<0.001	−0.5 [−0.6, −0.4]	<0.001	−0.26 [−0.44, −0.07]	0.006
ALSR$_{early}$	−0.44	−0.79 [−0.86, −0.72]	<0.001	−0.65 [−0.72, −0.55]	<0.001	−0.4 [−0.55, −0.25]	<0.001
LA$_{stiff}$	0.33	3.34 [2.92, 3.76]	<0.001	2.39 [1.97, 2.81]	<0.001	1.4 [0.63, 2.17]	<0.001

Multivariate model 1: adjusted by sex, systolic blood pressure, ALT, total cholesterol, high-density lipoprotein, glomerular filtration rate, history of hypertension, diabetes, hyperlipidemia, and smoking; Multivariate Model 2: Model 1 + EFV; * Since age and BMI are components of the NAFLD Fibrosis Score, they are not added to the models.

4. Discussion

In a large Asian population free from clinical HF and CVD, we demonstrated that NAFLD was associated with epicardial fat burden, systemic inflammation, insulin resistance, subclinical cardiac remodeling, diastolic dysfunction, and attenuated myocardial deformation. Moreover, diastolic function and most LA strain indices remained inversely correlated with NAFLD Fibrosis Score after correction for metabolic confounders and EFV.

Recently, the large population-based prospective CARDIA Study showed that NAFLD is longitudinally associated with subclinical LV remodeling, abnormal geometry, and impaired LV longitudinal strain after a five-year follow-up [15]. Several small studies have shown that NAFLD is associated with decreased LA strain indices [26,27]. There is a plethora of evidence that supports the adverse effects of NAFLD on diastolic function [28–30]. Although the pathogenesis of cardiac dysfunction in NAFLD is still unclear, insulin resistance, abnormal lipid metabolism, and systemic inflammation have been contributing factors. The cellular influx of free fatty acids may lead to myocardial lipid deposition, with consequent alterations in LV performance. Furthermore, hepatic steatosis is associated with hepatic insulin resistance, causing hyperglycemia and compensatory hyperinsulinemia, which may worsen both systemic and cardiac insulin resistance and subsequent myocardial dysfunction [31,32].

Several studies have demonstrated that HF with preserved ejection fraction (HFpEF) is highly prevalent in patients with underlying NAFLD [33,34]. The NAFLD Fibrosis Score is also associated with worse clinical outcomes among patients with HfpEF [35]. Thus, identifying predisposing factors for diastolic dysfunction is a pivotal first step toward implementing effective prevention strategies and treatment for HfpEF.

Consistent with our previous work based on epicardial fat thickness [36], one major finding of this study is that EFV was associated with LV diastolic dysfunction and LA contractile dysfunction independent of traditional risk factors and BMI. Previous epidemiological and clinical studies have consistently demonstrated that epicardial fat is related to the presence, severity, and recurrence of atrial fibrillation (AF) across various phenotypes [37]. Possible mechanisms include myocardial extracellular matrix turnover and fibrotic replacement, resulting in arrhythmogenic substrate formation [12]. Since LA strain is an established predictor of AF occurrence and recurrence [38], our findings may further support the usage of epicardial fat in AF risk evaluation. Interestingly, the association between EFV and LAV was attenuated after multivariate adjustment in our study, yet it did not appear to be masked by the effects of global obesity in terms of BMI.

Similarly, our study also showed that hepatic stiffness (predicted by NAFLD Fibrosis Score) was independently associated with LA contractile dysfunction, LA stiffness, and LV diastolic dysfunction, even after correction by EFV. This suggests a direct link between NAFLD severity and impaired LA/LV compliance, implying that hepatic fibrosis may be an additional risk factor in the development and progression of HfpEF and AF. Although $ALSR_{late}$ is higher in the low fibrosis group compared to normal group, this is expected, since LA booster pump function could be augmented as a compensatory mechanism for decreased early filling [39]. Additional prospective studies are needed to further assess the putative mechanisms between hepatic histology and myocardial mechanics.

There are several limitations to our study. First, our study had a male sex predominance, which may be somewhat biased. Secondly, this survey is retrospective and cross-sectional, without a longitudinal follow-up or validation with clinical outcomes. Thirdly, our diagnosis of fatty liver was not based on liver biopsy, so it may not be accurate. Lastly, the study population comprises asymptomatic participants who underwent a primary cardiovascular health survey, and may not be fully representative of the broader general population in daily outpatient clinics.

5. Conclusions

NAFLD may play a significant role in developing HFpEF and AF, and this pathway may be mediated by epicardial fat accumulation. In a large Asian community, we demonstrated that hepatic fibrosis in NAFLD is independently associated with LV diastolic dysfunction, impaired LA deformation, and LA stiffness. More studies are required to determine the exact mechanisms between fatty liver and clinical HF.

Supplementary Materials: The following supporting information can be downloaded at: https://www.mdpi.com/article/10.3390/diagnostics12040916/s1, Table S1: Baseline demographics, adiposity measures and biomarkers after excluding the youngest quartile from non-fatty liver group. Table S2: Echocardiographic parameters after excluding the youngest quartile from non-fatty liver group.

Author Contributions: Conceptualization, Y.-H.L. and C.-T.T.; methodology, C.-H.S. and T.-C.H.; software, C.-H.Y.; validation, C.-H.S.; formal analysis, Y.-H.L. and C.-L.H.; investigation, T.-C.H.; resources, C.-H.Y.; data curation, C.-L.H.; writing—original draft preparation, Y.-H.L.; writing—review and editing, C.-H.Y. and C.-T.T.; supervision, H.-I.Y. and C.-L.H. All authors have read and agreed to the published version of the manuscript.

Funding: This research was supported by the National Science Council (NSC) (101-2314-B-195-020, 103-2314-B-010-005-MY3, 103-2314-B-195-001-MY3, 101-2314-B-195-020–MY1), Ministry of Science and Technology (MOST) (103-2314-B-195-006-MY3, 106-2314-B-195-008-MY2, 108-2314-B-195-018-MY2, 110-2314-B-715-009-MY1, 109-2314-B-715-008) and MacKay Memorial Hospital (10271, 10248, 10220, 10253, 10375, 10358, E-102003,MMH-108-127, MMH-110-114, MMH-110-03).

Institutional Review Board Statement: This study conformed to the principles outlined in the Declaration of Helsinki, and the protocol was approved by the Institutional Review Board of MacKay Memorial Hospital (Project identification code-18MMHIS180e, Date of approval-8 January 2019).

Informed Consent Statement: Informed consent was waived for each participant owing to the retrospective study design.

Data Availability Statement: Owing to the local institutional regulation (which, in this study, was approved several years ago, and at that stage the authors did not apply for data spread or distribution out of the institution), together with the newly applied "Personal Information Protection Act" in Taiwan, the data will not be appropriate to be released in public place. The spread and data release will cause some concern from local ethical committees based on current institution regulations. Data are available from the "MacKay Memorial Hospital" Institutional Data Access/Ethics Committee for researchers who meet the criteria for access to confidential data. The contact information as follows:

Mackay Memorial Hospital, Address: No. 92, Sec. 2, Zhongshan N. Rd., Taipei City 10449, Taiwan, Tel: 02-25433535#3486~3488, Email: mmhirb82@gmail.com (Institutional Review Board).

Acknowledgments: The authors would like to express their gratitude to all the staff members and technicians of the Laboratory of Echocardiography at the MacKay Memorial Hospital, Taipei Branch, Taiwan, for the great support rendered in this study.

Conflicts of Interest: The authors declare no conflict of interest.

References

1. Eslam, M.; Newsome, P.N.; Sarin, S.K.; Anstee, Q.M.; Targher, G.; Romero-Gomez, M.; Zelber-Sagi, S.; Wong, V.W.-S.; Dufour, J.-F.; Schattenberg, J.M.; et al. A new definition for metabolic dysfunction-associated fatty liver disease: An international expert consensus statement. *J. Hepatol.* **2020**, *73*, 202–209. [CrossRef] [PubMed]
2. Younossi, Z.M.; Rinella, M.E.; Sanyal, A.J.; Harrison, S.A.; Brunt, E.M.; Goodman, Z.; Cohen, D.E.; Loomba, R. From NAFLD to MAFLD: Implications of a Premature Change in Terminology. *Hepatology* **2020**, *73*, 1194–1198. [CrossRef]
3. Anstee, Q.M.; Targher, G.; Day, C.P. Progression of NAFLD to diabetes mellitus, cardiovascular disease or cirrhosis. *Nat. Rev. Gastroenterol. Hepatol.* **2013**, *10*, 330–344. [CrossRef] [PubMed]
4. McPherson, S.; Hardy, T.; Henderson, E.; Burt, A.D.; Day, C.P.; Anstee, Q.M. Evidence of NAFLD progression from steatosis to fibrosing-steatohepatitis using paired biopsies: Implications for prognosis and clinical management. *J. Hepatol.* **2015**, *62*, 1148–1155. [CrossRef] [PubMed]
5. Adams, L.A.; Anstee, Q.M.; Tilg, H.; Targher, G. Non-alcoholic fatty liver disease and its relationship with cardiovascular disease and other extrahepatic diseases. *Gut* **2017**, *66*, 1138–1153. [CrossRef] [PubMed]
6. Francque, S.M.; van der Graaff, D.; Kwanten, W. Non-alcoholic fatty liver disease and cardiovascular risk: Pathophysiological mechanisms and implications. *J. Hepatol.* **2016**, *65*, 425–443. [CrossRef]
7. Sperling, L.S.; Mechanick, J.I.; Neeland, I.J.; Herrick, C.J.; Després, J.P.; Ndumele, C.E.; Vijayaraghavan, K.; Handelsman, Y.; Puckrein, G.A.; Araneta, M.R.; et al. The CardioMetabolic Health Alliance: Working toward a new care model for the metabolic syndrome. *J. Am. Coll. Cardiol.* **2015**, *66*, 1050–1067. [CrossRef]
8. Cusi, K. Role of obesity and lipotoxitcity in the development of nonalcoholic steatohepatitis: Pathophysiology and clinical implications. *Gastroenterology* **2012**, *142*, 711.e6–725.e6. [CrossRef]
9. Lai, Y.-H.; Yun, C.-H.; Yang, F.-S.; Liu, C.-C.; Wu, Y.-J.; Kuo, J.-Y.; Yeh, H.-I.; Lin, T.-Y.; Bezerra, H.G.; Shih, S.-C.; et al. Epicardial Adipose Tissue Relating to Anthropometrics, Metabolic Derangements and Fatty Liver Disease Independently Contributes to Serum High-Sensitivity C-Reactive Protein Beyond Body Fat Composition: A Study Validated with Computed Tomography. *J. Am. Soc. Echocardiogr.* **2012**, *25*, 234–241. [CrossRef]
10. Lai, Y.-H.; Hou, C.J.-Y.; Yun, C.-H.; Sung, K.-T.; Su, C.-H.; Wu, T.-H.; Yang, F.-S.; Hung, T.-C.; Hung, C.-L.; Bezerra, H.G.; et al. The association among MDCT-derived three-dimensional visceral adiposities on cardiac diastology and dyssynchrony in asymptomatic population. *BMC Cardiovasc. Disord.* **2015**, *15*, 142. [CrossRef]
11. Kankaanpää, M.; Lehto, H.R.; Pärkkä, J.P.; Komu, M.; Viljanen, A.; Ferrannini, E.; Knuuti, J.; Nuutila, P.; Parkkola, R.; Iozzo, P. Myocardial triglyceride content and epicardial adipose mass in human obesity: Relationship to left ventricular function and serum free fatty acid levels. *J. Clin. Endocrinol. Metab.* **2006**, *91*, 4689–4695. [CrossRef] [PubMed]
12. Fitzgibbons, T.P.; Czech, M.P. Epicardial and Perivascular Adipose Tissues and Their Influence on Cardiovascular Disease: Basic Mechanisms and Clinical Associations. *J. Am. Hear. Assoc.* **2014**, *3*, e000582. [CrossRef] [PubMed]
13. Obokata, M.; Reddy, Y.; Pislaru, S.; Melenovsky, V.; Borlaug, B.A. Evidence Supporting the Existence of a Distinct Obese Phenotype of Heart Failure with Preserved Ejection Fraction. *Circulation* **2017**, *136*, 6–19. [CrossRef] [PubMed]
14. VanWagner, L.B.; Wilcox, J.E.; Colangelo, L.A.; Lloyd-Jones, D.; Carr, J.J.; Lima, J.A.; Lewis, C.E.; Rinella, M.E.; Shah, S.J. Association of nonalcoholic fatty liver disease with subclinical myocardial remodeling and dysfunction: A population-based study. *Hepatology* **2015**, *62*, 773–783. [CrossRef] [PubMed]
15. VanWagner, L.B.; Wilcox, J.E.; Ning, H.; Lewis, C.E.; Carr, J.J.; Rinella, M.E.; Shah, S.J.; Lima, J.A.C.; Lloyd-Jones, D.M. Longitudinal association of non-alcoholic fatty liver disease with changes in myocardial structure and function: The CARDIA Study. *J. Am. Heart Assoc.* **2020**, *9*, e014279. [CrossRef] [PubMed]
16. Petta, S.; Argano, C.; Colomba, D.; Cammà, C.; Di Marco, V.; Cabibi, D.; Tuttolomondo, A.; Marchesini, G.; Pinto, A.; Licata, G.; et al. Epicardial fat, cardiac geometry and cardiac function in patients with non-alcoholic fatty liver disease: Association with the severity of liver disease. *J. Hepatol.* **2014**, *62*, 928–933. [CrossRef] [PubMed]
17. Pacifico, L.; Di Martino, M.; De Merulis, A.; Bezzi, M.; Osborn, J.F.; Catalano, C.; Chiesa, C. Left ventricular dysfunction in obese children and adolescents with nonalcoholic fatty liver disease. *Hepatology* **2013**, *59*, 461–470. [CrossRef]
18. Angulo, P.; Hui, J.M.; Marchesini, G.; Bugianesi, E.; George, J.; Farrell, G.C.; Enders, F.; Saksena, S.; Burt, A.D.; Bida, J.P.; et al. The NAFLD fibrosis score: A noninvasive system that identifies liver fibrosis in patients with NAFLD. *Hepatology* **2007**, *45*, 846–854. [CrossRef]
19. Zeb, I.; Li, D.; Budoff, M.J.; Katz, R.; Lloyd-Jones, D.; Agatston, A.; Blumenthal, R.S.; Blaha, M.J.; Blankstein, R.; Carr, J.; et al. Nonalcoholic fatty liver disease and incident cardiac events: The Multi-Ethnic Study of Atherosclerosis. *J. Am. Coll. Cardiol.* **2016**, *67*, 1965–1966. [CrossRef]

20. Kim, D.; Kim, W.R.; Kim, H.J.; Therneau, T.M. Association between noninvasive fibrosis markers and mortality among adults with nonalcoholic fatty liver disease in the United States. *Hepatology* **2012**, *57*, 1357–1365. [CrossRef]
21. Hung, C.-L.; Gonçalves, A.; Lai, Y.-J.; Lai, Y.-H.; Sung, K.-T.; Lo, C.-I.; Liu, C.-C.; Kuo, J.-Y.; Hou, C.J.-Y.; Chao, T.-F.; et al. Light to Moderate Habitual Alcohol Consumption Is Associated with Subclinical Ventricular and Left Atrial Mechanical Dysfunction in an Asymptomatic Population: Dose-Response and Propensity Analysis. *J. Am. Soc. Echocardiogr.* **2016**, *29*, 1043.e4–1051.e4. [CrossRef] [PubMed]
22. Osawa, H.; Mori, Y. Sonographic diagnosis of fatty liver using a histogram technique that compares liver and renal cortical echo amplitudes. *J. Clin. Ultrasound* **1996**, *24*, 25–29. [CrossRef]
23. Papadopoulos, N.; Vasileiadi, S.; Papavdi, M.; Sveroni, E.; Antonakaki, P.; Dellaporta, E.; Koutli, E.; Michalea, S.; Manolakopoulos, S.; Koskinas, J.; et al. Liver fibrosis staging with combination of APRI and FIB-4 scoring systems in chronic hepatitis C as an alternative to transient elastography. *Ann. Gastroenterol.* **2019**, *32*, 498–503. [CrossRef]
24. Yun, C.-H.; Lin, T.-Y.; Wu, Y.-J.; Liu, C.-C.; Kuo, J.-Y.; Yeh, H.-I.; Yang, F.-S.; Chen, S.-C.; Hou, C.J.-Y.; Bezerra, H.G.; et al. Pericardial and thoracic peri-aortic adipose tissues contribute to systemic inflammation and calcified coronary atherosclerosis independent of body fat composition, anthropometric measures and traditional cardiovascular risks. *Eur. J. Radiol.* **2012**, *81*, 749–756. [CrossRef] [PubMed]
25. Lang, R.M.; Badano, L.P.; Mor-Avi, V.; Afilalo, J.; Armstrong, A.; Ernande, L.; Flachskampf, F.A.; Foster, E.; Goldstein, S.A.; Kuznetsova, T.; et al. Recommendations for Cardiac Chamber Quantification by Echocardiography in Adults: An Update from the American Society of Echocardiography and the European Association of Cardiovascular Imaging. *J. Am. Soc. Echocardiogr.* **2015**, *28*, 1–39. [CrossRef]
26. Chang, W.; Wang, Y.; Sun, L.; Yu, N.; Li, Y.; Li, G. Evaluation of left atrial function in type 2 diabetes mellitus patients with nonalcoholic fatty liver disease by two-dimensional speckle tracking echocardiography. *Echocardiography* **2019**, *36*, 1290–1297. [CrossRef]
27. Kocabay, G.; Karabay, C.Y.; Colak, Y.; Oduncu, V.; Kalayci, A.; Akgun, T.; Guler, A.; Kirma, C. Left atrial deformation pa-rameters in patients with non-alcoholic fatty liver disease: A 2D speckle tracking imaging study. *Clin. Sci.* **2014**, *126*, 297–304. [CrossRef]
28. Wijarnpreecha, K.; Lou, S.; Panjawatanan, P.; Cheungpasitporn, W.; Pungpapong, S.; Lukens, F.J.; Ungprasert, P. Association between diastolic cardiac dysfunction and nonalcoholic fatty liver disease: A systematic review and meta-analysis. *Dig. Liver Dis.* **2018**, *50*, 1166–1175. [CrossRef]
29. Goland, S.; Shimoni, S.; Zornitzki, T.; Knobler, H.; Azoulai, O.; Lutaty, G.; Melzer, E.; Orr, A.; Caspi, A.; Malnick, S. Cardiac abnormalities as a new manifestation of nonalcoholic fatty liver disease: Echocardiographic and tissue Doppler imaging as-sessment. *J. Clin. Gastroenterol.* **2006**, *40*, 949–955. [CrossRef]
30. Fotbolcu, H.; Yakar, T.; Duman, D.; Karaahmet, T.; Tigen, K.; Cevik, C.; Kurtoglu, U.; Dindar, I. Impairment of the left ven-tricular systolic and diastolic function in patients with non-alcoholic fatty liver disease. *Cardiol. J.* **2010**, *17*, 457–463.
31. Singh, G.K.; Vitola, B.E.; Holland, M.R.; Sekarski, T.; Patterson, B.W.; Magkos, F.; Klein, S. Alterations in Ventricular Structure and Function in Obese Adolescents with Nonalcoholic Fatty Liver Disease. *J. Pediatr.* **2013**, *162*, 1160.e1–1168.e1. [CrossRef] [PubMed]
32. Bugianesi, E. Nonalcoholic fatty liver disease (NAFLD) and cardiac lipotoxicity: Another piece of the puzzle. *Hepatology* **2008**, *47*, 2–4. [CrossRef] [PubMed]
33. Itier, R.; Guillaume, M.; Ricci, J.; Roubille, F.; Delarche, N.; Picard, F.; Galinier, M.; Roncalli, J. Non-alcoholic fatty liver disease and heart failure with preserved ejection fraction: From pathophysiology to practical issues. *ESC Hear. Fail.* **2021**, *8*, 789–798. [CrossRef] [PubMed]
34. Packer, M. Atrial Fibrillation and Heart Failure with Preserved Ejection Fraction in Patients With Nonalcoholic Fatty Liver Disease. *Am. J. Med.* **2020**, *133*, 170–177. [CrossRef] [PubMed]
35. Yoshihisa, A.; Sato, Y.; Yokokawa, T.; Sato, T.; Suzuki, S.; Oikawa, M.; Kobayashi, A.; Yamaki, T.; Kunii, H.; Nakazato, K.; et al. Liver fibrosis score predicts mortality in heart failure patients with preserved ejection fraction. *ESC Hear. Fail.* **2018**, *5*, 262–270. [CrossRef] [PubMed]
36. Lai, Y.-H.; Liu, L.; Sung, K.-T.; Tsai, J.-P.; Huang, W.-H.; Yun, C.-H.; Lin, J.-L.; Chen, Y.-J.; Su, C.-H.; Hung, T.-C.; et al. Diverse Adiposity and Atrio-Ventricular Dysfunction across Obesity Phenotypes: Implication of Epicardial Fat Analysis. *Diagnostics* **2021**, *11*, 408. [CrossRef] [PubMed]
37. Wong, C.; Ganesan, A.; Selvanayagam, J.B. Epicardial fat and atrial fibrillation: Current evidence, potential mechanisms, clinical implications, and future directions. *Eur. Hear. J.* **2017**, *38*, ehw045–1302. [CrossRef]
38. Donal, E.; Galli, E.; Schnell, F. Left atrial strain: A must or a plus for routine clinical practice? *Circ. Cardiovasc. Imaging.* **2017**, *10*, e007023. [CrossRef]
39. Mehrzad, R.; Rajab, M.; Spodick, D.H. The Three Integrated Phases of Left Atrial Macrophysiology and Their Interactions. *Int. J. Mol. Sci.* **2014**, *15*, 15146–15160. [CrossRef]

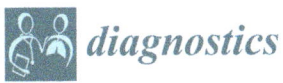

Review

Chronic Kidney Disease and Heart Failure–Everyday Diagnostic Challenges

Anna Adamska-Wełnicka [1], Marcin Wełnicki [2,*], Artur Mamcarz [2] and Ryszard Gellert [1]

1. Clinic of Nephrology and Internal Medicine, Centre of Postgraduate Medical Education, 01-813 Warsaw, Poland; anna.adamska-welnicka@cmkp.edu.pl (A.A.-W.); rgellert@cmkp.edu.pl (R.G.)
2. 3rd Department of Internal Medicine and Cardiology, Medical University of Warsaw, 02-091 Warsaw, Poland; artur.mamcarz@wum.edu.pl
* Correspondence: mwelnicki@wum.edu.pl

Abstract: Is advanced chronic kidney disease (CKD) a cardiac "no man's land"? Chronic heart failure (HF) is widely believed to be one of the most serious medical challenges of the 21st century. Moreover, the number of patients with CKD is increasing. To date, patients with estimated glomerular filtration rates <30 mL/min/1.73 m^2 have frequently been excluded from large, randomized clinical trials. Although this situation is slowly changing, in everyday practice we continue to struggle with problems that are not clearly addressed in the guidelines. This literature review was conducted by an interdisciplinary group, which comprised a nephrologist, internal medicine specialists, and cardiologist. In this review, we discuss the difficulties in ruling out HF for patients with advanced CKD and issues regarding the cardiotoxicity of dialysis fistulas and the occurrence of pulmonary hypertension in patients with CKD. Due to the recent publication of the new HF guidelines by the European Society of Cardiology, this is a good time to address these difficult issues. Contrary to appearances, these are not niche issues, but problems that affect many patients.

Keywords: heart failure; chronic kidney disease; pulmonary hypertension; arteriovenous fistulas; overhydration

1. Introduction

Chronic heart failure (HF) is one of the greatest medical challenges of the 21st century. It is estimated that HF currently affects 1–2% of the adult population in developed countries [1]. Moreover, the prevalence of HF rises significantly among people over 70, reaching 10% [2]. According to data from the European Society of Cardiology (ESC) Long-Term Registry, most outpatients with HF (60%) have a reduced left ventricle ejection fraction (LVEF), about one quarter (24%) have mildly reduced LVEF, and the remainder (16%) have preserved LVEF [3]. Chronic kidney disease (CKD) is also a very serious public health problem. The prevalence of CKD in the general population is estimated at about 9–16%, and it has increased by almost 30% over the last three decades [4]. HF and CKD frequently coexist; according to a meta-analysis by Damman et al., CKD is found in approximately half of patients with HF [5]. Similar observations were made by McAlister et al., who found features of kidney damage in 43% of patients with chronic HF and in 53% of patients with acute HF [6]. However, it would be difficult to determine how many patients with CKD have concurrent HF, because few studies report those specific numbers. In the guidelines for the diagnosis and treatment of HF, the section on CKD indicates that most studies conducted to date have used an estimated glomerulus filtration rate (eGFR) of <30 mL/min/1.73 m^2 as a criterion for excluding patients with HF [1]. Therefore, advanced CKD is a kind of "no man's land" for many of us in everyday clinical practice. Research has shown that the coexistence of HF and CKD doubles the risk of death. A sharp increase in mortality is observed when the eGFR value drops below 60 mL/min/1.73 m^2, and the highest mortality rates are found among patients with HF and end stage kidney disease, i.e., when the eGFR is <15 mL/min/1.73 m^2 [5,7]. The latter group also includes patients on dialysis. Therefore, there is no doubt that this population requires special attention. In practice, however, a patient with severe renal impairment presents a dual challenge: first, in the context of therapeutic decisions, and second, in the context of diagnosing HF. HF is described as a clinical syndrome consisting of major symptoms and signs: dyspnea, peripheral edema and pulmonary congestion. Echocardiography and plasma concentration of natriuretic peptides play a key role in HF diagnosis [1]. At the same time, overhydration in the course of advanced renal failure causes similar symptoms and signs, has an impact on the heart's function and structure, and makes it difficult to interpret natriuretic peptide concentration [8]. With the recent publication of the new ESC guidelines on HF, this is a good time to focus on the most difficult and debated issues at the interface between cardiology and nephrology.

2. Materials and Methods

We searched PubMed for articles with the key words "heart failure", "chronic kidney disease", "pulmonary hypertension", "arteriovenous fistula", "natriuretic peptides", "fluid overload", "end stage renal disease", and "hemodialysis". In particular, we used the following search terms and logic: "chronic kidney disease AND heart failure" OR pulmonary hypertension AND "chronic kidney disease OR heart failure" or "chronic kidney disease AND arteriovenous fistula AND cardiotoxicity". Additional studies were identified by examining the references of some articles. Articles were selected according to their title and abstract, based on eligibility criteria. We included English articles, adult populations, and all types of study, including narrative and systematic reviews, clinical studies, case reports, and expert opinions. Manuscripts published in a language other than English were excluded. In general, we excluded studies published earlier than in 2010, but we made single exceptions to this rule. The final analysis included 61 articles, which we selected, based on originality and relevance to the broader scope of our review. In the discussion of the basic issues concerning the pharmacotherapy of HF in the coexistence of advanced CKD, an additional 11 articles were cited, according to the subjective assessment of the authors of the review.

3. How to Confirm or Rule out HF in a Patient

According to the current diagnostic algorithm, we suspect HF on the basis of typical symptoms and signs in a patient with HF risk factors and an incorrect ECG [1]. A concentration of BNP $\geq$ 35 pg/mL or NT-proBNP $\geq$ 125 pg/mL and abnormal findings in echocardiography confirm the diagnosis. Echocardiography also allows determination of the HF phenotype [1]. HF and CKD share many risk factors. Among these, hypertension and diabetes are the most important. In practice, however, it is important to realize that HF can be both a cause and a consequence of renal failure. The basic pathophysiological mechanisms underlying this relationship are presented in Figure 1. To emphasize the frequent coexistence and close relationship between cardiovascular diseases and kidney diseases, the term "cardio–renal syndrome" was coined [8].

Nosologically, neither HF nor CKD are disease entities; instead, they are clinical syndromes. HF is currently defined as a "clinical syndrome consisting of cardinal symptoms (e.g., breathlessness, ankle swelling, and fatigue) that may be accompanied by signs (e.g., elevated jugular venous pressure, pulmonary crackles, and peripheral edema). HF is due to a structural and/or functional abnormality of the heart that results in elevated intracardiac pressures and/or inadequate cardiac output (CO) at rest and/or during exercise." [1]. The definition of CKD has not changed for almost a decade. CKD is diagnosed, when, for at least 3 months, we find one or both of the following signs:

1. A reduction in the eGFR to <60 mL/min/1.73 m^2;
2. Kidney damage in imaging, histopathology, or laboratory tests.

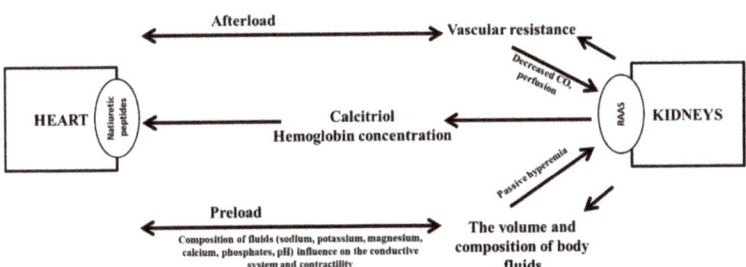

Figure 1. Basic mechanisms underlying the mutual dependencies of heart and kidney functions. CO, cardiac output; RAAS, renin-angiotensin-aldosterone system. A figure prepared by the authors on the basis of pathophysiological issues described by Rangaswami et al. [8]. The figure shows the influence of heart and kidney function on the afterload and preload values. The decrease in cardiac output due to heart failure causes renal hypoperfusion. The sympathetic nervous system, the renin-angiotensin-aldosterone system and the release of vasopressin are activated in order to increase systemic vascular resistance and circulating blood volume. Increased venous pressure causes renal congestion, which additionally impairs their function. A decrease in glomerular filtration causes not only hypervolemia (increased preload), but also unfavorable changes in ion concentrations, which affects the contractility of cardiomyocytes. In addition, along with the deteriorating kidney function, disturbances in calcium-phosphate metabolism increase and the synthesis of erythropoietin is impaired, which also adversely affects the function of blood vessels and the heart muscle.

Therefore, the diagnosis of CKD is determined by specific tests, not by clinical symptoms. According to the Kidney Disease: Improving Global Outcomes guidelines of 2012, there are five stages of CKD. A correct classification of the CKD stage requires assessments of GFR and albuminuria, and to determine the combination of causes; thus, the classification includes the GFR category (G1–G5), and albuminuria category (A1–A3), as proposed in the guidelines [9]. Hence, the diagnosis of CKD is straightforward in a patient with previously diagnosed HF. However, for patients with previously diagnosed CKD, the usefulness of the HF diagnostic algorithm currently proposed may be considered questionable [1] (Figure 2).

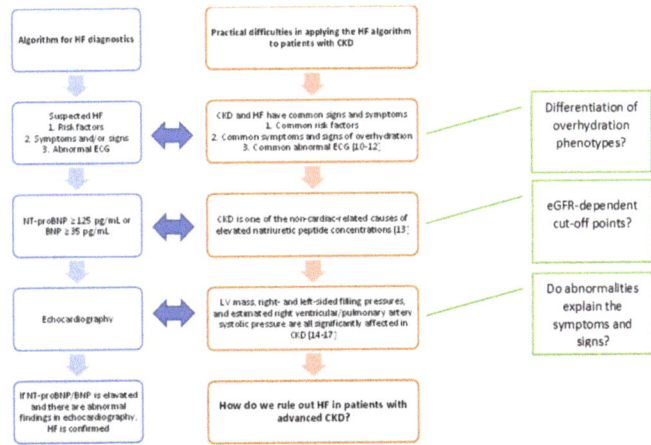

Figure 2. Difficulties in implementing the current diagnostic algorithm for HF for patients with CKD [1,10–17]. The HF diagnostic algorithm (left) includes symptoms that are common in patients with CKD, with or without HF (center). Ruling out HF in patients with CKD may require further differentiation; (right) some potential differentiation factors are proposed; For example, arterial

hypertension and diabetes are the primary risk factors for both CKD and HF. In a patient with a significantly reduced eGFR, dyspnea and oedema may be caused by both CKD and concomitant or occurring de novo HF. With the deteriorating renal function, the unequivocal interpretation of the elevated concentration of natriuretic peptides becomes troublesome and electrolyte disturbances may affect the ECG. In such a setting, it is difficult to conclude whether HF coexists with CKD or whether the deterioration of cardiac function is secondary to renal failure and therefore potentially reversible. This issue is discussed in detail later in the article; HF: heart failure; CKD: chronic kidney disease; ECG: electrocardiogram; BNP: brain natriuretic peptide; LV: left ventricular; eGFR: estimated glomerular filtration rate.

4. Is the Nature of Overhydration the Same in HF and CKD?

The circulatory system consists of four main compartments—venous, arterial, pulmonary, and systemic. The distribution of fluid volumes within these compartments is asymmetric. The arterial system comprises 20–30% and the venous system comprises 70–80% of the fluid volume. The structure and function of the heart contribute to the maintenance of this physiological asymmetry. When disorders in the heart's pumping function outweigh disorders of the return function, the cardiac muscle cannot generate an adequate CO, due to low stroke volume. The result is called forward failure. Conversely, when the return dysfunction is predominant, the result is called backward failure, and the predominant venous outflow results in organ congestion. Therefore, the consequence of HF is a redistribution of the intravascular volume, which leads to a permanent underfilling of the arterial compartment (10–15%) and displacement of the "extra" volume into the venous compartment (85–95%). Thus, ultimately, in HF, fluid overload is most often associated with hypovolemia. However, it should be emphasized that, in patients with CKD, fluid overload is associated with hypervolemia. As shown in Figure 1, in HF, hypovolemia is one of the causes of kidney damage (types 1 and 2 of the cardio-renal syndrome) [8]. Conversely, hypervolemia in the course of renal failure can cause HF (types 3 and 4 of the cardio-renal syndrome) [18]. The classification of cardio-renal syndromes systematizes knowledge; however, it is not easily translated into everyday practice [8]. Indeed, in everyday practice, it is sufficient to identify the coexistence of HF and renal dysfunction and to identify the initiating factor. Then, the initiating factor is the target of the therapy. Moreover, patients may not present with only one specific type of cardio-renal syndrome; they can change between types and even present two types at the same time [8].

A physical examination generally assesses the patient's signs and symptoms, and severity is graded with the New York Heart Association (NYHA) classification. The examination typically includes a blood pressure measurement and assessments of the presence and severity of peripheral edema and the detection of crackles over the pulmonary fields. However, these assessments are not sufficient to make a reliable assessment of the degree of fluid overload [19–21]. Moreover, it remains challenging to assess the correct hydration status in patients that require dialysis. Consequently, the medical examination results are objectified with additional methods; for example, the whole body electrical bioimpedance can be measured; ultrasound can be performed to assess inferior vena cava compliance; or ultrasound can be performed to assess pulmonary congestion [21]. Each of these methods has advantages and limitations (Table 1).

The use of additional assessment methods is time-consuming. Therefore, research is ongoing on the development of simplified diagnostic schemes. Among the biochemical markers for assessing hydration status, natriuretic peptide concentrations are often measured. Both brain natriuretic peptide (BNP) and the inactive N-terminal prohormone-BNP (NT-proBNP) are produced at high levels in HF. However, the results should be interpreted carefully.

Table 1. Benefits and limitations of additional study methods for evaluating overhydration.

Study Methods	Benefits	Limitations
Electrical bioimpedance	<ul><li>The method has been validated against the "gold standard"</li><li>Recommended method</li><li>Assessment of total body hydration</li><li>Non-invasive examination</li><li>Simple execution</li><li>Repeatability of measurements</li><li>Low cost</li><li>Short waiting time for the result</li><li>Performed "at the bedside"</li><li>Detection of subclinical forms of fluid overload</li></ul>	<ul><li>Numerous factors influence measurement accuracy</li><li>Parameters are assessed based on mathematical estimates of data from the population of healthy Caucasian people</li><li>It provides only a summary assessment of total body fluid overload</li><li>Limited sensitivity of fluid assessment in the so-called third space</li></ul>
Ultrasound evaluation of the inferior vena cava	<ul><li>Low cost</li><li>Performed "at the bedside"</li><li>Non-invasive</li><li>Possibility of multiple inspections</li><li>Results available immediately after the end of the test</li></ul>	<ul><li>Assesses blood volume only (intravascular fluid)</li><li>Requires cooperation from the patient</li><li>The abnormalities found may not be specific to overhydration alone</li><li>Possibility of multiple inspections</li></ul>
Lung Ultrasound	<ul><li>A simple, repeatable method</li><li>Favorable learning curve</li><li>Low cost</li><li>Wide availability</li><li>Low hardware requirements: any ultrasound head, use of portable devices</li><li>Preformed "at the bedside"</li><li>Non-invasive</li><li>Detection of subclinical forms of pulmonary congestion</li><li>Possible to make accurate assessments of pleural cavities</li><li>Results are available immediately after the end of the test</li></ul>	<ul><li>Requires differentiation of the causes of B-line artifacts, based on clinical data</li><li>Difficult to assess several things, including: the presence of a large amount of fluid in the pleural cavities; pneumonia; interstitial lung diseases</li></ul>

5. What Is the Practical Significance of BNP and NT-proBNP in Patients with Advanced CKD?

Normally when HF is suspected, BNP/NT-proBNP concentration is of key importance in the diagnostic algorithm [1]. They are also good prognostic markers [1]. However, the coexistence of renal failure may influence the diagnostic value of BNP/NT-proBNP. It is believed that, for stages 1–2 CKD, standard BNP cut-off thresholds can be used to diagnose HF. In the more advanced stages of kidney damage, research shows that the cut-off point must be adjusted. The NT-proBNP concentration is more dependent on kidney function than the BNP concentration [22]. In patients with a similar degree of LV dysfunction, natriuretic peptide concentrations are significantly higher in the presence of renal failure, and they are positively correlated with a reduction in the GFR [22]. A study by Vickery et al. showed that, for each 10 mL/min reduction in GFR, there was a 38% increase in the NT-pro-BNP concentration [23].

For patients with stage 3–5 CKD, the BNP threshold for diagnosing HF should be 200 pg/mL [13,24–26]. It has been suggested that, in patients with stage 4–5 CKD that exhibit symptoms of acute HF, very high levels of BNP indicate that the symptoms are related to an ischemic background. In this group of patients, a prospective study showed that, on admission, a BNP concentration >2907 pg/mL showed 71% sensitivity and 72% specificity for identifying an ischemic etiology of HF [27]. Moreover, in patients with stage 4–5 CKD, a BNP concentration >157 pg/mL was identified as an independent risk factor for a cardiovascular event; however, the sensitivity and specificity were only 65% and 56%, respectively [28]. It has also been shown that, in patients with end-stage renal failure, but without clinical symptoms of HF, the detection of BNP levels >150 pg/mL before starting renal replacement therapy was an independent risk factor for overt HF [29].

Deteriorating renal function affects the NT-proBNP concentration to a greater extent than the BNP concentration. In patients without CKD, these markers are equally important for the diagnosis of HF; however, in the context of a prognosis assessment, NT-proBNP has shown better value than BNP [1,13,26]. In patients with impaired renal function, the significance of high NT-proBNP concentrations in the diagnosis of acute HF was similar to its significance in the population of patients with eGFRs > 60 mL/min/1.73 m^2; however, that finding was based on the adoption of cut-off thresholds that were double the typical NT-proBNP thresholds used for diagnosing HF in different age groups [13]. A standardized natriuretic peptide cut-off threshold for diagnosing chronic HF has not been clearly established to date. This uncertainty is probably due to the difficulty in determining whether the chronic increase in NT-proBNP concentration is mainly caused by damage to the myocardium or by impaired glomerular filtration [22]. Many studies have shown that an elevated NT-proBNP concentration is a negative prognostic factor in patients with CKD; however, the cut-off threshold differs significantly for different CKD severities. For example, Horri et al. conducted a study involving over 1000 patients with CKD, including 85 patients with stage 4–5 CKD. They used NT-proBNP cut-off points of 5809.0 pg/mL, for patients with eGFRs < 30 mL/min/1.73 m^2, and 259.7 pg/mL for patients with eGFRs > 30 mL/min/1.73 m^2 [28]. Şimşek et al. analyzed data from patients with stage 3–4 CKD. They proposed NT-proBNP cut-off points of 197 pg/mL, for predicting an increased risk of death in patients with eGFRs > 60 mL/min/1.73 m^2, and 251 pg/mL for predicting cardiovascular death in patients with eGFRs < 60 mL/min/1.73 m^2 [30]. That study excluded patients with end-stage kidney disease [30]. Based on the cited data, the concentration of natriuretic peptides appears to change dynamically, between the 4th and 5th stages of CKD.

NT-proBNP is also an important prognostic factor in patients on dialysis [31]. Tsai et al. showed that NT-proBNP was an indicator of intravascular fluid status [32]. The NT-proBNP concentration depended on the fluid distribution between the intra- and extracellular compartments. In patients with advanced CKD that were undergoing dialysis, NT-proBNP was a marker of fluid overload [31]. Moreover, the coexistence of high NT-proBNP concentrations and the symptoms and signs of overhydration had a synergistic effect on the risk of death and the risk of cardiovascular events [32]. However, no specific cut-off points were determined. Additionally, in patients that require repeated hemodialysis, the natriuretic peptide concentration may be influenced by the type of membrane in the dialyzer. When low-flux membranes were used for hemodialysis, the patient's BNP concentration decreased, and the NT-proBNP concentration increased. However, when high-flux membranes were used, the patient's BNP concentration decreased and the NT-proBNP concentration remained unchanged [33,34]. Moreover, in patients undergoing hemodialysis, the use of arteriovenous fistulas (AVFs) can be cardiotoxic, which may cause additional difficulty in interpreting the significance of the BNP concentrations. Therefore, it is difficult to interpret the significance of high natriuretic peptide concentrations in patients with advanced CKD. The cut-off thresholds can be dramatically different in different stages of the disease, and the concentrations may be affected by dialysis. This situation is similar to the situation in patients with advanced, chronic HF, where it is difficult to interpret changes in the concentration of highly sensitive T troponins, due to the many influencing factors. Thus, it remains unclear when dynamic changes in natriuretic peptide concentrations should be considered important.

6. Cardiotoxicity of Arteriovenous Fistulas

The implantation of a venous catheter during hemodialysis is associated with an increased rate of infection and early mortality. Hence, the principle of "fistula first" has been widely promoted. However, although AVFs are associated with better clinical outcomes compared to other forms of vascular access, they are not without potential complications [35,36]. The first reports on the potential cardiotoxicity associated with AVFs appeared over 50 years ago. Currently, the suggested management strategy is often marked with the slogan "Patient first, not fistula first, but avoid a catheter if at all possible" [37].

When an AVF is generated, it causes an immediate decrease in systemic peripheral resistance and blood leaks through the low-resistance artificial arteriovenous junction. A decrease in systemic resistance increases sympathetic activity, which increases the CO to maintain blood pressure. Therefore, the first adaptive mechanism is the occurrence of hyperkinetic circulation [37,38], which results in an increase in venous return. Gradually, the increased venous return to the ventricles (functional hypervolemia) causes an increase in the stroke volume and tends to slow the heart rate. These changes occur in every patient that receives an AVF, but the changes are generally compensatory in nature. When fistula flow (Qa) is not high and the heart remains efficient, these changes compensate for the left-to-right leak [37,39,40]. Symptoms of HF typically appear when the Qa rises to 20–50% of the CO. Chronic maintenance of an elevated CO or periodic increases in CO, in response to exercise, are dependent on the heart reserves. Exceeding the heart reserve leads to structural changes in the heart, including muscle hypertrophy, ventricle dilatation, and the gradual development of HF [37]. The minute volume capacity generated by the damaged heart becomes insufficient for the needs of the body. As a result, hypertension develops in the systemic veins and pulmonary vessels. The first signs of dysfunction are a volume overload, compensatory vasoconstriction, and an increase in systemic pressure, which further exacerbates HF. An AVF requires a satisfactory access Qa to ensure adequate dialysis. However, the paradox is that, on one hand, a low Qa value indicates fistula dysfunction and, on the other hand, a high Qa results in HF with a high CO. It is worth noting that the relationship between the Qa and CO does not appear to be linear. At the end of the 20th century, Pandeya and Lindsay presented the concept of using the Qa/CO ratio (a measure of cardiopulmonary recirculation) to monitor AVF flow in patients undergoing hemodialysis [41]. Thus, the propensity to develop symptomatic HF is believed to be proportional to the Qa, with a proposed cut-off of 2.0 L/min. As a cut-off point, this value has 89% sensitivity and 100% specificity for the diagnosis of HF in patients with a high CO [42].

The therapeutic management of HF with a high CO is difficult. Standard pharmacological treatment does not seem to be particularly effective. In recent years, several case reports showed that a surgical fistula closure was associated with improved performance in HF [43–45]. However, the study by Gumus and Saricaoglu deserves special attention because they analyzed 81 patients to determine potential predictors of the occurrence of right ventricular (RV) HF symptoms after an AVF insertion [46]. Prior to creating the AVF, 74% of patients presented symptoms of grades II-III chronic HF, according to the NYHA classification. Independent predictors for RV HF after an AVF were a RV longitudinal strain (RVLS) in the free wall <−19% (odds ratio (OR): 2.31, 95% CI: 1.02–3.22) and tricuspid regurgitation jet velocity (TRJV) >2.5 m/s (OR: 5.68, 95% CI: 1.21–4.38). The areas under receiver operating curves were 0.86 (95% CI: 0.55–0.89, $p = 0.004$), for RVLS, and 0.81 (95% CI: 0.55–0.89, $p = 0.005$), for TRJV > 2.61 m/s [44]. It is worth noting that the groups with and without RV HF after AVF had similar Qa values (approximately 0.5 L/min) and NT-proBNP concentrations (approximately 850 pg/mL vs. approximately 940 pg/mL). Moreover, in both groups, these values were significantly above the norm expected for patients without CKD [46].

Additionally, it is worth noting that, in the Gumus and Saricaoglu study, the definition of RV HF included the natriuretic peptide concentrations and a number of echocardiographic parameters (i.e., central venous pressure or right atrial pressure >16 mm Hg; tricuspid annular plane systolic excursion <16 mm, or an RV fractional area change <35% or an RV basal end-diastolic diameter >41 mm; an inferior vena cava diameter >21 mm; and <50% inferior vena cava collapsibility); the presence of significant peripheral edema, ascites, or hepatomegaly; and laboratory markers of deteriorating liver or kidney function, compared to the state before the fistula creation [46]. The literature on this subject suggests that, in patients with end-stage renal failure and concomitant NYHA I-II HF, AVF dialysis therapy can be started, but distal vessels should be used for this purpose [47]. Moreover, in patients with NYHA III HF, the decision to select AVF must be carefully considered, and it should depend on echocardiographic parameters. In patients with an LVEF < 30%, a permanent catheter placement is recommended. In patients with NYHA IV HF, a permanent catheter is elective for venous access [47]. However, due to the practical difficulties (mentioned above) in making a definitive diagnosis of chronic HF in patients with end-stage renal disease, the functional classification available does not guarantee a correct diagnosis. Indeed, many patients with advanced CKD have a normal LVEF.

Currently, we know little about how to apply the existing knowledge about the cardiotoxic potential of AVF in practice [48,49]. Among the symptoms of RV HF, it is worth noting another difficult, and yet little known, problem frequently present in patients with advanced CKD—pulmonary hypertension.

7. Pulmonary Hypertension in Patients with CKD

Pulmonary hypertension is defined as a mean pulmonary artery pressure ≥25 mmHg at rest, based on a direct hemodynamic measurement. Pulmonary hypertension can occur secondary to many diseases of the heart, lungs, and pulmonary vessels. Classically, there are five groups of pulmonary hypertension. The fifth group includes: hematologic disorders, systemic diseases, metabolic disorders, chronic renal failure, and disorders leading to pulmonary vascular occlusion or compression. However, for patients with advanced renal failure, including those on dialysis, the pathophysiology of pulmonary hypertension is multifactorial. The pathophysiological mechanisms include:

- overhydration;
- pulmonary congestion, resulting from reduced LV compliance, and LV diastolic dysfunction (a consequence of arteriosclerosis and chronic hypertension);
- pulmonary vessel remodeling, caused by an increase in vasoactive factors (e.g., nitric oxide, prostacyclin, and endothelin);
- inflammation;
- coexisting lung disease (e.g., obstructive sleep apnea and chronic obstructive pulmonary disease);
- increased CO in the course of anemia, due to the presence of an AVF [17,50].

Ultimately, pulmonary hypertension affects 21–41% of patients with chronic kidney disease and up to 60% of patients treated with hemodialysis [50–56]. When pulmonary hypertension is suspected, echocardiography is the first diagnostic test performed. The probability of pulmonary hypertension is established based on an evaluation of the maximum velocity of the tricuspid regurgitation velocity (Table 2), taking into account the possible coexistence of other features of RV overload.

Table 2. Probability of pulmonary hypertension (PH), stratified by echocardiography results.

Maximum Velocity of the Tricuspid Regurgitation Velocity	Probability of PH
≤2.8 m/s (TVPG ≤ 31 mm Hg)	Low
2.9–3.4 m/s (TVPG 32–46 mm Hg)	Intermediate
>3.4 m/s	High

TVPG: tricuspid valve pressure gradient.

Depending on the probability of pulmonary hypertension, assessed by echocardiography and the clinical picture, indications for cardiac catheterization are determined. Cardiac catheterization is the only examination that determines the diagnosis of pulmonary hypertension. During right heart catheterization the pulmonary capillary wedge pressure, pulmonary arterial pressure, and pulmonary vascular resistance are determined. Based on these results, three pulmonary hypertension subtypes are distinguished: (1) pre-capillary, (2) post-capillary, and (3) combined pre- and post-capillary [17].

Concurrent CKD strongly influences both the pulmonary hypertension subtype and the associated mortality. Edmonston et al. showed that, among patients without CKD, the pre-capillary subtype was dominant, and was associated with the highest risk of death. In contrast, among patients with CKD, the combined pre- and post-capillary and isolated extra-capillary subtypes dominated [17]. The multifactorial nature of pulmonary hypertension in the course of CKD suggests that the cause may be, among others, pulmonary congestion, due to reduced LV compliance and LV diastolic dysfunction [17,50]. The coincidence of CKD and pulmonary hypertension is associated with a significant increase in patient mortality; therefore, it is important to understand the pathological mechanisms underlying pulmonary hypertension. However, currently, there are many hypotheses [57–61], including a chronic volume overload, which can accelerate pulmonary vascular remodeling. The role of nitric oxide was also suggested because nitric oxide regulates pulmonary vascular tone, and it is a frequent target of pharmacotherapy for pulmonary arterial hypertension. Moreover, CKD adversely affects many mediators of nitric oxide metabolism (e.g., L-arginine and homocysteine). Another postulated pathological mechanism for pulmonary hypertension is an increase in fibroblast growth factor-23 (FGF-23) concentration, which is observed in the course of CKD. FGF-23 is associated with, among other things, the occurrence of LV hypertrophy and HF. Moreover, the FGF-23 concentration is correlated with pulmonary artery pressure, in some populations; however, this relationship remains unclear in patients with CKD. In addition, progressive renal dysfunction and dialysis therapy promote the activation of the inflammatory system. In this context, researchers have examined the correlation between increasing concentrations of various factors (e.g., TGF-β, IL-6, or IL-10) and the presence of pulmonary hypertension [57–61]. Ultimately, despite the high prevalence and increased risk of mortality associated with pulmonary hypertension in patients with CKD, pulmonary hypertension remains insufficiently understood in patients with CKD [61].

8. Whether CKD Affects Basic Pharmacotherapy of HF?

The main topic of our review is the issue of diagnostic difficulties, but it is impossible not to refer to the issue of pharmacotherapy. Medications that can improve prognosis in HF with reduced LVEF are angiotensin-converting enzyme inhibitors (ACE), angiotensin II receptor blockers (ARB), angiotensin receptor neprilysin inhibitors (ARNI), b-blockers, and mineralocorticoid receptor antagonists (MRA). Recently sodium-glucose cotransporter 2 inhibitors (SGLT-2) have joined this group, and according to current ESC guidelines blockade of the renin-angiotensin-aldosterone system with ACE, ARNI or ARB, beta-blocker, SGLT-2 inhibitor and MRA should be started as soon as possible after the diagnosis of HF with reduced LVEF [1]. Until recently, it was considered that the coexistence of CKD did not affect the general principles of pharmacological management in HF [22]. However, the scientific evidence for the efficacy of conventional treatment of HF with decreased LVEF is lower the more advanced CKD is. The strongest evidence is for beta-blocker. The studies on bisoprolol, carvedilol and metoprolol have also shown an improvement in the prognosis of patients with HF in the case of concomitant CKD [62–64]. Although ACE and ARB can cause eGFR to decrease in patients with HF, the benefit of angiotensin blockade in terms of prognosis in patients with HF and reduced LVEF seems to be maintained [65,66]. Evidence for the efficacy of MRA in the treatment of patients with HF and advanced CKD are limited [67,68]. For decades another serious challenge was the management of HF with preserved LVEF, for which there was no treatment improving prognosis [22,69]. This situation changed with the publication of the results of the EMPEROR-Preserved trail. Empagliflozin is the first molecule to improve the prognosis of HF patients with preserved LVEF [70]. Considering the data on the nephroprotective effect of SGLT-2 inhibitors, and the prevalence of HF with preserved EF among CKD patients, the results of this study are particularly noteworthy [71,72]. However, a detailed discussion of the principles and doubts regarding the pharmacotherapy of HF in the coexistence of advanced CKD is beyond the scope of this review.

9. Conclusions

Among patients that first develop chronic progressive renal failure, it may be difficult to confirm concurrent HF. The clinical symptoms of HF and advanced CKD may be confusingly similar, particularly in patients on dialysis. The eGFR has a significant impact on natriuretic peptide concentrations—indeed, increases in these peptides result from both damage to the heart and their impaired elimination in the kidneys. Definitive cut-off points for BNP and/or NT-proBNP concentrations have not been established for diagnosing HF in patients with CKD. However, elevated levels of these peptides have been shown to have negative prognostic significance. Therefore, for patients with intermediate or preserved LVEF and CKD, there remains a need for new diagnostic criteria that can confirm or exclude HF as the primary cause of fluid overload. Moreover, the correct diagnosis of HF in patients classified as pre-dialysis may be a key issue in selecting the optimal vascular access. Despite the convincing pathophysiological basis, little evidence is available to support the potential cardiotoxicity of fistulas. However, new research has indicated that it may be possible to use an echocardiographic assessment of RV strain.

Author Contributions: Conceptualization, A.A.-W., M.W.; methodology, A.A.-W., M.W.; writing—original draft preparation, A.A.-W., M.W.; writing—review and editing, A.A.-W., M.W., A.M., R.G.; visualization, A.A.-W., M.W.; supervision, A.M., R.G. All authors have read and agreed to the published version of the manuscript.

Funding: The APC was funded by Centre of Postgraduate Medical Education, Warsaw, 01-813 Poland.

Institutional Review Board Statement: Not applicable.

Informed Consent Statement: Not applicable.

Data Availability Statement: Not applicable.

Conflicts of Interest: The authors declare no conflict of interest.

References

1. McDonagh, T.A.; Metra, M.; Adamo, M.; Gardner, R.S.; Baumbach, A.; Böhm, M.; Burri, H.; Butler, J.; Čelutkienė, J.; Chioncel, O.; et al. 2021 ESC Guidelines for the diagnosis and treatment of acute and chronic heart failure. ESC Clinical Practice Guidelines. *Eur. Heart J.* **2021**, *42*, 3599–3726. [CrossRef]
2. Van Riet, E.E.; Hoes, A.W.; Limburg, A.; Landman, M.A.; van der Hoeven, H.; Rutten, F.H. Prevalence of unrecognized heart failure in older persons with shortness of breath on exertion. *Eur. J. Heart Fail.* **2014**, *16*, 772–777. [CrossRef]
3. Chioncel, O.; Lainscak, M.; Seferovic, P.M.; Anker, S.D.; Crespo-Leiro, M.G.; Harjola, V.P.; Parissis, J.; Laroche, C.; Piepoli, M.F.; Fonseca, C.; et al. Epidemiology and one-year outcomes in patients with chronic heart failure and preserved, mid-range and reduced ejection fraction: An analysis of the ESC Heart Failure Long-Term Registry. *Eur. J. Heart Fail.* **2017**, *19*, 1574–1585. [CrossRef]
4. Gellert, R.; Kalinowska, A.; Prystacki, T.; Daniewska, D.; Polak, W. Treatment of anemia in patients with advanced chronic kidney disease in Poland. *Nefrol. Dial. Pol.* **2021**, *25*, 33–40.
5. Damman, K.; Valente, M.A.; Voors, A.A.; O'Connor, C.M.; van Veldhuisen, D.J.; Hillege, H.L. Renal impairment, worsening renal function, and outcome in patients with heart failure: An updated meta-analysis. *Eur. Heart J.* **2014**, *35*, 455–469. [CrossRef]
6. McAlister, F.A.; Ezekowitz, J.; Tarantini, L.; Squire, I.; Komajda, M.; Bayes-Genis, A.; Gotsman, I.; Whalley, G.; Earle, N.; Poppe, K.K.; et al. Renal dysfunction in patients with heart failure with preserved versus reduced ejection fraction: Impact of the new chronic kidney disease—Epidemiology collaboration group formula. *Circ. Heart Fail.* **2012**, *5*, 309–314. [CrossRef] [PubMed]
7. Damman, K.; Masson, S.; Lucci, D.; Gorini, M.; Urso, R.; Maggioni, A.P.; Tavazzi, L.; Tarantini, L.; Tognoni, G.; Voors, A.; et al. Progression of renal impairment and chronic kidney disease in chronic heart failure: An analysis from GISSI-HF. *J. Card. Fail.* **2017**, *23*, 2–9. [CrossRef]
8. Rangaswami, J.; Bhalla, V.; Blair, J.; Chang, T.I.; Costa, S.; Lentine, K.L.; Lerma, E.V.; Mezue, K.; Molitch, M.; Mullens, W.; et al. Cardiorenal syndrome: Classification, pathophysiology, diagnosis, and treatment strategies: A scientific statement from the american heart association. *Circulation* **2019**, *139*, e840–e878. [CrossRef]
9. Levin, A.; Stevens, P.E.; Bilous, R.W.; Coresh, J.; de Francisco, A.L.M.; de Jong, P.E.; Griffith, K.E.; Hemmelgarn, B.R.; Iseki, K.; Lamb, E.J.; et al. Kidney disease: Improving global outcomes (KDIGO) CKD work group. KDIGO 2012 clinical practice guideline for the evaluation and management of chronic kidney disease. *Kidney Int.* **2013**, *3*, 1–150.

10. Mulia, E.; Nugraha, R.A.; A'yun, M.Q.; Juwita, R.R.; Yofrido, F.M.; Julario, R.; Alkaff, F.F. Electrocardiographic abnormalities among late-stage non-dialysis chronic kidney disease patients. *J. Basic Clin. Physiol. Pharmacol.* **2020**, *32*, 155–162. [CrossRef]
11. Heo, N.J.; Rhee, S.Y.; Waalen, J.; Steinhubl, S. Chronic kidney disease and undiagnosed atrial fibrillation in individuals with diabetes. *Cardiovasc. Diabetol.* **2020**, *19*, 157. [CrossRef] [PubMed]
12. Ajam, F.; Akoluk, A.; Alrefaee, A.; Campbell, N.; Masud, A.; Mehandru, S.; Patel, M.; Asif, A.; Carson, M.P. Prevalence of abnormalities in electrocardiogram conduction in dialysis patients: A comparative study. *J. Bras. Nefrol.* **2020**, *42*, 448–453. [CrossRef]
13. Han, X.; Zhang, S.; Chen, Z.; Adhikari, B.K.; Zhang, Y.; Zhang, J.; Sun, J.; Wang, Y. Cardiac biomarkers of heart failure in chronic kidney disease. *Clin. Chim. Acta* **2020**, *510*, 298–310. [CrossRef]
14. Whalley, G.A.; Marwick, T.H.; Doughty, R.N.; Cooper, B.A.; Johnson, D.W.; Pilmore, A.; Harris, D.C.; Pollock, C.A.; Collins, J.F.; IDEAL Echo Substudy Investigators. Effect of early initiation of dialysis on cardiac structure and function: Results from the echo substudy of the IDEAL trial. *Am. J. Kidney Dis.* **2013**, *61*, 262–270. [CrossRef]
15. Park, M.; Hsu, C.Y.; Li, Y.; Mishra, R.K.; Keane, M.; Rosas, S.E.; Dries, D.; Xie, D.; Chen, J.; He, J.; et al. Associations between kidney function and subclinical cardiac abnormalities in CKD. *J. Am. Soc. Nephrol.* **2012**, *23*, 1725–1734. [CrossRef]
16. Shroff, G.R.; Herzog, C.A. Echocardiography: Providing additional insights into cardiovascular structural and functional abnormalities in advanced CKD. *Clin. J. Am. Soc. Nephrol.* **2013**, *8*, 339–341. [CrossRef]
17. Edmonston, D.L.; Rajagopal, S.; Wolf, M. Echocardiography to screen for pulmonary hypertension in CKD. *Kidney Int. Rep.* **2020**, *5*, 2275–2283. [CrossRef] [PubMed]
18. Ronco, C.; Haapio, M.; House, A.A.; Anavekar, N.; Bellomo, R. Cardiorenal syndrome. *J. Am. Coll. Cardiol.* **2008**, *52*, 1527–1539. [CrossRef] [PubMed]
19. Voroneanu, L.; Cusai, C.; Hogas, S.; Ardeleanu, S.; Onofriescu, M.; Nistor, I.; Prisada, O.; Sascau, R.; Goldsmith, D.; Covic, A. The relationship between chronic volume overload and elevated blood pressure in hemodialysis patients: Use of bioimpedance provides a different perspective from echocardiography and biomarker methodologies. *Int. Urol. Nephrol.* **2010**, *42*, 789–797. [CrossRef]
20. Agarwal, R.; Andersen, M.J.; Pratt, J.H. On the importance of pedal edema in hemodialysis patients. *Clin. J. Am. Soc. Nephrol.* **2008**, *3*, 153–158. [CrossRef] [PubMed]
21. Adamska-Wełnicka, A.; Wełnicki, M.; Krzesiński, P.; Niemczyk, S.; Lubas, A. Multi-method complex approach for hydration assessment does not detect a hydration difference in hemodialysis versus peritoneal dialysis patient. *Diagnostics* **2020**, *10*, 767. [CrossRef] [PubMed]
22. House, A.A.; Wanner, C.; Sarnak, M.J.; Piña, I.L.; McIntyre, C.W.; Komenda, P.; Kasiske, B.L.; Deswal, A.; deFilippi, C.R.; Cleland, J.; et al. Heart failure in chronic kidney disease: Conclusions from a kidney disease: Improving Global Outcomes (KDIGO) Controversies Conference. *Kidney Int.* **2019**, *95*, 1304–1317. [CrossRef] [PubMed]
23. Vickery, S.; Price, C.P.; John, R.I.; Abbas, N.A.; Webb, M.C.; Kempson, M.E.; Lamb, E.J. B-type natriuretic peptide (BNP) and amino-terminal proBNP in patients with CKD: Relationship to renal function and left ventricular hypertrophy. *Am. J. Kidney Dis. Off. J. Natl. Kidney Found.* **2005**, *46*, 610–620. [CrossRef]
24. Sato, Y. Diagnostic and prognostic property of NT-proBNP in patients with renal dysfunction. *J. Cardiol.* **2013**, *61*, 446–447. [CrossRef]
25. McCullough, P.A.; Duc, P.; Omland, T.; McCord, J.; Nowak, R.M.; Hollander, J.E.; Herrmann, H.C.; Steg, P.G.; Westheim, A.; Knudsen, C.W.; et al. B-type natriuretic peptide and renal function in the diagnosis of heart failure: An analysis from the breathing not properly multinational study. *Am. J. Kidney Dis.* **2003**, *41*, 571–579. [CrossRef]
26. Mueller, C.; McDonald, K.; de Boer, R.A.; Maisel, A.; Cleland, J.; Kozhuharov, N.; Coats, A.; Metra, M.; Mebazaa, A.; Ruschitzka, F.; et al. Heart Failure Association of the European Society of Cardiology practical guidance on the use of natriuretic peptide concentrations. *Eur. J. Heart Fail.* **2019**, *21*, 715–731. [CrossRef]
27. Kim, S.E.; Park, S.; Kim, J.K.; Kim, S.G.; Kim, H.J.; Song, Y.R. B-type natriuretic peptide predicts an ischemic etiology of acute heart failure in patients with stage 4-5 chronic kidney disease. *Clin. Biochem.* **2014**, *47*, 344–348. [CrossRef] [PubMed]
28. Horii, M.; Matsumoto, T.; Uemura, S.; Sugawara, Y.; Takitsume, A.; Ueda, T.; Nakagawa, H.; Nishida, T.; Soeda, T.; Okayama, S.; et al. Prognostic value of B-type natriuretic peptide and its amino-terminal proBNP fragment for cardiovascular events with stratification by renal function. *J. Cardiol.* **2013**, *61*, 410–416. [CrossRef] [PubMed]
29. Hayashi, T.; Yasuda, K.; Kimura, T.; Sasaki, K.; Shimada, K.; Hashimoto, N.; Isaka, Y. Prognostic significance of asymptomatic brain natriuretic peptide elevation at nephrology referral in patients with chronic kidney disease. *Am. J. Nephrol.* **2018**, *48*, 205–213. [CrossRef]
30. Şimşek, M.A.; Değertekin, M.; Türer Cabbar, A.; Hünük, B.; Aktürk, S.; Erdoğmuş, S.; Mutlu, B.; Kozan, Ö. NT-proBNP level in stage 3-4 chronic kidney disease and mortality in long-term follow-up: HAPPY study subgroup analysis. *Turk. Kardiyol. Dern. Ars.* **2020**, *48*, 454–460. [CrossRef]
31. Hickman, P.E.; McGill, D.A.; Talaulikar, G.; Hiremagalur, B.; Bromley, J.; Rahman, A.; Koerbin, G.; Southcott, E.; Potter, J.M. Prognostic efficacy of cardiac biomarkers for mortality in dialysis patients. *Intern. Med. J.* **2009**, *39*, 812–818. [CrossRef]
32. Tsai, Y.C.; Tsai, H.J.; Lee, C.S.; Chiu, Y.W.; Kuo, H.T.; Lee, S.C.; Chen, T.H.; Kuo, M.C. The interaction between N-terminal pro-brain natriuretic peptide and fluid status in adverse clinical outcomes of late stages of chronic kidney disease. *PLoS ONE* **2018**, *13*, e0202733. [CrossRef]

33. Scheen, V.; Bhalla, V.; Tulua Tata, A. The use of B-type natriuretic peptide to assess volume status in patients with end-stage renal disease. *Am. Heart J.* **2007**, *153*, 244.e1–244.e5. [CrossRef]
34. Somer, C.; Heckle, S.; Schwenger, V. Cardiac biomarkers are influenced by dialysis characteristics. *Clin. Nephrol.* **2007**, *68*, 392–400. [CrossRef]
35. Kalloo, S.; Blake, P.G.; Wish, J. A patient centered approach to hemodialysis vascular access in the era of fistula first. *Semin. Dial.* **2016**, *29*, 148–157. [CrossRef] [PubMed]
36. Collins, A.J.; Foley, R.N.; Gilbertson, D.T.; Chen, S.C. The state of chronic kidney disease, ESRD, and morbidity and mortality in the first year of dialysis. *Clin. J. Am. Soc. Nephrol.* **2009**, *4*, S5–S11. [CrossRef] [PubMed]
37. Basile, C.; Lomonte, C.; Vernaglione, L.; Casucci, F.; Antonelli, M.; Losurdo, N. The relationship between the flow of arteriovenous fistula and cardiac output in haemodialysis patients. *Nephrol. Dial. Transplant.* **2007**, *23*, 282–287. [CrossRef]
38. Korsheed, S.; Eldehni, M.T.; John, S.G.; Fluck, R.J.; McIntyre, C.W. Effects of arteriovenous fistula formation on arterial stiffness and cardiovascular performance and function. *Nephrol. Dial. Transplant.* **2011**, *26*, 3296–3302. [CrossRef]
39. Reddy, Y.; Obokata, M.; Dean, P.G.; Melenovsky, V.; Nath, K.A.; Borlaug, B. A Long term cardiovascular changes following creation of arteriovenous fistula in patients with end stage renal disease. *Eur. Heart J.* **2017**, *38*, 1913–1923. [CrossRef] [PubMed]
40. Iwashima, Y.; Horio, T.; Takami, Y.; Inenaga, T.; Nishikimi, T.; Takishita, S.; Kawano, Y. Effects of the creation of arteriovenous fistula for hemodialysis on cardiac function and natriuretic peptide levels in CRF. *Am. J. Kidney Dis.* **2002**, *40*, 974–982. [CrossRef]
41. Pandeya, S.; Lindsay, R.M. The relationship between cardiac output and access flow during hemodialysis. *ASAIO J.* **1999**, *45*, 135–138. [CrossRef]
42. Wasse, H.; Singapuri, M.S. High output heart failure: How to define it, when to treat it, and how to treat it. *Semin. Nephrol.* **2012**, *32*, 551–557. [CrossRef]
43. Raza, F.; Alkhouli, M.; Rogers, F.; Vaidya, A.; Forfia, P. Case series of 5 patients with end stage renal disease with reversible dyspnea, heart failure, and pulmonary hypertension related to arteriovenous dialysis access. *Pulm. Circ.* **2015**, *5*, 398–406. [CrossRef] [PubMed]
44. Turner, A.D.; Chen, M.; Dahl, N.; Scoutt, L.; Dardik, A.; Ochoa Chaar, C.I. Intraoperative ultrasound guidance for banding of an arteriovenous fistula causing high cardiac output heart failure. *Ann. Vasc. Surg.* **2020**, *66*, 665.e5–665.e8. [CrossRef]
45. Rao, N.; Worthley, M.; Disney, P.; Faull, R. Dramatic improvement in decompensated right heart failure due to severe tricuspid regurgitation following ligation of arteriovenous fistula in a renal transplant recipient. *Semin. Dial.* **2014**, *27*, E24–E26. [CrossRef]
46. Gumus, F.; Saricaoglu, M.C. Assessment of right heart functions in the patients with arteriovenous fistula for hemodialysis access: Right ventricular free wall strain and tricuspid regurgitation jet velocity as the predictors of right heart failure. *Vascular* **2020**, *28*, 96–103. [CrossRef]
47. Roca-Tey, R. Permanent arteriovenous fistula or catheter dialysis for heart failure patients. *J. Vasc. Access* **2016**, *17*, S23–S29. [CrossRef] [PubMed]
48. Faull, R.; Rao, N.; Worthley, M. Do arteriovenous fistulas increase cardiac risk? *Semin. Dial.* **2018**, *31*, 357–361. [CrossRef]
49. Pietryga, J.A.; Little, M.D.; Robbin, M.L. Sonography of arteriovenous fistulas and grafts. *Semin. Dial.* **2017**, *30*, 309–318. [CrossRef] [PubMed]
50. Sise, M.E.; Courtwright, A.M.; Channick, R.N. Pulmonary hypertension in patients with chronic and end stage kidney disease. *Kidney Int.* **2013**, *84*, 682–692. [CrossRef]
51. Tedford, R.J.; Forfia, P. Hemodynamic evaluation of pulmonary hypertension in chronic kidney disease. *Adv. Pulm. Hypertens.* **2013**, *12*, 82. [CrossRef]
52. Delgado, J.F. Pulmonary circulation in heart failure. *Rev. Esp. Cardiol.* **2010**, *63*, 334–345. [CrossRef]
53. Zhang, Q.; Wang, L.; Zeng, H.; Lv, Y.; Huang, Y. Epidemiology and risk factors in CKD patients with pulmonary hypertension: A retrospective study. *BMC Nephrol.* **2018**, *19*, 70. [CrossRef] [PubMed]
54. Tang, M.; Batty, J.A.; Lin, C.; Fan, X.; Chan, K.E.; Kalim, S. Pulmonary hypertension, mortality, and cardiovascular disease in ckd and esrd patients: A systematic review and meta-analysis. *Am. J. Kidney Dis.* **2018**, *72*, 75–83. [CrossRef] [PubMed]
55. Selvaraj, S.; Shah, S.J.; Ommerborn, M.J.; Clark, C.R.; Hall, M.E.; Mentz, R.J.; Qazi, S.; Robbins, J.M.; Skelton, T.N.; Chen, J.; et al. Pulmonary hypertension is associated with a higher risk of heart failure hospitalization and mortality in patients with chronic kidney disease: The Jackson heart study. circulation. *Heart Fail.* **2017**, *10*, e003940. [CrossRef]
56. Reque, J.; Garcia-Prieto, A.; Linares, T.; Vega, A.; Abad, S.; Panizo, N.; Quiroga, B.; Collado Boira, E.J.; López-Gómez, J.M. Pulmonary hypertension is associated with mortality and cardiovascular events in chronic kidney disease patients. *Am. J. Nephrol.* **2017**, *45*, 107–114. [CrossRef]
57. Guazzi, M.; Naeije, R. Pulmonary hypertension in heart failure: Pathophysiology, pathobiology, and emerging clinical perspectives. *J. Am. Coll. Cardiol.* **2017**, *69*, 1718–1734. [CrossRef]
58. Sandqvist, A.; Schneede, J.; Kylhammar, D.; Henrohn, D.; Lundgren, J.; Hedeland, M.; Bondesson, U.; Rådegran, G.; Wikström, G. Plasma L arginine levels distinguish pulmonary arterial hypertension from left ventricular systolic dysfunction. *Heart Vessels* **2018**, *33*, 255–263. [CrossRef] [PubMed]
59. Petropoulos, T.E.; Ramirez, M.E.; Granton, J.; Licht, C.; John, R.; Moayedi, Y.; Morel, C.F.; McQuillan, R.F. Renal thrombotic microangiopathy and pulmonary arterial hypertension in a patient with late onset cobalamin C deficiency. *Clin. Kidney J.* **2018**, *11*, 310–314. [CrossRef]

60. Imazu, M.; Takahama, H.; Amaki, M.; Sugano, Y.; Ohara, T.; Hasegawa, T.; Kanzaki, H.; Anzai, T.; Mochizuki, N.; Asanuma, H.; et al. Use of serum fibroblast growth factor 23 vs. plasma B type natriuretic peptide levels in assessing the pathophysiology of patients with heart failure. *Hypertens. Res.* **2017**, *40*, 181–188. [CrossRef]
61. Walther, C.P.; Nambi, V.; Hanania, N.A.; Navaneethan, S.D. Diagnosis and management of pulmonary hypertension in patients with ckd. *Am. J. Kidney Dis.* **2020**, *75*, 935–945. [CrossRef]
62. Ghali, J.K.; Wikstrand, J.; Van Veldhuisen, D.J.; Fagerberg, B.; Goldstein, S.; Hjalmarson, A.; Johansson, P.; Kjekshus, J.; Ohlsson, L.; Samuelsson, O.; et al. The influence of renal function on clinical outcome and response to beta-blockade in systolic heart failure: Insights from metoprolol CR/XL randomized intervention trial in chronic HF (MERIT-HF). *J. Card Fail.* **2009**, *15*, 310–318. [CrossRef] [PubMed]
63. CIBIS-II Investigators. The cardiac insufficiency bisoprolol study II (CIBISII): A randomised trial. *Lancet* **1999**, *353*, 9–13. [CrossRef]
64. Cice, G.; Ferrara, L.; D'Andrea, A.; D'Isa, S.; Di Benedetto, A.; Cittadini, A.; Russo, P.E.; Golino, P.; Calabrò, R. Carvedilol increases two-year survival in dialysis patients with dilated cardiomyopathy: A prospective, placebo-controlled trial. *J. Am. Coll. Cardiol.* **2003**, *41*, 1438–1444. [CrossRef]
65. Clark, H.; Krum, H.; Hopper, I. Worsening renal function during renin angiotensin aldosterone system inhibitor initiation and long term outcomes in patients with left ventricular systolic dysfunction. *Eur. J. Heart Fail* **2014**, *16*, 41–48. [CrossRef] [PubMed]
66. Edner, M.; Benson, L.; Dahlström, U.; Lund, L.H. Association between renin-angiotensin system antagonist use and mortality in heart failure with severe renal insufficiency: A prospective propensity score-matched cohort study. *Eur. Heart J.* **2015**, *36*, 2318–2326. [CrossRef]
67. Quach, K.; Lvtvyn, L.; Baigent, C.; Bueti, J.; Garg, A.X.; Hawley, C.; Haynes, R.; Manns, B.; Perkovic, V.; Rabbat, C.G.; et al. The Safety and efficacy of mineralocorticoid receptor antagonists in patients who require dialysis: A systematic review and meta-analysis. *Am. J. Kidney Dis. Off. J. Natl. Kidney Found.* **2016**, *68*, 591–598. [CrossRef] [PubMed]
68. Tseng, W.C.; Liu, J.S.; Hung, S.C.; Kuo, K.L.; Chen, Y.H.; Tarng, D.C.; Hsu, C.C. Effect of spironolactone on the risks of mortality and hospitalization for heart failure in pre-dialysis advanced chronic kidney disease: A nationwide population-based study. *Int. J. Cardiol.* **2017**, *238*, 72–78. [CrossRef]
69. Pfeffer, M.A.; Shah, A.M.; Borlaug, B.A. Heart failure with preserved ejection fraction in perspective. *Circ. Res.* **2019**, *124*, 1598–1617. [CrossRef]
70. Anker, S.D.; Butler, J.; Filippatos, G.; Ferreira, J.P.; Bocchi, E.; Böhm, M.; Brunner-La Rocca, H.P.; Choi, D.J.; Chopra, V.; Chuquiure-Valenzuela, E.; et al. Empagliflozin in heart failure with a preserved ejection fraction. *N. Engl. J. Med.* **2021**, *385*, 1451–1461. [CrossRef]
71. Packer, M.; Anker, S.D.; Butler, J.; Filippatos, G.; Pocock, S.J.; Carson, P.; Januzzi, J.; Verma, S.; Tsutsui, H.; Brueckmann, M.; et al. Cardiovascular and renal outcomes with empagliflozin in heart failure. *N. Engl. J. Med.* **2020**, *383*, 1413–1424. [CrossRef] [PubMed]
72. Heerspink, H.; Stefánsson, B.V.; Correa-Rotter, R.; Chertow, G.M.; Greene, T.; DAPA-CKD Trial Committees and Investigators. Dapagliflozin in patients with chronic kidney disease. *N. Engl. J. Med.* **2020**, *383*, 1436–1446. [CrossRef] [PubMed]

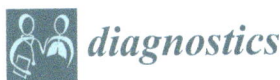

Article

The Interrelationship between Ventilatory Inefficiency and Left Ventricular Ejection Fraction in Terms of Cardiovascular Outcomes in Heart Failure Outpatients

Shyh-Ming Chen [1,*], Lin-Yi Wang [2], Po-Jui Wu [1], Mei-Yun Liaw [2], Yung-Lung Chen [1], An-Ni Chen [3], Tzu-Hsien Tsai [1], Chi-Ling Hang [1] and Meng-Chih Lin [4]

1. Section of Cardiology, Department of Internal Medicine, Kaohsiung Chang Gung Memorial Hospital and Chang Gung University College of Medicine, Kaohsiung 83301, Taiwan; sky1021@cgmh.org.tw (P.-J.W.); feymanchen@yahoo.com.tw (Y.-L.C.); garytsai@adm.cgmh.org.tw (T.-H.T.); samuelhang@hotmail.com (C.-L.H.)
2. Department of Physical Medicine and Rehabilitation, Kaohsiung Chang Gung Memorial Hospital and Chang Gung University College of Medicine, Kaohsiung 83301, Taiwan; s801121@cgmh.org.tw (L.-Y.W.); meiynliaw@cgmh.org.tw (M.-Y.L.)
3. Department of Physical Therapy, Kaohsiung Chang Gung Memorial Hospital, Kaohsiung 83301, Taiwan; anni@cgmh.org.tw
4. Section of Pulmonary and Critical Care Medicine, Department of Internal Medicine and Chang Gung University College of Medicine, Kaohsiung Chang Gung Memorial Hospital, Kaohsiung 83301, Taiwan; mengchih@cgmh.org.tw
* Correspondence: syming99@gmail.com; Tel.: +886-7-731-7123 (ext. 8300)

Received: 16 June 2020; Accepted: 8 July 2020; Published: 10 July 2020

Abstract: The relationship between left ventricular ejection fraction (LVEF) and cardiovascular (CV) outcome is documented in patients with low LVEF. Ventilatory inefficiency is an important prognostic predictor. We hypothesized that the presence of ventilatory inefficiency influences the prognostic predictability of LVEF in heart failure (HF) outpatients. In total, 169 HF outpatients underwent the cardiopulmonary exercise test (CPET) and were followed up for a median of 9.25 years. Subjects were divided into five groups of similar size according to baseline LVEF (≤39%, 40–58%, 59–68%, 69–74%, and ≥75%). The primary endpoints were CV mortality and first HF hospitalization. The Cox proportional hazard model was used for simple and multiple regression analyses to evaluate the interrelationship between LVEF and ventilatory inefficiency (ventilatory equivalent for carbon dioxide (VE/VCO2) at anaerobic threshold (AT) >34.3, optimized cut-point). Only LVEF and VE/VCO2 at AT were significant predictors of major CV events. The lower LVEF subgroup (LVEF ≤ 39%) was associated with an increased risk of CV events, relative to the LVEF ≥75% subgroup, except for patients with ventilatory inefficiency ($p = 0.400$). In conclusion, ventilatory inefficiency influenced the prognostic predictability of LVEF in reduced LVEF outpatients. Ventilatory inefficiency can be used as a therapeutic target in HF management.

Keywords: heart failure; mortality; ejection fraction; cardiopulmonary exercise test; ventilatory inefficiency

1. Introduction

Heart failure (HF) is a leading cause of cardiovascular (CV) mortality and hospitalization. Preventing hospitalization in HF patients, such as using a multidisciplinary treatment strategy, has become a great priority for clinicians, researchers, and policymakers [1]. In addition to clinical demographic risk factors, left ventricular ejection fraction (LVEF) determined by echocardiography is the most commonly used parameter for the diagnosis and management of stable chronic HF patients [2,3]. The relationship between LVEF and CV outcome is well documented in patients with low LVEF HF [4]. However, LVEF is less useful as a prognostic indicator when it is >45% [5,6]. Thus, reliable assessment of prognosis and risk stratification remain challenges in HF outpatients across the full spectrum of LVEF.

The cardiopulmonary exercise test (CPET) is a useful tool in all stages of HF patient management, from diagnosis to risk assessment [7]. In the past several decades, the peak oxygen uptake (peak VO2/kg) from CPET was considered as the best predictor of 1- to 3-year event-free survival after HF [8]. In some patients, ventilatory inefficiency during exercise may be a superior predictor of prognosis compared to peak VO2/kg [9,10].

Pulmonary abnormalities, such as impaired lung mechanics and abnormal alveolar-capillary gas exchange, may be caused by respiratory comorbidities or HF itself [11]. In stable HF outpatients, whether the relationship between LVEF and CV outcome is affected by ventilatory inefficiency remains unknown. In this study, we hypothesized that the presence of ventilatory inefficiency influences the prognostic predictability of LVEF in stable chronic HF patients.

2. Materials and Methods

2.1. Subjects

A retrospective cohort of 169 HF outpatients with exercise intolerance took the CPET at a tertiary referral center between May, 2007, and July, 2010. Patients with concurrent signs and symptoms of HF (New York Heart Association functional class II–IV) and evidence of structural heart disease (increased left atrial size or left ventricle hypertrophy) were recruited consecutively. Diagnosis was established by the attending physicians with elevated cardiac biomarker (BNP > 100 pg/mL). Ischemic cardiomyopathy was defined as HF with the presence of severe coronary artery disease or a history of myocardial infarction. Valvular cardiomyopathy was defined as HF caused by primary disease of one of the four heart valves. Dilated cardiomyopathy was defined as dilation and impaired left ventricle contraction, in which primary and secondary causes of heart disease (e.g., coronary artery disease and myocarditis) were excluded. Patients who had a history of HF hospitalization within 6 months or were unable to perform an exercise test were excluded from the study. The patients were followed up at a median of 9.25 years (interquartile range (IQR), 7.48–10.32 years) since the administration of CPET. LVEF was assessed by quantitative echocardiography using the biplane Simpson method. This study was approved by the Institutional Review Board of the Kaohsiung Chang Gung Memorial Hospital (201701459B0, 13th October 2017) and was conducted in accordance with the Helsinki Declaration of 1975 (as revised in 1983). This study was registered at ClinicalTrials.gov (identifier: NCT04141345). Informed consent was obtained prior to CPET administration in all subjects.

2.2. CPET Procedures

Patients performed an upright graded bicycle exercise using an individualized protocol. The heart rate was continuously monitored by electrocardiography at rest and during exercise. Blood pressure was measured using an electronic sphygmomanometer (SunTech Medical, Morrisville, NC, USA) every 2 min and as needed. The minute ventilation (VE), oxygen consumption (VO2), and carbon dioxide production (VCO2) were continuously recorded every 1 min using a respiratory mass spectrometer (Vmax Encore, VIASYS, Yorba Linda, CA, USA). Prior to each respiratory gas analysis study, the mass spectrometer was calibrated with a standard gas of known concentration. The peak VO2/kg and the peak respiratory exchange ratio (RER) were defined as the highest 30-s average value obtained during exercise. The anaerobic threshold (AT) was determined using the V-slope method. The VE/VCO2 at AT was calculated as the average VE/VCO2 for 1 min during AT and immediately after AT. If the AT could not be determined, the lowest VE/VCO2 was determined by averaging the three lowest consecutive

0.5-min data points. Since the variability of VE/VCO2 at AT is slightly lower than the variability of the slope of VE versus VCO2 below the ventilatory compensatory point [12,13], this study used VE/VCO2 at AT as a marker of ventilatory efficiency. Spirometric measurements included lung vital capacity, forced vital capacity, forced expiratory volume in 1 s, and maximal voluntary ventilation.

The criteria for discontinuing the test were as follows: request by the subject, threatened arrhythmia, peak RER >1.1, and ≥2.0 mm of horizontal or downslope ST segment depression during progressive exercise. The CPET exams were conducted by a qualified physical therapist under the supervision of a physician.

2.3. Outcome Analysis

Defined time-dependent CV outcomes included CV mortality and first HF hospitalization, which were the primary endpoints of the analysis. Study subjects were followed until the end of 2018. HF hospitalization was defined as an unplanned hospitalization due to new or worsening HF requiring the use of intravenous diuretics, inotropes, or vasodilators.

2.4. Statistical Analyses

Subjects were divided into five groups of similar size according to baseline LVEF (≤39%, 40–58%, 59–68%, 69–74%, and ≥75%) by each 20-percentile sample size to evaluate the relationship between LVEF and CV outcomes. Comparisons between LVEF groups were analyzed using Pearson's chi-square test or Fisher's exact test for categorical variables. Continuous variables were expressed as median (IQR). Comparisons between LVEF groups were analyzed using the Kruskal–Wallis test and multiple comparisons for continuous variables. The Kolmogorov–Smirnov test was used to test for normality. For the univariate and multivariable analyses, the hazard ratio and 95% confidence interval were computed using the Cox proportional hazard model. The variables in which p value was <0.1 by univariate analysis were included on multivariate analysis and stepwise method. The primary endpoint was defined as CV mortality or the first HF hospitalization. The comparative results of primary endpoints between patients with LVEF ≥50% (HFpEF–i.e., HF with preserved ejection fraction (EF)) and those with LVEF <50% (non-HFpEF–i.e., mid-range (LVEF 40–49%) and reduced EF (LVEF < 40%)) were analyzed. The various CPET parameters were evaluated as predictors of primary endpoints by performing time-dependent receiver operating characteristic curve (ROC) analyses. Optimized threshold values for VE/VCO2 at AT were identified via ROC analysis and the Youden index. The Cox proportional hazard model was used for simple and multiple regression analyses to evaluate the interrelationship between LVEF and ventilatory inefficiency (defined as VE/VCO2 at AT >34.3, optimized cutoff point). The interaction term "ventilatory inefficiency multiplied by LVEF category" was introduced to the previous model. Kaplan–Meier survival curves were constructed for five groups of patients according to baseline LVEF. Data were analyzed using R v3.6.1 software using "time ROC" and "survival" package and SPSS 22.0 (SPSS Inc., Chicago, IL, USA). In all analyses, a p value of less than 0.05 was considered statistically significant.

3. Results

3.1. Baseline Clinical and Pharmacological Characteristics by LVEF

The mean LVEF in our HF outpatients was 64.0 ± 18.6%. The baseline clinical demographic and pharmacological characteristics according to LVEF are shown in Table 1. Patients with higher EF were more often female and were more likely to have a history of hypertension. Patients with lower EF were more likely to have a history of smoking, ischemic cardiomyopathy, and/or received percutaneous coronary intervention (PCI). Patients who suffered from dilated cardiomyopathy had lower EF. The incidence of diabetes, valvular heart disease, and ischemic stroke did not differ across these LVEF subgroups. The distribution of age also did not differ significantly across the LVEF subgroups. The proportion of patients who received beta-blockers, angiotensin-converting enzyme inhibitors (ACEIs), angiotensin-receptor blockers (ARB), loop diuretics, and mineralocorticoid receptor antagonists (MRAs) increased in the lower EF patients. In contrast, the proportion of patients who received dihydropyridine (DHP) calcium (Ca^+) channel blockers increased in the higher EF patients. The CPET parameters including peak VO2/kg, AT, ΔVO2/ΔWR and VE/VCO2 at AT had a significant difference across the spectrum of LVEF (Table 1).

Table 1. Baseline clinical and pharmacological characteristics by LVEF.

Variables	All Patients (n = 169)	LVEF ≤39% (37)	LVEF 40–58% (31)	LVEF 59–68% (38)	LVEF 69–74% (32)	LVEF ≥75% (31)	p Value
Age	55.7 ± 13.5	50.9 ± 14.7	59.6 ± 12.3	54.3 ± 12.8	57.1 ± 14.6	57.7 ± 11.7	0.097
Male	121 (71.6%)	34 (91.9%)	23 (74.2%)	27 (71.1%)	17 (53.1%)	20 (64.5%)	0.008
Lung disease Both (%)	79 (46.7%)	20 (54.1%)	17 (54.8%)	15 (39.5%)	15 (46.9%)	12 (38.7%)	0.522
Obstructive lung (%)	13 (7.7%)	4 (10.8%)	4 (12.9%)	1 (2.6%)	3 (9.4%)	1 (3.2%)	0.396
Restrictive lung (%)	66 (39.1%)	16 (43.2%)	13 (41.9%)	14 (36.8%)	12 (37.5%)	11 (35.5%)	0.956
Hypertension (%)	99 (58.6%)	13 (35.1%)	23 (74.2%)	23 (60.5%)	19 (65.5%)	21 (72.4%)	0.006
Diabetes (%)	37 (22.7%)	9 (24.3%)	10 (32.3%)	10 (26.3%)	4 (13.8%)	4 (14.3%)	0.355
Smoking (%)	39 (23.5%)	16 (43.2%)	8 (25.8%)	7 (18.4)	5 (16.1%)	3 (10.3%)	0.015
Ischemic stroke (%)	9 (5.6%)	0 (0%)	1(3.2%)	2 (5.3%)	2 (6.9%)	4 (14.3%)	0.158
Ischemic CM (%)	33 (19.5%)	15 (40.5%)	10 (32.3%)	2 (5.3%)	4 (12.5%)	2 (6.5%)	<0.0001
Valvular CM (%)	22 (13.0%)	3 (8.1%)	6 (19.4%)	4 (10.5%)	3 (9.4%)	6 (19.4%)	0.497
Dilated CM (%)	24 (14.2%)	15 (40.5%)	7 (22.6%)	2 (5.3%)	0 (0%)	0 (0%)	<0.0001
Prior PCI (%)	29 (17.2%)	13 (35.1%)	9 (29.0%)	2 (5.3%)	4 (12.5%)	1 (3.2%)	0.001
Medication							
Beta-blocker (%)	97 (58.4%)	30 (81.1%)	25 (80.6%)	19 (50.0%)	12 (38.7%)	11 (37.9%)	<0.0001
ACEI/ARB (%)	114 (67.5%)	32 (86.5%)	28 (90.3%)	21 (55.3%)	15 (46.9%)	18 (58.1%)	<0.0001
DHP Ca^+ channel blocker (%)	36 (21.7%)	1 (2.7%)	10 (32.3%)	5 (13.2%)	11 (35.5%)	9 (31.0%)	0.002
Loop diuretic (%)	43 (25.9%)	22 (59.5%)	13 (41.9%)	3 (7.9%)	4 (12.9%)	1 (3.4%)	<0.0001
MRA (%)	21 (12.4%)	13 (35.1%)	5 (16.1%)	2 (5.3%)	1 (3.2%)	0 (0%)	<0.0001
Statin (%)	53 (31.9%)	13 (35.1%)	9 (29.0%)	12 (31.6%)	10 (32.3%)	9 (31.0%)	0.989
Parameters of CPET							
Peak O2 pulse (mL/beat)	11.9 (9.64–14.89)	11.04 (9.18–15.99)	10.97 (7.78–13.76)	12.16 (9.93–14.92)	12.11 (9.42–15.1)	12.12 (10.11–14.90)	0.303
Peak VO2/kg (mL/kg/min)	22.9 (18.2–28.4)	20.0 (15.9–26.0)	21.3 (16.8–25.1)	25.1 (19.1–29.7)	23.4 (19.5–29.0)	25.5 (19.4–31.9)	0.045
Peak VE (L/min)	54.0 (43.0–65.0)	60.0 (44.5–71.0)	52.0 (37.0–63.0)	59.0 (45.8–68.8)	49.0 (41.0–60.5)	49.0 (43.0–65.0)	0.159
AT (% of VO2 max)	54.9 (45.8–66.2)	50.0 (41.2–60.7)	51.0 (45.7–57.8)	58.2 (49.2–66.4)	56.4 (44.6–73.5)	61.7 (52.2–74.2)	0.007
VE/VCO2 at AT	32.3 (29.2–35.8)	33.4 (29.9–38.1)	34.8 (29.8–37.9)	31.7 (28.8–35.8)	32.0 (28.9–34.1)	30.9 (27.7–33.1)	0.036
Peak RER	1.04 (0.98–1.09)	1.05 (1.02–1.12)	1.02 (0.97–1.09)	1.05 (1.0–1.12)	1.03 (0.96–1.07)	1.04 (0.95–1.07)	0.118
ΔVO2/ΔWR (mL/min/W)	11.6 (9.9–14.3)	10.4 (8.1–12.6)	11.2 (10.2–13.2)	11.8 (9.9–14.4)	11.4 (10.1–14.3)	14.0 (10.8–16.0)	0.015
Peak VO2 (L/min)	1600 (1233–2074)	1528 (1101–2217)	1461 (980–1676)	1668 (1352–2114)	1609 (1245–1982)	1706 (1339–2117)	0.152
Peak Work (Watts)	119.0 (77.5–161.5)	135.0 (69.0–193.5)	96.0 (74.0–125.0)	125.5 (88.5–162.3)	115.5 (79.8–158.5)	123.0 (69.0–158.0)	0.353
Breathing Reserve (L)	28.9 (15.1–42.0)	34.0 (12.8–44.2)	26.2 (10.6–40.0)	30.9 (22.0–42.9)	20.2 (8.5–35.6)	33.2 (18.2–41.6)	0.221

LVEF: left ventricle ejection fraction; CM: cardiomyopathy; PCI: percutaneous coronary intervention; ACEI: angiotensin-converting enzyme inhibitor; ARB: angiotensin receptor blocker; DHP: dihydropyridine; MRA: mineralocorticoid receptor antagonist; CPET: cardiopulmonary exercise test; VO2/kg: oxygen consumption per kilogram; VE: minute ventilation; AT: anaerobic threshold; VE/VCO2 at AT: ventilatory equivalent for carbon dioxide at anaerobic threshold; RER: respiratory exchange ratio; ΔVO2/ΔWR: the ratio of increase in oxygen uptake to increase in work rate.

3.2. Outcomes by LVEF

Within a median follow-up period of 9.25 years (IQR, 7.48–10.32 years), 49 patients achieved our primary endpoints. The relationship between LVEF and the primary endpoints, including CV mortality, is shown in Table 2A. The risk of primary endpoints and CV mortality was increased in the lower LVEF subgroups ($p = 0.002$ and 0.001, respectively). HFpEF patients had better CV outcomes compared with non-HFpEF patients (primary endpoints and CV mortality: $p = <0.0001$ and 0.001, respectively). There were similar CV outcomes of HFpEF who had ventilatory inefficiency and those with non-HFpEF (primary endpoints and CV mortality: $p = 0.792$ and 0.358, respectively) (Table 2B).

Table 2. (**A**) Outcomes by LVEF (5 groups); (**B**) outcomes between HFpEF and non-HFpEF without or with ventilatory inefficiency.

(A)

Variables	All Patients (n = 169)	LVEF ≤39%	LVEF 40–58%	LVEF 59–68%	LVEF 69–74%	LVEF ≥75%	p Value
Primary endpoints	49 (29%)	20 (54.1%)	10 (32.3%)	8 (21.1%)	6 (18.8%)	5 (16.1%)	0.002
Cardiovascular mortality	18 (10.7%)	10 (27.0%)	5 (16.1%)	2 (5.3%)	0 (0%)	1 (3.2%)	0.001

(B)

Variables	Non-HFpEF	HFpEF	p Value	Non-HFpEF with Ventilatory Inefficiency	HFpEF with Ventilatory Inefficiency	p Value
Primary endpoints	27 (48.2%)	22 (19.5%)	<0.0001	17 (58.6%)	15 (51.7%)	0.792
Cardiovascular mortality	12 (21.4%)	6 (5.3%)	0.001	9 (31.0%)	5 (17.2%)	0.358

LVEF: left ventricular ejection fraction; HFpEF: heart failure with preserve ejection fraction (LVEF ≥ 50%); non-HFpEF: heart failure with LVEF <50% (i.e., mid-range (LVEF 40–49%) and reduced ejection fraction (LVEF < 40%); ventilatory inefficiency: VE/VCO2 at AT (ventilatory equivalent for carbon dioxide at anaerobic threshold) >34.3.

3.3. Univariate and Multivariate Analysis of Predictors of Major Cardiovascular Events

Table 3 shows that, according to the univariate Cox regression analysis, the significant predictors of major CV events included comorbidities with lung disease, diabetes, LVEF, or dilated cardiomyopathy, a history of smoking, and treatments with beta-blockers, loop diuretics, or MRAs. The CPET parameters, including VE/VCO2 at AT, ΔVO2/ΔWR, peak O2 pulse, peak VO2, peak VO2/kg, peak work, and AT, were significant predictors for major CV events, based on the univariate analysis. In the multivariate Cox regression analyses and stepwise method, which included those variables in which p was <0.1 by univariate analysis, only LVEF and VE/VCO2 at AT were found to be significant predictors of major CV events in our cohort study (Table 3). The optimized threshold value of VE/VCO2 at AT was identified by ROC analysis. For predicting primary endpoints in all patients, the best cutoff point for VE/VCO2 at AT was 34.3 (64.3 sensitivity and 78.0% specificity, Youden index = 0.42) (Figure 1).

3.4. Adjust Hazard Ratio Associated with LVEF for Major Cardiovascular Events by Baseline LVEF Category Relative to LVEF ≥ 75

As presented in Figure 2, the relationship between LVEF and major CV events was not linear. We defined ventilatory inefficiency as VE/VCO2 at AT >34.3. To characterize the relationship between LVEF and the risk of CV mortality or HF hospitalization among patients with ventilatory inefficiency, subjects were divided into five subgroups according to baseline LVEF. Figure 3 shows the relationship between LVEF and major CV events in patients with ventilatory inefficiency (VE/VCO2 at AT >34.3) and in patients without ventilatory inefficiency (VE/VCO2 at AT ≤34.3). After multivariable adjustment, the Cox proportional hazard model showed that the lower LVEF subgroup (LVEF ≤ 39%) was associated with a significantly increased risk of CV mortality or HF hospitalization relative to the LVEF ≥75% subgroup among patients without ventilatory inefficiency (VE/VCO2 at AT ≤34.3) ($p = 0.019$) and among all patients ($p = 0.002$) (Table 4). Conversely, there was no prognostic predictability relative to low EF (LVEF ≤ 39%) among patients with ventilatory inefficiency (VE/VCO2 at AT >34.3) ($p = 0.400$). However, the interaction effect between LVEF and ventilatory inefficiency in predicting CV major events was not significant ($p = 0.579$). Figure 4 showed the results of Kaplan–Meier analysis of five groups of patients with different LVEF. Among them, only the LVEF ≤39% group showed a significant survival difference ($p = 0.047$ vs. LVEF 40–58%, $p = 0.002$ vs. LVEF 59–68%, $p = 0.001$ vs. LVEF 69–74%, and $p = 0.001$ vs. LVEF ≥75%).

Table 3. Univariate and multivariate analysis of predictors of major cardiovascular events.

Independent Variable	Univariate Analysis			Multivariate Analysis		
	HR	(95% CI)	p Value	HR	(95% CI)	p Value
Age at CPET	1.0	(0.99–1.02)	0.966			
Male	1.66	(0.83–3.33)	0.152			
Lung Disease						
Obstructive	1.45	(0.57–3.65)	0.433			
Restrictive	1.73	(0.99–3.02)	0.057			
Both	1.92	(1.09–3.40)	0.025			
Ischemic stroke	1.56	(0.56–4.44)	0.392			
Myocardial infarction	1.31	(0.66–2.63)	0.442			
Hypertension	0.66	(0.37–1.15)	0.139			
Prior PCI	1.74	(0.91–3.34)	0.096			
Diabetes	2.06	(1.14–3.71)	0.016			
Smoking	1.97	(1.10–3.56)	0.024			
LVEF	0.97	(0.96–0.98)	<0.001	0.98	(0.96–0.99)	0.002
Ischemic cardiomyopathy	1.65	(0.88–3.11)	0.122			
Dilated cardiomyopathy	2.03	(1.04–3.98)	0.039			
Valvular cardiomyopathy	1.37	(0.64–2.92)	0.416			
Beta-blocker	2.24	(1.19–4.22)	0.013			
ACEI/ARB	1.88	(0.96–3.69)	0.064			
DHP Ca^+ channel blocker	0.88	(0.44–1.76)	0.718			
Loop diuretic	3.39	(1.93–5.96)	<0.001			
MRA	4.10	(2.17–7.77)	<0.001			
Statin	1.57	(0.89–2.78)	0.121			
VE/VCO2 at AT	1.19	(1.14–1.25)	<0.001	1.17	(1.12–1.23)	<0.001
ΔVO2/ΔWR (mL/min/W)	1.04	(1.01–1.07)	0.008			
Peak O2 pulse (mL/beat)	0.90	(0.83–0.97)	0.009			
Peak VO2 (L/min)	1.0	(0.99–1.0)	0.001			
Peak RER	0.27	(0.01–5.60)	0.395			
Breathing reserve (mL)	1.00	(0.99–1.01)	0.934			
Peak VE (L/mins)	1.0	(0.98–1.01)	0.731			
Peak VO2/kg (mL/kg/mins)	0.90	(0.85–0.95)	<0.001			
Peak work (Watts)	0.99	(0.99–1.0)	0.009			
Anaerobic threshold	0.95	(0.93–0.97)	<0.001			

Method = forward stepwise selection. HR: hazard ratio; CI: confidence interval; CPET: cardiac pulmonary exercise test; PCI: percutaneous coronary intervention; ACEI: angiotensin-converting enzyme inhibitor; ARB: angiotensin receptor blocker; DHP: dihydropyridine; MRA: mineralocorticoid receptor antagonist; VE/VCO$_2$ at AT: ventilatory equivalent for carbon dioxide at anaerobic threshold; ΔVO2/ΔWR: the ratio of increase in oxygen uptake to increase in work rate; peak VO2: peak oxygen consumption; RER: respiratory exchange ratio; VE: minute ventilation; VO2/kg: oxygen consumption per kilogram; AT: anaerobic threshold.

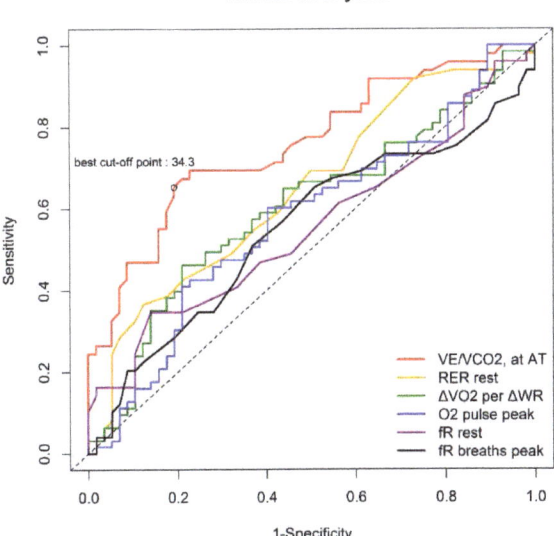

Figure 1. In ROC analyses of different CPET parameters, the only significant predictor of heart failure hospitalization was the VE/VCO2 at AT. Best cut-off point: 34.3, AUROC: 0.756. VE/VCO2 at AT: ventilatory equivalent for carbon dioxide at anaerobic threshold; RER: respiratory exchange ratio; ΔVO2/ΔWR: the ratio of increase in oxygen uptake to increase in work rate; fR rest: resting breathing rate; fR breath peak: peak exercise breathing rate; AUROC: area under receiver operating characteristic curve; CPET: cardiopulmonary exercise test.

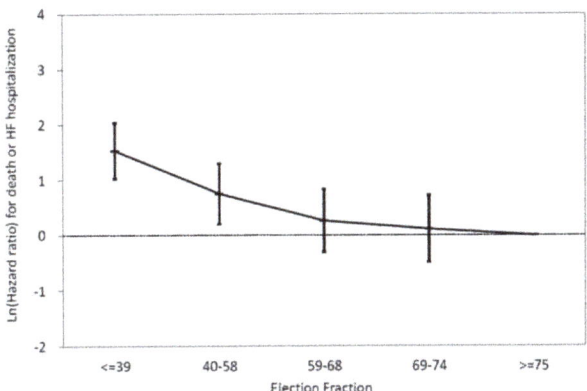

Figure 2. The relationship between LVEF and CV outcomes in all patients. This relationship was not linear. The lower LVEF subgroup (LVEF ≤ 39%) was associated with a significantly increased risk of CV mortality or HF hospitalization relative to the LVEF ≥75% subgroup. ($p = 0.002$). LVEF: left ventricular ejection fraction; CV: cardiovascular; HF: heart failure.

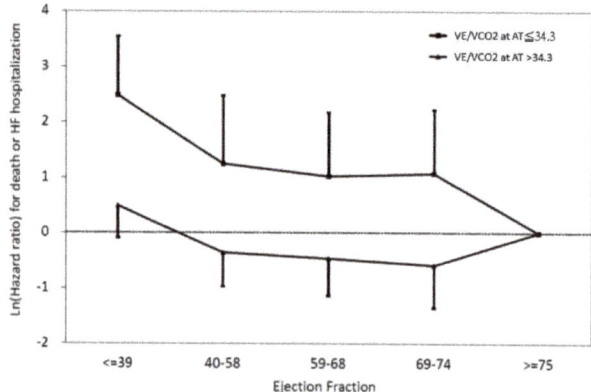

Figure 3. The relationship between LVEF and CV outcomes in patients with ventilatory inefficiency (VE/VCO2 at AT >34.3) and in patients without ventilatory inefficiency (VE/VCO2 at AT ≤34.3). The lower LVEF subgroup (LVEF ≤ 39%) was associated with a significantly increased risk of CV mortality or HF hospitalization relative to the LVEF ≥75% subgroup among patients without ventilatory inefficiency ($p = 0.019$). There was no prognostic predictability relative to low EF (LVEF ≤ 39%) among patients with ventilatory inefficiency ($p = 0.400$). LVEF: left ventricular ejection fraction, CV: cardiovascular, VE/VCO2 at AT: ventilatory equivalent for carbon dioxide at anaerobic threshold, HF: heart failure.

Table 4. Adjust hazard ratio associated with LVEF for major cardiovascular events by baseline LVEF category relative to LVEF ≥75.

LVEF Group	VE/VCO2 at AT ≤34.3 HR (95% CI)	p Value	VE/VCO2 at AT >34.3 HR (95% CI)	p Value	All HR (95% CI)	p Value
≤39	12.00 (1.50–96.01)	0.019	1.63 (0.52–5.08)	0.400	4.63 (1.74–12.35)	0.002
40–58	3.49 (0.32–38.48)	0.308	0.70 (0.21–2.33)	0.561	2.12 (0.73–6.22)	0.169
59–68	2.78 (0.29–26.74)	0.376	0.63 (0.17–2.35)	0.492	1.30 (0.42–3.97)	0.647
69–74	2.92 (0.30–28.11)	0.353	0.56 (0.12–2.50)	0.445	1.12 (0.34–3.66)	0.854
≥75	1		1		1	

Interaction term: p value = 0.579. LVEF: left ventricular ejection fraction; HR: hazard ratio; VE/VCO2 at AT: ventilatory equivalent for carbon dioxide at anaerobic threshold.

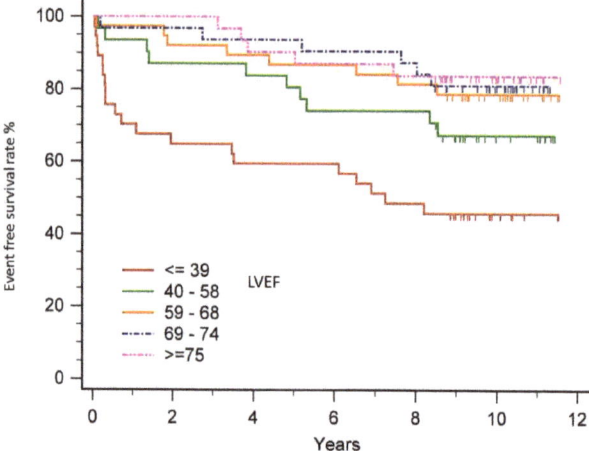

Figure 4. The Kaplan–Meier analysis of five groups of patients with different LVEF. Only patients with LVEF ≤39 had significant survival difference when compared with other groups. LVEF: left ventricular ejection fraction.

4. Discussion

In chronic HF outpatients followed for a median of 9.25 years, LVEF and VE/VCO2 at AT were both found to be significant independent predictors of increased risk of CV mortality or HF hospitalization. LVEF was a poor predictor in patients with ventilatory inefficiency and in those with LVEF >40%. Although our study showed that the interaction effect between LVEF and VE/VCO2 at AT was not significant, the prognostic predictability of LVEF was decreased in the HF with reduced LVEF (HFrEF, LVEF ≤39%) population in the ventilatory inefficiency group. As demonstrated in the CHARM Program [5], the relationship between LVEF and CV outcomes was not linear. We also demonstrated a similar finding in chronic HF outpatients. This relationship was further diminished in the ventilatory inefficiency group. This phenomenon revealed that HFpEF patients who had ventilatory inefficiency had similar CV outcomes as that of their HFrEF counterparts.

This study showed that the ventilation efficiency variable, in addition to LVEF, was a significant prognostic predictor in HF outpatients. Ventilatory inefficiency reflects the adverse effects of HF on lung mechanics and diffusion capacity [14], as HF also augments ventilatory drive and increases hemodynamic demand associated with breathing work [15]. Ergoreceptors stimulate ventilation and activate sympathetic hormones in response to work. The ergoreflex in the muscle also affects ventilatory effort. In response to carbon dioxide and pulmonary J receptors (which likely respond to congestion and alveolar stiffness), central and pulmonary chemoreceptors contribute to the ergoreflex and result in excess ventilation [16]. In HF patients, a high ventilatory drive can reduce the partial pressure of CO_2 (PaCO2) [17]. Consequently, a reduced PaCO2 and increased fractional dead space cause abnormally high VE/VCO2 at AT, i.e., ventilatory inefficiency [18,19].

The mechanism of ventilatory inefficiency influences the outcomes of HF patients differently between the HFrEF and HFpEF patients. A study analyzed the ventilatory inefficiency between 24 HFrEF patients and 33 HFpEF patients [20]. It demonstrated the loss of cardiac output augmentation related to ventilatory inefficiency regardless of LVEF; however, lung congestion parameters (echocardiographic parameter: e' and E/e') correlated with ventilatory inefficiency only in HFpEF. In another study, ventilatory inefficiency appeared to be influenced by mechanisms regulating PaCO2 in HFrEF. In contrast, dead space to tidal volume ratio (VD/VT) played a more important role in developing ventilatory inefficiency in HFpEF [21]. HFpEF and HFrEF may be two distinct entities in terms of ventilatory response to exercise; this study provides evidence that ventilatory inefficiency plays a critical role in HFpEF.

CPET-based measurements of ventilatory inefficiency provide unique physiologic information clinically relevant to contemporary treatment for HF. Several therapeutic interventions for HF affect ventilatory abnormalities both at rest and during exercise. For example, ACEI improves pulmonary diffusion, removes interstitial fluid, and improves pulmonary hemodynamic status [22]. Carvedilol, but not bisoprolol, improves ventilatory efficiency during exercise (reduction of VE/VCO2 slope and increase in maximum end-tidal CO_2 pressure) [23]. Carvedilol may have direct effects on respiratory chemoreceptor activity based on the CARNEBI (CARvedilol vs. NEbivolol vs. BIsoprolol in moderate heart failure) trial [24]. Carvedilol and bisoprolol are both beta-blockers in this study. CPET can be served as a practical guide for the best selection of different beta-blockers. As ventilatory inefficiency is a significant prognostic predictor across the spectrum of LVEF, we should consider ventilatory abnormalities during exercise as therapeutic targets and treat them accordingly. Therapeutic interventions, such as rehabilitation training (isolated quadriceps training) [25], device-guided paced breathing [26], yoga mantras [27], and reduction of afferent stimuli from ergopulmonary and cardiopulmonary receptors [28,29], might all alleviate ventilatory inefficiency. The use of CPET-derived variables to guide therapy and improve outcomes deserves further investigation.

LVEF has proven largely inadequate in correlating HF patients' mortality in heart transplant candidate [30]. However, LVEF is still a good predictor of incident HF in outpatient setting. In the CARE trial, LVEF was the significant predictor of HF attack in 3860 long-term survivors of myocardial infarction [31]. In chronic stable condition, LVEF is a prognostic indicator, as shown in our study.

However, this discriminatory effect of LVEF in predicting morbidity and mortality was limited in HFpEF and patients with ventilatory inefficiency.

This study has some limitations. First, the sample size was relatively small compared to those in other epidemiological studies. However, our study had a longer follow-up period than those of previous works. Second, patients were only recruited from outpatient clinics, which may have caused selection bias. The findings of this study may need further validation in other populations of patients with HF. Third, this study did not analyze other CPET variables that have been used to predict HF outcomes, e.g., oscillatory ventilation, end-tidal CO_2 pressure, VO2 kinetics during exercise, oxygen uptake efficiency slope, and heart rate recovery. Therefore, whether the predictive accuracy of these variables can be increased by combining them with VE/VCO2 at AT requires further investigation. The subgroup of HF patients who had improved LVEF had a more favorable prognosis compared with patients whose LVEF had not changed [32]. However, this study focused on clinically assessed LVEF at baseline, which is the actual measurement used to guide patient care and its relationship with outcomes. The change of LVEF was not used as a variable in our analysis.

5. Conclusions

Ventilatory inefficiency influenced the prognostic predictability of LVEF in HFrEF patients when compared to patients with LVEF ≥75%. The CPET-derived variable (VE/VCO2 at AT) can be used as a therapeutic target in HF management. However, the interaction effect between LVEF and ventilatory inefficiency in predicting CV outcomes was not significant.

Author Contributions: S.-M.C. led the conception and design of study, and revised the draft of the manuscript. L.-Y.W. collected the research data and prepared the draft of the manuscript. P.-J.W., M.-Y.L., and A.-N.C. performed clinical works and organized the collected data. Y.-L.C. and T.-H.T. performed the statistical analysis and drafted the manuscript. C.-L.H. and M.-C.L. supervised and validated the clinical works and results. All authors have read and agreed to the published version of the manuscript.

Funding: This study was supported by a program grant from Chang Gung Medical Foundation (Grant number: CMRPG8H1271).

Acknowledgments: We thank Hsin-Yi Chien, Chih-Yun Lin, and the Biostatistics Center, Kaohsiung Chang Gung Memorial Hospital for statistics work.

Conflicts of Interest: The authors declare that the research was conducted in the absence of any commercial or financial relationships that could be construed as a potential conflict of interests.

References

1. Chen, S.M.; Fang, Y.N.; Wang, L.Y.; Wu, M.K.; Wu, P.J.; Yang, T.H.; Chen, Y.L.; Hang, C.L. Impact of multi-disciplinary treatment strategy on systolic heart failure outcome. *BMC Cardiovasc. Disord.* **2019**, *19*, 220. [CrossRef] [PubMed]
2. Ponikowski, P.; Voors, A.A.; Anker, S.D.; Bueno, H.; Cleland, J.G.; Coats, A.J.; Falk, V.; González-Juanatey, J.R.; Harjola, V.P.; Jankowska, E.A.; et al. 2016 ESC Guidelines for the diagnosis and treatment of acute and chronic heart failure: The Task Force for the diagnosis and treatment of acute and chronic heart failure of the European Society of Cardiology (ESC). Developed with the special contribution of the Heart Failure Association (HFA) of the ESC. *Eur. J. Heart Fail.* **2016**, *18*, 891–975. [CrossRef] [PubMed]
3. Yancy, C.W.; Jessup, M.; Bozkurt, B.; Butler, J.; Casey, D.E.; Drazner, M.H.; Fonarow, G.C.; Geraci, S.A.; Horwich, T.; Januzzi, J.L.; et al. 2013 ACCF/AHA guideline for the management of heart failure: Executive summary: A report of the American College of Cardiology Foundation/American Heart Association Task Force on practice guidelines. *Circulation* **2013**, *128*, 1810–1852. [CrossRef] [PubMed]
4. McDermott, M.M.; Feinglass, J.; Lee, P.I.; Mehta, S.; Schmitt, B.; Lefevre, F.; Gheorghiade, M. Systolic function, readmission rates, and survival among consecutively hospitalized patients with congestive heart failure. *Am. Heart J.* **1997**, *134*, 728–736. [CrossRef]
5. Solomon, S.D.; Anavekar, N.; Skali, H.; McMurray, J.J.; Swedberg, K.; Yusuf, S.; Granger, C.B.; Michelson, E.L.; Wang, D.; Pocock, S.; et al. Influence of ejection fraction on cardiovascular outcomes in a broad spectrum of heart failure patients. *Circulation* **2005**, *112*, 3738–3744. [CrossRef]

6. Pocock, S.J.; Wang, D.; Pfeffer, M.A.; Yusuf, S.; McMurray, J.J.; Swedberg, K.B.; Ostergren, J.; Michelson, E.L.; Pieper, K.S.; Granger, C.B. Predictors of mortality and morbidity in patients with chronic heart failure. *Eur. Heart J.* **2006**, *27*, 65–75. [CrossRef]
7. Paolillo, S.; Agostoni, P. Prognostic Role of Cardiopulmonary Exercise Testing in Clinical Practice. *Ann. Am. Thorac. Soc.* **2017**, *14*, S53–S58. [CrossRef]
8. Mehra, M.R.; Canter, C.E.; Hannan, M.M.; Semigran, M.J.; Uber, P.A.; Baran, D.A.; Danziger-Isakov, L.; Kirklin, J.K.; Kirk, R.; Kushwaha, S.S.; et al. The 2016 International Society for Heart Lung Transplantation listing criteria for heart transplantation: A 10-year update. *J. Heart. Lung Transplant.* **2016**, *35*, 1–23. [CrossRef]
9. Poggio, R.; Arazi, H.C.; Giorgi, M.; Miriuka, S.G. Prediction of severe cardiovascular events by VE/VCO2 slope versus peak VO2 in systolic heart failure: A meta-analysis of the published literature. *Am. Heart J.* **2010**, *160*, 1004–1014. [CrossRef]
10. Kleber, F.X.; Vietzke, G.; Wernecke, K.D.; Bauer, U.; Opitz, C.; Wensel, R.; Sperfeld, A.; Glaser, S. Impairment of ventilatory efficiency in heart failure: Prognostic impact. *Circulation* **2000**, *101*, 2803–2809. [CrossRef]
11. Wasserman, K.; Zhang, Y.Y.; Gitt, A.; Belardinelli, R.; Koike, A.; Lubarsky, L.; Agostoni, P.G. Lung function and exercise gas exchange in chronic heart failure. *Circulation* **1997**, *96*, 2221–2227. [CrossRef]
12. Sun, X.G.; Hansen, J.E.; Garatachea, N.; Storer, T.W.; Wasserman, K. Ventilatory efficiency during exercise in healthy subjects. *Am. J. Respir. Crit. Care Med.* **2002**, *166*, 1443–1448. [CrossRef] [PubMed]
13. Guazzi, M.; Adams, V.; Conraads, V.; Halle, M.; Mezzani, A.; Vanhees, L.; Arena, R.; Fletcher, G.F.; Forman, D.E.; Kitzman, D.W.; et al. EACPR/AHA Scientific Statement. Clinical recommendations for cardiopulmonary exercise testing data assessment in specific patient populations. *Circulation* **2012**, *126*, 2261–2274. [CrossRef] [PubMed]
14. Myers, J.; Arena, R.; Cahalin, L.P.; Labate, V.; Guazzi, M. Cardiopulmonary Exercise Testing in Heart Failure. *Curr. Probl. Cardiol.* **2015**, *40*, 322–372. [CrossRef] [PubMed]
15. Olson, T.P.; Snyder, E.M.; Johnson, B.D. Exercise-disordered breathing in chronic heart failure. *Exerc. Sport Sci. Rev.* **2006**, *34*, 194–201. [CrossRef]
16. Goodlin, S.J. Palliative care in congestive heart failure. *J. Am. Coll. Cardiol.* **2009**, *54*, 386–396. [CrossRef] [PubMed]
17. Rocha, A.; Arbex, F.F.; Sperandio, P.A.; Souza, A.; Biazzim, L.; Mancuso, F.; Berton, D.C.; Hochhegger, B.; Alencar, M.C.N.; Nery, L.E.; et al. Excess Ventilation in Chronic Obstructive Pulmonary Disease-Heart Failure Overlap. Implications for Dyspnea and Exercise Intolerance. *Am. J. Respir. Crit. Care Med.* **2017**, *196*, 1264–1274. [CrossRef] [PubMed]
18. Johnson, R.L., Jr. Gas exchange efficiency in congestive heart failure II. *Circulation* **2001**, *103*, 916–918. [CrossRef]
19. Johnson, R.L., Jr. Gas exchange efficiency in congestive heart failure. *Circulation* **2000**, *101*, 2774–2776. [CrossRef]
20. Tsujinaga, S.; Iwano, H.; Chiba, Y.; Ishizaka, S.; Sarashina, M.; Murayama, M.; Nakabachi, M.; Nishino, H.; Yokoyama, S.; Okada, K.; et al. Heart Failure With Preserved Ejection Fraction vs. Reduced Ejection Fraction—Mechanisms of Ventilatory Inefficiency During Exercise in Heart Failure—. *Circ. Rep.* **2020**. [CrossRef]
21. Van Iterson, E.H.; Johnson, B.D.; Borlaug, B.A.; Olson, T.P. Physiological dead space and arterial carbon dioxide contributions to exercise ventilatory inefficiency in patients with reduced or preserved ejection fraction heart failure. *Eur. J. Heart Fail.* **2017**, *19*, 1675–1685. [CrossRef] [PubMed]
22. Guazzi, M.; Marenzi, G.; Alimento, M.; Contini, M.; Agostoni, P. Improvement of alveolar-capillary membrane diffusing capacity with enalapril in chronic heart failure and counteracting effect of aspirin. *Circulation* **1997**, *95*, 1930–1936. [CrossRef] [PubMed]
23. Agostoni, P.; Apostolo, A.; Cattadori, G.; Salvioni, E.; Berna, G.; Antonioli, L.; Vignati, C.; Schina, M.; Sciomer, S.; Bussotti, M.; et al. Effects of beta-blockers on ventilation efficiency in heart failure. *Am. Heart J.* **2010**, *159*, 1067–1073. [CrossRef] [PubMed]
24. Contini, M.; Apostolo, A.; Cattadori, G.; Paolillo, S.; Iorio, A.; Bertella, E.; Salvioni, E.; Alimento, M.; Farina, S.; Palermo, P.; et al. Multiparametric comparison of CARvedilol, vs. NEbivolol, vs. BIsoprolol in moderate heart failure: The CARNEBI trial. *Int. J. Cardiol.* **2013**, *168*, 2134–2140. [CrossRef] [PubMed]

25. Esposito, F.; Reese, V.; Shabetai, R.; Wagner, P.D.; Richardson, R.S. Isolated quadriceps training increases maximal exercise capacity in chronic heart failure: The role of skeletal muscle convective and diffusive oxygen transport. *J. Am. Coll. Cardiol.* **2011**, *58*, 1353–1362. [CrossRef] [PubMed]
26. Parati, G.; Malfatto, G.; Boarin, S.; Branzi, G.; Caldara, G.; Giglio, A.; Bilo, G.; Ongaro, G.; Alter, A.; Gavish, B.; et al. Device-guided paced breathing in the home setting: Effects on exercise capacity, pulmonary and ventricular function in patients with chronic heart failure: A pilot study. *Circ. Heart Fail.* **2008**, *1*, 178–183. [CrossRef]
27. Bernardi, L.; Sleight, P.; Bandinelli, G.; Cencetti, S.; Fattorini, L.; Wdowczyc-Szulc, J.; Lagi, A. Effect of rosary prayer and yoga mantras on autonomic cardiovascular rhythms: Comparative study. *BMJ* **2001**, *323*, 1446–1449. [CrossRef]
28. Chua, T.P.; Ponikowski, P.P.; Harrington, D.; Chambers, J.; Coats, A.J. Contribution of peripheral chemoreceptors to ventilation and the effects of their suppression on exercise tolerance in chronic heart failure. *Heart* **1996**, *76*, 483–489. [CrossRef]
29. Wensel, R.; Georgiadou, P.; Francis, D.P.; Bayne, S.; Scott, A.C.; Genth-Zotz, S.; Anker, S.D.; Coats, A.J.; Piepoli, M.F. Differential contribution of dead space ventilation and low arterial pCO2 to exercise hyperpnea in patients with chronic heart failure secondary to ischemic or idiopathic dilated cardiomyopathy. *Am. J. Cardiol.* **2004**, *93*, 318–323. [CrossRef]
30. Mehra, M.R.; Kobashigawa, J.; Starling, R.; Russell, S.; Uber, P.A.; Parameshwar, J.; Mohacsi, P.; Augustine, S.; Aaronson, K.; Barr, M. Listing criteria for heart transplantation: International Society for Heart and Lung Transplantation guidelines for the care of cardiac transplant candidates–2006. *J. Heart. Lung Transplant.* **2006**, *25*, 1024–1042. [CrossRef]
31. Lewis, E.F.; Moye, L.A.; Rouleau, J.L.; Sacks, F.M.; Arnold, J.M.; Warnica, J.W.; Flaker, G.C.; Braunwald, E.; Pfeffer, M.A.; Study, C. Predictors of late development of heart failure in stable survivors of myocardial infarction: The CARE study. *J. Am. Coll. Cardiol.* **2003**, *42*, 1446–1453. [CrossRef]
32. Lupón, J.; Díez-López, C.; de Antonio, M.; Domingo, M.; Zamora, E.; Moliner, P.; González, B.; Santesmases, J.; Troya, M.I.; Bayés-Genís, A. Recovered heart failure with reduced ejection fraction and outcomes: A prospective study. *Eur. J. Heart Fail.* **2017**, *19*, 1615–1623. [CrossRef] [PubMed]

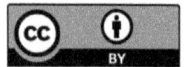

© 2020 by the authors. Licensee MDPI, Basel, Switzerland. This article is an open access article distributed under the terms and conditions of the Creative Commons Attribution (CC BY) license (http://creativecommons.org/licenses/by/4.0/).

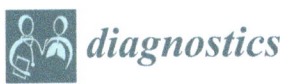

Review

Pulmonary Congestion Assessment in Heart Failure: Traditional and New Tools

Filippo Pirrotta [1], Benedetto Mazza [2], Luigi Gennari [1] and Alberto Palazzuoli [2],*

- [1] Department of Medicine, Surgery and Neurosciences, University of Siena, 53100 Siena, Italy; pirrotta@student.unisi.it (F.P.); luigi.gennari@unisi.it (L.G.)
- [2] Cardiovascular Diseases Unit, Department of Medical Sciences, Le Scotte Hospital, University of Siena, 53100 Siena, Italy; b.mazza@student.unisi.it
- * Correspondence: palazzuoli2@unisi.it; Tel.: +39-577-585-363 or +39-577-585-461; Fax: +39-577-233-480

Abstract: Congestion related to cardiac pressure and/or volume overload plays a central role in the pathophysiology, presentation, and prognosis of heart failure (HF). Most HF exacerbations are related to a progressive rise in cardiac filling pressures that precipitate pulmonary congestion and symptomatic decompensation. Furthermore, persistent symptoms and signs of congestion at discharge or among outpatients are strong predictors of an adverse outcome. Pulmonary congestion is also one of the most important diagnostic and therapeutic targets in chronic heart failure. The aim of this review is to analyze the importance of clinical, instrumental, and biochemical evaluation of congestion in HF by describing old and new tools. Lung ultrasonography (LUS) is an emerging method to assess pulmonary congestion. Accordingly, we describe the additive prognostic role of chest ultrasound with respect to traditional clinical and X-ray assessment in acute and chronic HF setting.

Keywords: heart failure; congestion; clinical assessment

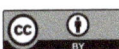

1. Introduction

Congestion occurrence is the primary cause of acute HF (AHF) decompensation, and it is considered the main cause of hospitalization [1]. The clinical assessment evaluating peripheral and central signs of congestion is not accurate enough, and all clinical congestion scores proposed have demonstrated modest accuracy [2,3]. The real challenge is to render an early diagnosis of pulmonary congestion before symptom deterioration in order to reduce the hospitalizations. Traditionally, the most used tools behind clinical evaluation are chest radiography (CRx) and natriuretic peptides (NPs) measurement. However, both methods are poorly available to the general medical practitioner at a patient's home, and they need access to a laboratory or specific clinical wards. Conversely, chest lung ultrasound (LUS) can be performed using a simple echograph with either linear or convex probe, and it does not require a specific skill. B-line counts represent a simple and reliable method to assess pulmonary congestion and to evaluate effective water retention in the lung. A B-line artefact is defined as a laser-like hyperechogenic reverberation arising from the pleural line up to the screen bottom, moving vertically and in synchrony with lung sliding in a way that is similar to that of a comet [4]. Although the screening is relatively simple, there are different methods and approaches to counting the whole number of comets. Some studies used a detailed methodology evaluating 14 different zones for each hemithorax. Other simpler approaches comprise eight- or four-spaces techniques for each chest side [4]. Currently, there is not a gold standard; the examination is usually performed alongside a traditional echocardiographic exam, and the examination depends on the physician's or ultrasound technician's experience and amount of time allocated to spend with each patient. Overall, lung ultrasonography is an emerging tool for evaluating congestion in acute and chronic settings, one that could change the current traditional assessment.

2. Clinical Examination

Physical examination is the first step for the detection of congestion and severity. The search for signs and symptoms, such as jugular vein distention, pulmonary crackles, hepatomegaly, dyspnea at rest, presence of peripheral edema, and additional cardiac sound can reveal the presence of central and systemic congestion. Clinical evaluation is important in the identification of pulmonary congestion, but the specificity and sometimes the sensitivity of the signs and symptoms of pulmonary congestion are often scarce [5]. Dyspnea is the principal symptom that can predict the presence of congestion, but it is common among cardiac, respiratory, and systemic diseases. Indeed, its sensitivity and specificity are very low (66% and 52%, respectively). Peripheral edema is a common consequence of hypoproteinemia: malabsorption and hepatic and renal disorders may configure a similar picture due to low albumin levels and oncotic pressure decrease. Some drugs such as dyidropiridine, a calcium channel blocker, or alpha blockers can lead to a bilateral leg edema. Auscultation of rales or crackles may indicate interstitial pulmonary edema, but it is not present during early phases of decompensation and during chronic pulmonary venous congestion. Therefore, other pulmonary diseases such as interstitial fibrosis or pneumonia may include these signs. Crackles could be found in other pulmonary conditions such as chronic bronchitis, asthma, and emphysema, which can affect lungs at the same time [6]. According to previous studies, combining and grading together all signs and symptoms in a Congestion Score algorithm allows a notable improvement of the diagnostic process. Even though clinical symptoms and signs are late manifestations of congestion, clinical examination is a good approach for predicting 6-month event-free survival in patients with acute decompensation [7–9]. Among patients developing acute decompensated HF, pulmonary congestion (characterized by interstitial and alveolar edema) precedes clinical symptoms and manifestations of congestion. While clinical congestion may be quickly resolved with treatment, pulmonary congestion may persist for longer, and its resolution during hospitalization may be delayed or incomplete despite aggressive diuretics. Furthermore, decompensation could be clinically silent in some patients with chronic heart failure (CHF), and it could remain unrecognized until the occurrence of relevant symptoms requires hospitalization [10]. For these reasons, a more accurate evaluation through the combination of different imaging methods appears the most reliable solution (Figure 1).

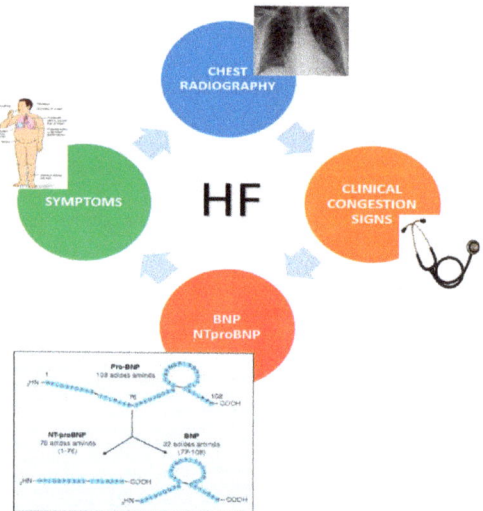

Figure 1. Traditional diagnostic screening for congestion detection in HF: current criteria are based on signs and symptoms, NPs measurement, and chest radiography.

3. Chest Radiography

Chest radiography (CRx) is a fast and inexpensive method performed especially in the Emergency Department (ED) as a first-line diagnostic imaging modality in patients with acute dyspnea [11–13]. However, its diagnostic accuracy for HF has been reported to be relatively low [14,15]. In particular, diagnosing HF in patients with concomitant lung diseases, such as chronic obstructive pulmonary disease (COPD) and pneumonia, still remains challenging. Moreover, the radiographic resolution of the images in some population, such as patients with obesity or bedridden elderly, is significantly reduced. The role of CRx changes in relation to clinical presentation and timing: in a patient with de novo HF, its accuracy remains high, whereas in those with repetitive episodes and recurrence of CHF, in which a chronic pulmonary vein hypertension has occurred, the diagnostic power is less accurate. Similarly, in AHF and CHF, the diagnostic value is debated. Killip's classification is one of the most used modalities to assess heart failure severity in symptomatic patients, and it is used as prognostic scale. CRx allows evaluation of only the most severe Killip classes (III, IV, rarely also II). This demonstrates that the isolated approach with CRx in patients with AHF is useful for the evaluation of the most advanced stages, but it does not recognize the earliest classes, resulting in a delayed diagnosis and possible mistreatment. Although it is useful for detecting pulmonary edema, the absence of other radiological evidence in chronic outpatients does not exclude elevated filling pressure [16]. A serial assessment of a large population admitted in the ED with dyspnea was conducted, and 18% had a negative CRx, while approximately 1 of every 5 subjects with AHF did not demonstrate signs of chest congestion [17]. Therefore, serial CRxs are not recommended in the assessment of pulmonary congestion in CHF. Further limitations of CRx are exposure to radiation, operator-dependent quality, interobserver [18,19] variability, and the detection of only the most extreme extravascular pulmonary water variations [18–20]. For these reasons, supplementary laboratory and diagnostic tests may be warranted.

4. Natriuretic Peptides

B-type natriuretic peptide (BNP) was initially described by Japanese researchers in 1988. An early study, published in 1994, showed that this biomarker could help distinguish between cardiac and non-cardiac causes of dyspnea. Since the initial studies showing the usefulness of NPs for HF diagnosis, a vast number of other clinical applications for these neurohormones have emerged. NPs are now being used in outpatient heart failure clinics, for screening programs, and for risk-prediction algorithms in various settings. Over last 10 years, NPs measurement significantly increased diagnostic sensitivity, and it reduced the diagnostic time process in patients with dyspnea [21]. For these reasons, American and European guidelines introduced these biomarkers into the diagnostic algorithm of patients presenting with AHF. Because of their diagnostic and prognostic power, NPs assays are now also used in chronic setting to evaluate disease status, congestion degree, and response to therapy [22].

These hormones have a very high negative predictive value that allows dyspnea of cardiogenic origin to be ruled out when values are in the normal range. In particular, their contribution is important in the assessment of new-onset heart failure [23]. NPs are not only important for the diagnostic accuracy of HF, but they also provide relevant prognostic information. An elevated cutoff value of NPs at discharge is one of the best mortality predictors. In hospitalized patients, a reduction in NT-proBNP from treatment entry to discharge of less than 30% has been related to an increased probability of rehospitalization and death [24]. Serial BNP measurement was also demonstrated to be an important marker for risk stratification in patients with CHF [25]. Elevated levels are associated with a higher incidence of recurrent episodes of heart failure or sudden death [26]. Plasma NPs values range according to the type of HF and the presence of associated diseases: among patients with similar NYHA class, hormones are reduced in patients with heart failure and preserved ejection fraction (HFpEF) compared with those with heart failure and reduced ejection fraction (HFrEF), but they remain still higher than in controls [27].

NPs elevations are closely related to high cardiac filling pressure values, parietal stress, and distension, which are the most important triggers for hormone release. Throughton et al. [28] evaluated the changes in serum levels of NPs in stable patients with ventricular systolic dysfunction in relation to some echocardiographic parameters including the degree of diastolic dysfunction, the degree of right ventricular dysfunction, and the severity of mitral regurgitation. BNP values were closely correlated with some indices of diastolic dysfunction, such as deceleration time (DT), E/e', and the velocity of the transmitral flow—all the parameters that reflect an increase in filling pressures. Serum levels of NPs increased significantly in accordance with the degree of diastolic dysfunction. Furthermore, the increase in NPs is closely correlated with systolic dysfunction, left ventricle filling pressure pulmonary, hypertension, and right ventricular dysfunction [29,30]. The importance of NPs in the detection of pulmonary congestion must be emphasized, particularly in the forms in which the clinical signs of congestion are scarcely recognizable. Several studies showed that enrolled patients with either AHF or CHF had NPs values at admission, despite the symptoms' absence and negative clinical assessment. Therefore, numerous studies have focused their attention on the correlation between NPs and echocardiography in pulmonary congestion recognition [28,31,32].

Although these blood tests have a very high sensitivity, their specificity remains relatively low. In fact, several features may influence baseline levels: chronic kidney disease, atrial fibrillation, and ischemic heart disease tend to increase the value, whereas other conditions such as obesity and HFpEF showed lower levels. In patients with acute renal failure, NPs levels may be increased independently of the presence of cardiac dysfunction; therefore, diagnosing CHF in this population should rely on more standard criteria. Despite these findings, NT-proBNP has recently been demonstrated to be useful both in diagnosing and excluding CHF across a wide spectrum of renal function, but higher cutoff points may be applied [33].

5. Emerging Role of Chest Ultrasound in HF Diagnosis

Lung ultrasonography (LUS) is a quantitative, simple, economic, and rapid method to assess pulmonary congestion [4]. This diagnostic tool is widely available, particularly in acute settings, while in outpatient primary care it is less practicable due to the limited experience of general doctors and the lack of ultrasounds machines' distribution. Therefore, LUS requires some experience in an accredited echo lab. The association of this tool with clinical and NPs evaluation has greatly increased the diagnostic accuracy of heart failure. LUS consists of the measurement of discrete laser-like vertical hyperechoic reverberation artifacts arising from the pleural line, extending to the bottom of the screen without fading, and moving synchronously with lung sliding [4]. These artifacts are defined as "B-lines" by scanning along the intercostal spaces using either a phased array or curvilinear transducer.

After critical analysis of previous studies, we can discern between two different methods quantifying B-lines: a score approach and a count-based method. The former method considers a minimum number of B-lines for each space as a "positive" zone (typically at least three B-lines) and then adds up the number of positive zones [34,35]. The latter method consists of counting B-lines in each zone and summarizing all B-lines for each lung [36,37]; when comets are confluent between two different zones, their number can be estimated from the percentage of space they occupy on the screen below the pleural line, divided by 10 (i.e., if about 70% of the screen below the pleural line is occupied by B-lines, it would conventionally count as 7 B-lines, up to a maximum of 10 per zone) [38].

The subdivisions of the chest into 8 zones and 28 sub-zones permits the best quantification of B-line count. The eight zones of interest are the anterior and lateral hemi-thoraxes, scanning along the parasternal, midclavicular, anterior axillary, and medium axillary line from the second to the fifth intercostal space on the right hemithorax, and from the second to the fourth intercostal space on the left hemithorax. Each of the mentioned areas are in turn subdivided into four further zones. The subspaces belonging to the fifth left intercostal space are excluded from the count [4].

Nevertheless, the role of congestion in diagnosis of HF has been emerging over last 10 years. Different approaches in different populations and settings and the analysis of patients with various clinical characteristics and different congestion status has led to diversity in terms of cutoffs and scan procedures. The first pioneering study analyzing the additive diagnostic role of chest ultrasound in ambulatory outpatients reported a significant correlation among B-line congestion scores and NPs levels. Therefore, a B-line cutoff >15 was described as a reliable threshold for pulmonary congestion. That report was the first to demonstrate that LUS assessment was a simple and relatively accurate method to assess decompensation [39]. Other studies demonstrated that a total amount of ≤5 B-lines was defined as a normal echographic chest pattern, as it has been reported that healthy patients may have a small number of comets, especially confined laterally to the last intercostal spaces above the diaphragm [40]. Despite these findings, another study of 195 ambulatory patients comparing LUS with clinical congestion evaluation found that a number of >3 B-lines was associated with increased risk of hospitalization or death [37]. Therefore 80% of patients in higher LUS terciles did not show any signs of congestion during clinical examination, and only 19% had crackles at auscultation [37]. Current discrepancies confirm that there are not uniform criteria and that better standardization appears desirable in order to provide a consistent message to clinicians.

Since the diagnostic role and exact threshold in outpatients is debated, LUS assessment in acute care settings is probably much more accurate. Indeed, Coiro et al. describe sixty consecutive acute care patients who underwent clinical echocardiographic and LUS examinations, in which B-lines >30 was associated with improved diagnostic accuracy and predicted a combined end point during 3-month follow-up [41].

In a direct comparison between AHF with either reduced or with preserved ejection fraction, we found a similar number of B-lines in both HF subtypes; although it was slightly higher in those with reduced ejection fraction, the correlation with the other echo parameters of congestion remained similar. Therefore, a cutoff value >32 was predictive of poor outcome. Pellicori et al. showed that a cutoff value of ≥3 B-lines in at least two zones per hemithorax (of six to eight evaluated zones in total) had substantial sensitivity (94–97%) and specificity (96–97%) in patients with AHF—higher than in physical examination, CRx, and NT-proBNP) (sensitivity 85%, specificity 89–90%) [42]. Finally, the last meta-analysis comparing LUS with CRx suggests that B-line counts are more sensitive than radiography in detecting pulmonary edema and that it should be included as an additional modality in patients presenting with acute dyspnea [14].

The role of B-lines in guiding therapy is another interesting field because in theory the serial LUS examination during hospitalization could help in treatment tailoring and congestion grading before discharge. The simple difference between B-line counts at admission and before discharge could guide physicians in therapy optimization. Similarly, in a study conducted by Cortellaro et al., LUS analysis was applied for assessing the effective determination of pulmonary congestion and diuretic response after diuretic therapy during the first 24 h after admission. Significant B-line differences between admission and ongoing treatment was associated with good diuretic response and relevant decongestion [43]. As reported in Platz et al., studying the evaluation of the B-lines at 3 h from admission and from the beginning of therapy showed an improvement in pulmonary congestion, intended as a reduction of the B-lines, and this fact provides a real-time approach to therapy, allowing a better titration of therapy that is based on the type of patient and the severity of the acute congestion. Although in this study a cutoff of 3 h was considered, as far as we know from previous studies, there is no exact cutoff time to evaluate the effect of therapy [44]. The ability to perform a rapid evaluation and to compare the first findings with a subsequent scan is one of the main practical advantages of LUS detection in HF (Table 1) [35,38,42–44].

Table 1. Diagnostic accuracy of different LUS analyses in pulmonary congestion evaluations compared with clinical congestion evaluation NPs measurements and relationship with echocardiographic parameters.

Author of the study	N. patients	B-lines number/score	Congestion signs, n (%)	NT-proBNP/BNP (pg/mL)	Eco parameters admission	Accuracy
			AHF			
Coiro et al. (2015) [41]	60	Assessed on 8 and 28 chest zones. Method: score and count. Score ≥ 3 zone: positive zones. Count: sum of B-lines in all zones > 30	Crackles: 18 (30%); Leg edema: 11 (18%)	BNP: 575 (228.5–1147)	E/E′: 19.11 ± 9.5; IVC diameter (mm): 19.71 ± 5.16; TAPSE (mm): 17.26 ± 3.8; EF (%): 37.5% ± 15	Outcome: composite: 3-month HF hospitalization or death. ≥30 B-lines (HR 5.66, 95% CI 1.74–18.39, $p = 0.04$)
Gargani et al. (2015) [40]	100	Assessed on 28 chest zones. Method: score and count. Score: mild: 6–15 B-lines; moderate: 16–30 B-lines; severe: > 30 B-lines. Count: sum of B-lines in all zones	Not assessed	NT-proBNP: 5291 ± 5877	Pseudonormal pattern 11%; Restrictive pattern 23%; PAPs (mmHg): 49 ± 15; TAPSE (mm): 16.5 ± 4.7	Outcome: composite HF hospitalization or death (mean follow-up 159 days). >15 B-lines- readmission for HF. Sens: 100% spec: 64.8%. >20 B-lines- readmission for HF. Sens: 100% spec: 74.7% NPV: 100%
Cogliati et al. (2016) [45]	149	Assessed on 8 and 28 chest zones. Method: Score (8 zones) Count (28 zones). Score: ≥3 B-lines per zone: positive zone. Count: sum of B-lines in all zones. Count: total B-lines > 15; Total B-lines > 30	Peripheral edema, JVT (jugular vein turgescence) and pulmonary crackles.	NT-proBNP: 2407 ± 1400	E/E′ > 15. 41.6% pz (49) TAPSE (mm): 16.5	Outcome: composite 100-day HF hospitalization or all-cause death. Correlation between the sonographic score and event occurrence (HR 1.19; CI 1.05 to 1.34; $p = 0.005$) increase of 24% the risk of outcome.
Cortellaro et al. (2016) [43]	41	Assessed on 11 chest zones. Method: Score. <3 B-lines in a zone (0 points); ≥3 B-lines in ≥1 zone (1 point); multiple/confluent B-lines (2 points)	Dyspnea, orthopnea, paroxysmal nocturnal dyspnea, rales	NTproBNP: 5867 ± 6112	After therapy: IVC diameter (cm): 1.9 ± 0.5 TAPSE (mm) 20.0 ± 3.5 PAPs (mmHg) 37.2 ± 9.8 E/E′: 14.8 ± 5.2	Mean B-score significantly decreased at T3 (from 1.59 ± 0.40 to 0.73 ± 0.44, $p < 0.001$) and between T3 and T 24 (from 0.73 ± 0.44 to 0.38 ± 0.33, $p < 0.001$).
Palazzuoli et al. (2018) [46]	162	B-line count > 22	Crackles: 140 (86%) Hepatomegaly: 56 (35%) 3th tone: 48 (41%) JVD: 68 (42%) Leg edema: 102 (63%)	BNP HFrEF: 1164 ± 420 BNP HFpEF: 889 ± 130	E/e′: 16 ± 4 TAPSE (mm) 20 ± 4	Sens: 70%; spec: 81%; accuracy: 76%

Table 1. Cont.

			CHF			
Author of the study	N. patients	B-lines number/score	Congestion signs, n (%)	NT-proBNP/ BNP (pg/mL)	Eco parameters admission	Accuracy
Miglioranza et al. (2013) [39]	97	Score $\geq$ 3 zone: positive zone > 15	CCS > 2: 44 (66.7%) s3–s4: 7 (7%)	NT-proBNP: 3070 ± 3100	E/e': 23 ± 16; PAPm: 39.1 ± 10.9;	Combining NT-proBNP > 1000 pg/mL and/or E/e' > 15: yielded a C-statistic of 0.89 for LUS spec: 83.3%; sens: 84.9%; AUC delta: 0.194, 95% CI 0.147, 0.315; p = 0.001 primary outcome
Platz et al. (2016) [37]	185	Assessed on 8 chest zones. Method: count. Sum of B-lines in all zones Score $\geq$ 3 zone: positive zone > 15	Crackles: 35 (19%) JVD: 68 (37%) Leg edema: 65 (35%)	NT-proBNP: 5086 (3023–9248)	EF < or $\geq$ 45%	Outcome: composite: 6-month HF hospitalization or all-cause mortality. AUC delta: 0.132, 95% CI 0.078, 0.213; p < 0.001
Gustafsson et al. (2015) [47]	104	Assessed on 5 chest zones. Method: count and score. Score: $\geq$ 3 B-lines in one zone. Count sum of B-lines in all zones.	Not assessed	NT-proBNP: 1820 ± 1000	IVC diameter (mm): 18 ± 4	Outcome: composite 6-month HF hospitalization or all-cause mortality. B-lines cox proportional HR adjusted for age > 72, NT-proBNP and LV function. B-lines > 3 (HR 2.9 (1.3–6.6), p = 0.11, HR 3.5 (1.5–7.9), 0.003; Age > 72 HR 0.3 (0.2–0.8), p = 14; EF <40% HR 0.7 (0.3–1.6) p = 0.70; NT-proBNP HR 3.5 (1.5–8.5) p = 0.005
Pellicori et al. (2019) [48]	342	Assessed on 28 chest zones. Method: count. B-lines ($\geq$14)	Crackles: 40 (11.7%) JVP: 55 (16.1%) peripheral edema: 103 (30.1%) No signs of congestion: 205 (59.9%)	NT-ProBNP HFrEF: 1494 (684–3502) HFmrEF: 1330 (382–2881) HFpEF: 1100 (354–1994)	JVD RATIO mediana: 5.3 TAPSE (mm) mediana: 19 E/e' lat: mediana: 11 IVC diameter (cm): 2.0	Outcome: (Composite of all-cause mortality or heart failure hospitalization). B-lines-HR: 1.02 (1.01–1.03); Chi2: 26.3; p < 0.001

6. Prognostic Role of Chest Ultrasound

A high number of B-lines at the time of discharge from a hospitalization for AHF or in ambulatory patients with CHF identifies those at high risk of subsequent HF readmissions or death in observational studies [42].

Over the years, several studies have been conducted in order to establish the effectiveness of B-lines in the prognostic evaluation of patients with HF. Gustafsson et al., found that a high number of B-lines assessed by a five-zone method adjusted for age, systolic function, and NT-proBNP identified an increased risk of death or hospitalization after 6-month follow-up [47].

Gargani et al. [40] showed that patients with persistent sonographic pulmonary congestion have an increased risk for rehospitalization for HF in the next 6 months. Patients with ≤15 B-lines before discharge presented a very low risk of rehospitalization. Platz et al. [44] reported that ambulatory HF patients ≥3 B-lines in eight chest zones were at higher risk for HF hospitalization or death over follow-up period of 180 days. Additionally, Coiro et al. showed that in AHF patients LUS examination together with NYHA class and baseline log-BNP was capable of identifying patients with higher risk for rehospitalization [41]. A cutoff ≥30 B-lines at discharge was a very powerful predictor of post-discharge outcome in terms of risk of death, HF hospitalization, and the combined endpoint during 3-month follow-up. Compared with ≥15 B-lines at discharge, Coiro et al. proposed ≥30 B-lines at discharge as the best B-line predictor of outcome, assessed by multivariate analysis [41]. Similarly, Cogliati et al. found that a 1-point increase in the ultrasound score of the B-lines was associated with an approximately 24% adverse event risk increase within 100 days [45]. Current findings highlight the importance of assessing subclinical pulmonary congestion as a potential reason to modify treatment and to reduce the risk of HF hospitalization [40–42,44,45].

In our previous study [46], we identified that a cutoff point of >22 B-lines at discharge did not show significant differences between patients with HFrEF and HFpEF. These threshold differences may have been a result of the time frame of the scan and the effective type of HF congestion that appeared during examination and the start of treatment. Therefore, some associated diseases and comorbidities may affect B-line count. We demonstrated that patients with increased body mass index (BMI) experienced a lower cutoff value compared with those with normal weight [46]. Other situations potentially influencing LUS examination are contemporary presence of pneumonia, interstitial lung disease, or cachectic status with low plasma protein level, in which B-line count could be misinterpreted and overestimated. Thus, although the comet count is a good parameter to estimate the congestion situation [39,41,42], LUS must be contextualized in each specific patient situation. According to current assumptions, it would be useful to outline different profiles based on the variations of B-lines in each patient, evaluating the number of comets at admission, during hospitalization, and at discharge. Establishing a precise timing would also allow better standardization of the scores. Interestingly, a low B-line number is relevant in order to rule out HF diagnosis and congestion: a number <5 B-lines can be a good negative predictor of the presence of pulmonary congestion [40]. However, the opposite is not true.

7. Relevance of Lung Ultrasound in Different Settings

B-LINES IN PRIMARY CARE—Early diagnosis of HF can reduce the number of hospitalizations with related consequences on quality of life and risk. An early diagnosis could be performed in the setting's general population by a specific diagnostic screening, including clinical assessment and rapid ultrasound chest and abdominal scan. Indeed, in primary care (PC), HF diagnosis by simple check-up is difficult because of the symptoms' non-specificity and the late onset of clinical signs of congestion. For this reason, LUS can be an additive, easy, and rapid method for ruling-in patients with a new diagnosis of HF. A recent study evaluating LUS in primary care showed that the evaluation of B-lines in anterior, lateral, and posterior areas demonstrated a positive predictive value (92%) to accurately rule-in HF patients [49]. Associating this value with the negative predictive value of NPs can significantly reduce the diagnostic delay that may lead to treatment delay. Considering that the availability of the NPs assay is not always guaranteed in PC clinics, LUS appears an alternative tool for physicians, and its application may be extended for initial screening of the general population.

B-LINES IN CHF OUTPATIENTS—Since almost 90% of HF recurrence is related to congestion, the presence of pulmonary congestion may identify patients with high risk of HF hospitalization and death [44]. For this reason, lung congestion quantification permits a better stratification of risk in chronic HF patients and can permit the appropriate control and management of CHF patients at follow-up. A recent study including 577 patients showed the importance of B-line count as an independent prognostic factor. Quantifying B-line number in quartiles identifies patients at high risk—in particular, a high number of B-lines identified patients with a 2.6× increased risk of death and rehospitalization [50]. Like PC, outpatients who are followed-up with LUS can achieve a relevant improvement of prognostic stratification by a tailored treatment focused on decongestive therapy optimization that is LUS-guided.

B-LINES AS GUIDE FOR TREATMENT—Treatment with diuretics—in particular, loop diuretics—in patients with HF plays an important role in reducing pulmonary congestion. Because LUS reflects the dynamic variation in pulmonary water content, a serial and repetitive screening could be of relevance in both acute HF and chronic HF patients prone to multiple rehospitalization (Frequent Flyers). Assessment and quantification of pulmonary congestion may help to guide treatment in patients with HF and help to improve their prognosis [51]. Rivas-Lasarte et al. conducted a case-control study, considering 123 patients, divided in a LUS group and a control group. A LUS-guided diuretic therapy titration was performed in the former [52]. Considering hospitalization for worsening HF and all-cause death as primary end points, this study showed a reduced number of decompensations in the LUS group versus an increase of number of urgent visits for those with decompensated HF in control group. Accordingly, another report, found significant improvement of walking capacity observed by the 6 min test in patients monitored by LUS [53]. Diuretic tailoring of dose by a guided-LUS approach can significantly reduce the episodes of HF decompensation, avoiding redundant hospitalization with improvement of quality of life together with diuretic titration optimization.

8. Current GAPS and Potential Applications

Despite the elevated sensitivity of B-line findings in pulmonary congestion assessment, B-line number could change when patients assume different positions: the traditional position for LUS acquisition is a semi-supine standing that allows both the posterior and anterior chest zones to be viewed. This is not always possible in patients with acute dyspnea who cannot assume such a forced position. Another weakness is related to the exam specificity: B-line occurrences are not only proper for use in HF, but they are relevant for use in several pulmonary disease, such as pulmonary fibrosis and COPD, acute respiratory distress syndrome (ARDS) and interstitial pneumonia [40]. A recent new application of chest ultrasound scan has been proposed in COVID-19 patients in order recognize the side and extent of pulmonary infection. Some regions adopted the pulmonary scan for SARS-CoV patient screening and hospitalization decisions. Moreover, in hospitalized patients, the chest scan became an additional tool alongside CRx for chest tomography. However, in these patients, B-lines demonstrated specific characteristics; being mainly located in the subpleural area, the diagnostic differentiation of patients with suspected HF is complex, and it requires additional laboratory and imaging tools [54]. Other concerns are related to BMI. Because higher BMI is associated with more thoracic sub-cutaneous adipose tissue and greater distance between the probe and pleural line, the correct B-lines identification during chest examination can be difficult, and it could result in underestimation. Similar to the NPs, B-line counts tend to decline with increasing BMI [48]. A more universal approach should be recommended; indeed, published research has applied various methodologies with different scan windows and chest areas. This differentiation led to a lack of uniformity and results discrepancies, creating confusion for clinicians and resulting in diagnostic algorithms that are not standardized.

Current weakness may be bypassed using an integrated approach that includes different imaging tools. As reported in a recent study, B-line analysis together with BNP and cava vein distention lead to a more accurate diagnosis and better risk stratification [48]. Current ESC guidelines do not recommend the contemporary use of LUS and inferior cava vein (IVC) diameter for the assessment of volume status; conversely, a toolbox for congestion determination should comprise LUS, central congestion evaluation by echocardiographic assessment, and vascular ultrasound analysis. Recently, some papers have suggested the application of a complete ultrasound score, including a detailed analysis of echo parameters for non-invasive estimation: E/e' is a good mirror of increased left ventricular filling pressure, tricuspid regurgitation is closely related to invasive measurement of systolic pulmonary pressure, integral velocity time of pulmonary flow is related to mean pulmonary artery pressure, and cava vein diameter is a good marker of central vein pressure [55,56]. Thus, the contemporary measurement of all these variables may better define the effective central and peripheral congestion for each patient affected by HF (Figure 2) [34].

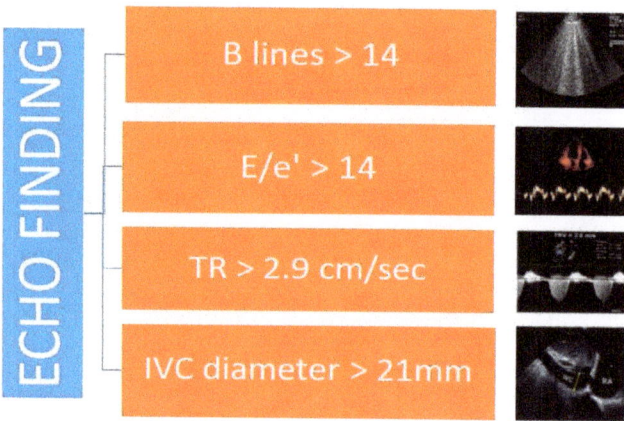

Figure 2. Echographic findings in HF.

Although this diagnostic algorithm may reduce misdiagnosis and the number of false positives, it is only partially applicable in the emergency setting and in ambulatory patients because it requires a specific experience and cardiology competence.

9. Conclusions

Clinical congestion plays a central role in HF exacerbation and in its detection during early-phase avoidance of recurrent hospitalization and functional deterioration. Thus, congestion detection before HF-related symptom occurrence remains a goal for clinical management. Typically, clinical assessment mainly reveals peripheral water retention and increased central venous signs, but it is less specific in the detection of pulmonary congestion. Similarly, the traditional CRx has good accuracy in AHF and in more advanced stages, but it is less accurate in chronic settings. In this framework, LUS demonstrated optimal diagnostic power and good prognostic relevance. Some gaps remain with regard to the different methods and applications as well as to the diagnostic cutoff capable of ruling-in an HF diagnosis. The contemporary assessment of some echocardiographic findings of congestion with B-line assessment may facilitate HF diagnosis and monitoring. The future challenge is to recognize the best available imaging variables of congestion and to apply a standardized algorithm in clinical practice.

Author Contributions: Conceptualization and methodology were carried out by A.P. Validation, writing—review and supervision were made by L.G. Images creation and writing review Resources B.M., data curation, writing—original draft preparation was made by F.P. All authors have read and agreed to the published version of the manuscript.

Funding: This research received no external funding.

Institutional Review Board Statement: Not applicable.

Informed Consent Statement: Not applicable.

Data Availability Statement: Not applicable.

Conflicts of Interest: The authors declare no conflict of interest.

Abbreviations

AHF	Acute Heart Failure
ARDS	Acute Respiratory Distress Syndrome
BNP	Brain Natriuretic Peptide
CHF	Chronic Heart Failure
COPD	Chronic Obstructive Pulmonary Disease
CRX	Chest X-ray
HF	Heart Failure
HFpEF	Heart Failure with Preserved Ejection Fraction
HFrEF	Heart Failure with Reduced Ejection Fraction
IVC	Inferior Cava Vein (IVC)
LUS	Lung Ultrasounds
NPs	Natriuretics Peptides

References

1. Mentz, R.J.; Stevens, S.R.; DeVore, A.D.; Lala, A.; Vader, J.M.; AbouEzzeddine, O.F.; Khazanie, P.; Redfield, M.M.; Stevenson, L.W.; O'Connor, C.M.; et al. Decongestion strategies and renin–angiotensin–aldosterone system activation in acute heart failure. *JACC Heart Fail.* **2015**, *3*, 97–107. [CrossRef]
2. Lok, C.; Morgan, C.D.; Ranganathan, N. The Accuracy and Interobserver Agreement in Detecting the 'Gallop Sounds' by Cardiac Auscultation. *Chest* **1998**, *114*, 1283–1288. [CrossRef]
3. Ambrosy, A.P.; Pang, P.; Khan, S.; Konstam, M.A.; Fonarow, G.; Traver, B.; Maggioni, A.P.; Cook, T.; Swedberg, K.; Burnett, J.C.; et al. Clinical course and predictive value of congestion during hospitalization in patients admitted for worsening signs and symptoms of heart failure with reduced ejection fraction: Findings from the EVEREST trial. *Eur. Heart J.* **2013**, *34*, 835–843. [CrossRef]
4. Volpicelli, G.; Elbarbary, M.; Blaivas, M.; Lichtenstein, D.A.; Mathis, G.; Kirkpatrick, A.W.; Melniker, L.; Gargani, L.; Noble, V.E.; International Liaison Committee on Lung Ultrasound (ILC-LUS) for the International Consensus Conference on Lung Ultrasound (ICC-LUS); et al. International evidence-based recommendations for point-of-care lung ultrasound. *Intensiv. Care Med.* **2012**, *38*, 577–591. [CrossRef]
5. Remes, J.; Mlettinen, H.; Reunanen, A.; Pyörälä, K. Validity of clinical diagnosis of heart failure in primary health care. *Eur. Heart J.* **1991**, *12*, 315–321. [CrossRef] [PubMed]
6. Gheorghiade, M.; Follath, F.; Ponikowski, P.; Barsuk, J.; Blair, J.E.; Cleland, J.G.; Dickstein, K.; Drazner, M.H.; Fonarow, G.; Jaarsma, T.; et al. Assessing and grading congestion in acute heart failure: A scientific statement from the Acute Heart Failure Committee of the Heart Failure Association of the European Society of Cardiology and endorsed by the European Society of Intensive Care Medicine. *Eur. J. Heart Fail.* **2010**, *12*, 423–433. [CrossRef]
7. Beck da Silva, L.; Mielniczuk, L.; Laberge, M.; Anselm, A.; Fraser, M.; Williams, K.; Haddad, H. Persistent orthopnea and the prognosis of patients in the heart failure clinic. *Congest. Heart Fail.* **2004**, *10*, 177–180. [CrossRef] [PubMed]
8. Breidthardt, T.; Moreno-Weidmann, Z.; Uthoff, H.; Sabti, Z.; Aeppli, S.; Puelacher, C.; Stallone, F.; Twerenbold, R.; Wildi, K.; Kozhuharov, N.; et al. How accurate is clinical assessment of neck veins in the estimation of central venous pressure in acute heart failure? Insights from a prospective study. *Eur. J. Heart Fail.* **2018**, *20*, 1160–1162. [CrossRef] [PubMed]
9. Rohde, L.E.; da Silva, L.B.; Goldraich, L.; Grazziotin, T.C.; Palombini, D.V.; Polanczyk, C.A.; Clausell, N. Reliability and prognostic value of traditional signs and symptoms in outpatients with congestive heart failure. *Can. J. Cardiol.* **2004**, *20*, 697–702.
10. Gheorghiade, M.; Filippatos, G.; De Luca, L.; Burnett, J. Congestion in Acute Heart Failure Syndromes: An Essential Target of Evaluation and Treatment. *Am. J. Med.* **2006**, *119*, S3–S10. [CrossRef]

11. Girerd, N.; Seronde, M.F.; Coiro, S.; Chouihed, T.; Bilbault, P.; Braun, F.; Kenizou, D.; Maillier, B.; Nazeyrollas, P.; Roul, G.; et al. Integrative Assessment of Congestion in Heart Failure Throughout the Patient Journey. *JACC Heart Fail.* **2018**, *6*, 273–285. [CrossRef]
12. Chouihed, T.; Manzo-Silberman, S.; Peschanski, N.; Charpentier, S.; Elbaz, M.; Savary, D.; Bonnefoy-Cudraz, E.; Laribi, S.; Henry, P.; Girerd, N.; et al. Management of suspected acute heart failure dyspnea in the emergency department: Results from the French prospective multicenter DeFSSICA survey. *Scand. J. Trauma Resusc. Emerg. Med.* **2016**, *24*, 112. [CrossRef] [PubMed]
13. Ponikowski, P.; Voors, A.A.; Anker, S.D.; Bueno, H.; Cleland, J.G.; Coats, A.J.; Falk, V.; González-Juanatey, J.R.; Harjola, V.P.; Jankowska, E.A.; et al. 2016 ESC Guidelines for the diagnosis and treatment of acute and chronic heart failure: The Task Force for the diagnosis and treatment of acute and chronic heart failure of the European Society of Cardiology (ESC). Developed with the special contribution of the Heart Failure Association (HFA) of the ESC. *Eur. J. Heart Fail.* **2016**, *18*, 891–975. [PubMed]
14. Maw, A.M.; Hassanin, A.; Ho, P.M.; McInnes, M.D.F.; Moss, A.; Juarez-Colunga, E.; Soni, N.J.; Miglioranza, M.H.; Platz, E.; DeSanto, K.; et al. Diagnostic accuracy of point-of-care lung ultrasonography and chest radiography in adults with symptoms suggestive of acute decompensated heart failure: A systematic review and meta-analysis. *JAMA Netw. Open* **2019**, *2*, e190703. [CrossRef]
15. Mueller-Lenke, N.; Rudez, J.; Staub, D.; Laule-Kilian, K.; Klima, T.; Perruchoud, A.P.; Mueller, C. Use of chest radiography in the emergency diagnosis of acute congestive heart failure. *Heart* **2006**, *92*, 695–696. [CrossRef] [PubMed]
16. Chakko, S.; Woska, D.; Martinez, H.; de Marchena, E.; Futterman, L.; Kessler, K.M.; Myerberg, R.J. Clinical, radiographic, and hemodynamic correlations in chronic congestive heart failure: Conflicting results may lead to inappropriate care. *Am. J. Med.* **1991**, *90*, 353–359. [CrossRef]
17. Collins, S.P.; Lindsell, C.; Storrow, A.B.; Abraham, W.T. Prevalence of Negative Chest Radiography Results in the Emergency Department Patient with Decompensated Heart Failure. *Ann. Emerg. Med.* **2006**, *47*, 13–18. [CrossRef]
18. Picano, E. Sustainability of medical imaging. *BMJ* **2004**, *328*, 578–580. [CrossRef] [PubMed]
19. Nieminen, M.S.; Bohm, M.; Cowie, M.R.; Drexler, H.; Filippatos, G.S.; Jondeau, G.; Hasin, Y.; Lopez-Sendon, J.; Mebazaa, A.; Metra, M.; et al. Executive summary of the guidelines on the diagnosis and treatment of acute heart failure: The taskforce on acute heart failure of the European Society of Cardiology. *Eur. Heart J.* **2005**, *26*, 384–416.
20. Hunt, S.A.; Abraham, W.T.; Chin, M.H.; Feldman, A.M.; Francis, G.S.; Ganiats, T.G.; Jessup, M.; Konstam, M.A.; Mancini, D.M.; Keith, K.; et al. ACC/AHA 2005 guideline update for the diagnosis and management of chronic heart failure in the adult. A report of the American College of Cardiology/American heart association task force on practice guidelines (Writing Committee to update the 2001 guidelines for the evaluation and management of heart failure). *J. Am. Coll. Cardiol.* **2005**, *46*, e1–e82.
21. Alan, S.; Maisel, L.; Daniels, B. Breathing Not Properly 10 Years Later: What We Have Learned and What We Still Need to Learn. *J. Am. Coll. Cardiol.* **2012**, *60*, 277–282.
22. Silver, M.A.; Maisel, A.; Yancy, C.W.; McCullough, P.A.; Burnett, J.C., Jr.; Francis, G.S.; Mehra, M.R.; Peacock, W.F., IV; Fonarow, G.; Gibler, W.B.; et al. BNP Consensus Panel 2004: A clinical approach for the diagnostic, prognostic, screening, treatment monitoring, and therapeutic roles of natriuretic peptides in cardiovascular diseases. *Congest Heart Fail.* **2004**, *10*, 1–30. [CrossRef] [PubMed]
23. Palmer, S.C.; Yandle, T.; Nicholls, M.G.; Frampton, C.M.; Richards, A.M. Regional clearance of amino-terminal pro-brain natriuretic peptide from human plasma. *Eur. J. Heart Fail.* **2009**, *11*, 832–839. [CrossRef] [PubMed]
24. Chow, S.L.; Alan, S.M.; Inder, A.; Biykem, B.; de Boer, A.; Felker, M.; Fonarow, G.; Greenberg, B.; Januzzi, J.; Kiernan, M.S.; et al. Role of Biomarkers for the Prevention, Assessment, and Management of Heart Failure. A Scientific Statement from the American Heart Association. *Circulation* **2017**, *30*, 135. [CrossRef] [PubMed]
25. Koglin, J.; Pehlivanli, S.; Schwaiblmair, M.; Vogeser, M.; Cremer, P.; Vonscheidt, W. Role of brain natriuretic peptide in risk stratification of patients with congestive heart failure. *J. Am. Coll. Cardiol.* **2001**, *38*, 1934–1941. [CrossRef]
26. Berger, R.; Huelsman, M.; Strecker, K.; Bojic, A.; Moser, P.; Stanek, B.; Pacher, R. B-Type Natriuretic Peptide Predicts Sudden Death in Patients with Chronic Heart Failure. *Circulation* **2002**, *105*, 2392–2397. [CrossRef] [PubMed]
27. Mueller, C.; Scholer, A.A.; Laule-Kilian, K.; Martina, B.; Schindler, C.; Buser, P.; Pfisterer, M.; Perruchoud, A.P. Use of B-Type Natriuretic Peptide in the Evaluation and Management of Acute Dyspnea. *N. Engl. J. Med.* **2004**, *350*, 647–654. [CrossRef]
28. Troughton, R.W.; Richards, A.M. B-type natriuretic peptides and echocardiographic measures of cardiac structure and function. *JACC Cardiovasc. Imaging* **2009**, *2*, 216–225. [CrossRef]
29. Troisi, F.; Greco, S.; Brunetti, N.D.; Di Biase, M. Right heart dysfunction assessed with echography, B-type natriuretic peptide and cardiopulmonary test in patients with chronic heart failure. *J. Cardiovasc. Med.* **2008**, *9*, 672–676. [CrossRef]
30. Goto, K.; Arai, M.; Watanabe, A.; Hasegawa, A.; Nakano, A.; Kurabayashi, M. Utility of echocardiography versus BNP level for the prediction of pulmonary arterial pressure in patients with pulmonary arterial hypertension. *Int. Heart J.* **2010**, *51*, 343–347. [CrossRef]
31. Palazzuoli, A.; Beltrami, M.; Ruocco, G.; Franci, B.; Campagna, M.S.; Nuti, R. Diagnostic utility of contemporary echo and BNP assessment in patients with acute heart failure during early hospitalization. *Eur. J. Intern. Med.* **2016**, *30*, 43–48. [CrossRef] [PubMed]
32. Dokainish, H.; Zoghbi, W.A.; Lakkis, N.; Al-Bakshy, F.; Dhir, M.; Quinones, M.; Nagueh, S. Optimal Noninvasive Assessment of Left. Ventricular Filling Pressures A Comparison of Tissue Doppler Echocardiography and B-Type Natriuretic Peptide in Patients with Pulmonary Artery Catheters. *Circulation* **2004**, *109*, 2432–2439. [CrossRef] [PubMed]

33. Anwaruddin, S.; Lloyd-Jones, D.M.; Baggish, A.; Chen, A.; Krauser, D.; Tung, R.; Chae, C.; Januzzi, J.L.J. Renal function, congestive heart failure, and amino-terminal pro-brain natriuretic peptide measurement: Results from the Pro-BNP Investigation of Dyspnea in the Emergency Department (PRIDE) Study. *J. Am. Coll. Cardiol.* **2006**, *47*, 91–97. [CrossRef] [PubMed]
34. Pivetta, E.; Baldassa, F.; Masellis, S.; Bovaro, F.; Lupia, E.; Maule, M.M. Sources of Variability in the Detection of B-Lines, Using Lung Ultrasound. *Ultrasound Med. Biol.* **2018**, *44*, 1212–1216. [CrossRef]
35. Pivetta, E.; Goffi, A.; Lupia, E.; Tizzani, M.; Porrino, G.; Ferreri, E.; Volpicelli, G.; Balzaretti, P.; Banderali, A.; Iacobucci, A.; et al. Lung Ultrasound-Implemented Diagnosis of Acute Decompensated Heart Failure in the ED: A SIMEU Multicenter Study. *Chest* **2015**, *148*, 202–210. [CrossRef]
36. Platz, E.; Campbell, R.T.; Claggett, B.; Lewis, E.F.; Groarke, J.D.; Docherty, K.F.; Lee, M.M.Y.; Merz, A.A.; Silverman, M.; Swamy, V.; et al. Lung Ultrasound in Acute Heart Failure: Prevalence of Pulmonary Congestion and Short- and Long-Term Outcomes. *JACC Heart Fail.* **2019**, *7*, 849–858. [CrossRef]
37. Platz, E.; Lewis, E.F.; Uno, H.; Peck, J.; Pivetta, E.; Merz, A.; Hempel, D.; Wilson, C.; Frasure, S.E.; Jhund, P.; et al. Detection and prognostic value of pulmonary congestion by lung ultrasound in ambulatory heart failure patients. *Eur. Heart J.* **2016**, *37*, 1244–1251. [CrossRef]
38. Gargani, L. Ultrasound of the Lungs: More than a Room with a View. *Heart Fail. Clin.* **2019**, *15*, 297–303. [CrossRef]
39. Miglioranza, M.H.; Gargani, L.; Sant'Anna, R.T.; Rover, M.M.; Martins, V.M.; Mantovani, A.; Weber, C.; Moraes, M.A.; Feldman, C.J.; Kalil, R.A.; et al. Lung ultrasound for the evaluation of pulmonary congestion in outpatients: A comparison with clinical assessment, natriuretic peptides, and echocardiography. *JACC Cardiovasc. Imaging* **2013**, *6*, 1141–1151. [CrossRef]
40. Gargani, L.; Pang, P.; Frassi, F.; Miglioranza, M.; Dini, F.L.; Landi, P.; Picano, E. Persistent pulmonary congestion before discharge predicts rehospitalization in heart failure: A lung ultrasound study. *Cardiovasc. Ultrasound* **2015**, *13*, 40. [CrossRef]
41. Coiro, S.; Rossignol, P.; Ambrosio, G.; Carluccio, E.; Alunni, G.; Murrone, A.; Tritto, I.; Zannad, F.; Girerd, N. Prognostic value of residual pulmonary congestion at discharge assessed by lung ultrasound imaging in heart failure. *Eur. J. Heart Fail.* **2015**, *17*, 1172–1181. [CrossRef]
42. Pellicori, P.; Platz, E.; Dauw, J.; ter Maaten, J.M.; Martens, P.; Pivetta, E.; Cleland, J.G.; McMurray, J.J.; Mullens, W.; Solomon, S.D.; et al. Ultrasound imaging of congestion in heart failure: Examinations beyond the heart. *Eur. J. Heart Fail.* **2020**, *23*, 703–712. [CrossRef] [PubMed]
43. Cortellaro, F.; Ceriani, E.; Spinelli, M.; Campanella, C.; Bossi, I.; Coen, D.; Casazza, G.; Cogliati, C. Lung ultrasound for monitoring cardiogenic pulmonary edema. *Intern. Emerg. Med.* **2016**, *12*, 1011–1017. [CrossRef]
44. Platz, E.; Merz, A.; Jhund, P.; Vazir, A.; Campbell, R.; Mcmurray, J. Dynamic changes and prognostic value of pulmonary congestion by lung ultrasound in acute and chronic heart failure: A systematic review. *Eur. J. Heart Fail.* **2017**, *19*, 1154–1163. [CrossRef]
45. Cogliati, C.; Casazza, G.; Ceriani, E.; Torzillo, D.; Furlotti, S.; Bossi, I.; Vago, T.; Costantino, G.; Montano, N. Lung ultrasound and short-term prognosis in heart failure patients. *Int. J. Cardiol.* **2016**, *218*, 104–108. [CrossRef]
46. Palazzuoli, A.; Ruocco, G.; Beltrami, M.; Nuti, R.; Cleland, J.G. Combined use of lung ultrasound, B-type natriuretic peptide, and echocardiography for outcome prediction in patients with acute HFrEF and HFpEF. *Clin. Res. Cardiol.* **2018**, *107*, 586–596. [CrossRef]
47. Gustafsson, M.; Alehagen, U.; Johansson, P. Imaging Congestion with a Pocket Ultrasound Device: Prognostic Implications in Patients with Chronic Heart Failure. *J. Card. Fail.* **2015**, *21*, 548–554. [CrossRef]
48. Pellicori, P.; Shah, P.; Cuthbert, J.; Urbinati, A.; Zhang, J.; Kallvikbacka-Bennett, A.; Clark, A.L.; Cleland, J.G. Prevalence, pattern and clinical relevance of ultrasound indices of congestion in outpatients with heart failure. *Eur. J. Heart Fail.* **2019**, *21*, 904–916. [CrossRef]
49. Conangla, L.; Domingo, M.; Lupón, J.; Wilke, A.; Juncà, G.; Tejedor, X.; Volpicelli, G.; Evangelista, L.; Pera, G.; Toran, P.; et al. Lung Ultrasound for Heart Failure Diagnosis in Primary Care. *J. Card. Fail.* **2020**, *26*, 824–831. [CrossRef]
50. Domingo, M.; Conangla, L.; Lupón, J.; De Antonio, M.; Moliner, P.; Santiago-Vacas, E.; Codina, P.; Zamora, E.; Cediel, G.; González, B.; et al. Prognostic value of lung ultrasound in chronic stable ambulatory heart failure patients. *Rev. Esp. Cardiol.* **2020**. [CrossRef]
51. Hman, J.; Harjola, V.P.; Karjalainen, P.; Lassus, J. Focused echocardiography and lung ultrasound protocol for guiding treatment in acute heart failure. *ESC Heart Fail.* **2018**, *5*, 120–128.
52. Rivas-Lasarte, M.; Alvarez-Garcia, J.; Fernández-Martínez, J.; Maestro, A.; López-López, L.; Gonzalez, E.S.; Pirla, M.J.; Mesado, N.; Mirabet, S.; Fluvià, P.; et al. Lung ultrasound-guided treatment in ambulatory patients with heart failure: A randomized controlled clinical trial (LUS-HF study). *Eur. J. Heart Fail.* **2019**, *21*, 1605–1613. [CrossRef] [PubMed]
53. Lomoro, P.; Verde, F.; Zerboni, F.; Simonetti, I.; Borghi, C.; Fachinetti, C.; Natalizi, A.; Martegani, A. COVID-19 pneumonia manifestations at the admission on chest ultrasound, radiographs, and CT: Single-center study and comprehensive radiologic literature review. *Eur. J. Radiol. Open* **2020**, *7*, 100231. [CrossRef] [PubMed]
54. Palazzuoli, A.; Ruocco, G.; Franci, B.; Evangelista, I.; Lucani, B.; Nuti, R.; Pellicori, P. Ultrasound indices of congestion in patients with acute heart failure according to body mass index. *Clin. Res. Cardiol.* **2020**, *109*, 1423–1433. [CrossRef] [PubMed]

55. Carluccio, E.; Dini, F.L.; Biagioli, P.; Lauciello, R.; Simioniuc, A.; Zuchi, C.; Alunni, G.; Reboldi, G.; Marzilli, M.; Ambrosio, G. The 'Echo Heart Failure Score': An echocardiographic risk prediction score of mortality in systolic heart failure. *Eur. J. Heart Fail.* **2013**, *15*, 868–876. [CrossRef]
56. Bonios, M.J.; Kyrzopoulos, S.; Tsiapras, D.; Adamopoulos, S.N. Ultrasound guidance for volume management in patients with heart failure. *Heart Fail. Rev.* **2019**, *25*, 927–935. [CrossRef]

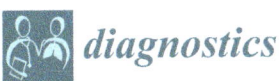

Review

Sodium-Glucose Cotransporter-2 Inhibitors Improve Heart Failure with Reduced Ejection Fraction Outcomes by Reducing Edema and Congestion

Michelle Hernandez [1,2], Ryan D. Sullivan [1], Mariana E. McCune [1], Guy L. Reed [1] and Inna P. Gladysheva [1,*]

[1] Department of Medicine, College of Medicine-Phoenix, University of Arizona, Phoenix, AZ 85004, USA; hernandez.michelle@edu.uag.mx (M.H.); ryansullivan@arizona.edu (R.D.S.); marianamccune@email.arizona.edu (M.E.M.); guyreed@arizona.edu (G.L.R.)
[2] School of Medicine, Universidad Autónoma de Guadalajara, Zapopan 45129, Mexico
* Correspondence: innagladysheva@arizona.edu; Tel.: +1-(602)-827-2919

Abstract: Pathological sodium-water retention or edema/congestion is a primary cause of heart failure (HF) decompensation, clinical symptoms, hospitalization, reduced quality of life, and premature mortality. Sodium-glucose cotransporter-2 inhibitors (SGLT-2i) based therapies reduce hospitalization due to HF, improve functional status, quality, and duration of life in patients with HF with reduced ejection fraction (HFrEF) independently of their glycemic status. The pathophysiologic mechanisms and molecular pathways responsible for the benefits of SGLT-2i in HFrEF remain inconclusive, but SGLT-2i may help HFrEF by normalizing salt-water homeostasis to prevent clinical edema/congestion. In HFrEF, edema and congestion are related to compromised cardiac function. Edema and congestion are further aggravated by renal and pulmonary abnormalities. Treatment of HFrEF patients with SGLT-2i enhances natriuresis/diuresis, improves cardiac function, and reduces natriuretic peptide plasma levels. In this review, we summarize current clinical research studies related to outcomes of SGLT-2i treatment in HFrEF with a specific focus on their contribution to relieving or preventing edema and congestion, slowing HF progression, and decreasing the rate of rehospitalization and cardiovascular mortality.

Keywords: HFrEF; edema; congestion; dilated cardiomyopathy; fluid management; endothelial dysfunction

Citation: Hernandez, M.; Sullivan, R.D.; McCune, M.E.; Reed, G.L.; Gladysheva, I.P. Sodium-Glucose Cotransporter-2 Inhibitors Improve Heart Failure with Reduced Ejection Fraction Outcomes by Reducing Edema and Congestion. *Diagnostics* **2022**, *12*, 989. https://doi.org/10.3390/diagnostics12040989

Academic Editor: Consolato M. Sergi

Received: 6 March 2022
Accepted: 12 April 2022
Published: 14 April 2022

Publisher's Note: MDPI stays neutral with regard to jurisdictional claims in published maps and institutional affiliations.

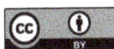

Copyright: © 2022 by the authors. Licensee MDPI, Basel, Switzerland. This article is an open access article distributed under the terms and conditions of the Creative Commons Attribution (CC BY) license (https://creativecommons.org/licenses/by/4.0/).

1. Introduction

Heart failure with reduced ejection fraction (HFrEF) is a complex and progressive clinical syndrome that results from structural or functional impairments of cardiac function (with left ventricular ejection fraction, LVEF ≤ 40%); it is typically associated with elevated natriuretic peptide (NP) levels and objective evidence of pulmonary or systemic edema or congestion [1–3]. Major clinical manifestations of HFrEF include dyspnea, fatigue and, malaise that linked to pulmonary and/or splanchnic congestion and/or peripheral edema [1–10]. HFrEF is a progressive disease ranging from pre-symptomatic stages A (at-risk for HF), B (pre-HF: decline in systolic function); to symptomatic stages C (true HF) and D (advanced HF) [1–3,6,10,11].

Despite progress in management, symptomatic HFrEF remains an irreversible condition that leads inexorably to a poor quality of life, disability and nearly 50% mortality within five years of diagnosis; mechanical circulatory support or heart transplantation being the only definitive curative measures [1–3].

In addition to regulating the neurohumoral system (sympathetic nervous system, SNS; renin-angiotensin-aldosterone system, RAAS; and natriuretic peptides, NPs) [12,13], recent advances in the pharmacological management of HFrEF include sodium-glucose cotransporter-2 inhibitors (SGLT-2i: canagliflozin, dapagliflozin, empagliflozin) [1–3,14,15].

SGLT-2i are a new class of hypoglycemic agents that were FDA-approved for the management of New York Heart Association (NYHA) class II-IV HFrEF, with or without type 2 diabetes mellitus (T2DM) [15]. SGLT-2i function by inhibiting the reabsorption of sodium (Na^+) and glucose in the proximal convoluted tubules of the kidney by SGLT2, thereby increasing urinary excretion of sodium and glucose in a 1:1 ratio and subsequently extracellular water [16,17]. Data from multiple clinical trials including post-hoc, meta and cross-trial analyses, showed that HFrEF patients receiving guideline-directed pharmacological therapy with SGLT-2i had improved cardiovascular outcomes with a significant reduction in the combined risk of cardiovascular death or HF-related hospitalization (HHF) and renal outcomes regardless of T2DM status [18–35]. These improvements were independent from co-administration of guideline-directed HF therapy [32,36]. The glucosuria and reduced glycemic levels are insufficient to explain the overwhelming benefits of SGLT-2i on cardiovascular outcomes, HHF and survival benefits in HFrEF. The pathophysiologic mechanisms and molecular pathways underlying the benefits of SGLT-2i in HFrEF are complex and have yet to be elucidated [15–17,37–48].

Symptomatic HF is characterized in part by excessive sodium and fluid retention in the interstitial space (interstitium or 'third' space) leading to clinically evident edema/congestion in the lungs (pulmonary edema), or the thoracic cavity (pleural effusion), the abdomen (ascites) and/or dependent extremities (peripheral edema). These clinical manifestations of fluid overload are the primary cause of patient HHF and are associated with significant morbidity and premature mortality [6–9,49–59]. The primary goals of HF management include maintaining normal fluid homeostasis by managing sodium intake, use of HF medication(s) and pharmacological treatment of edema [59].

The aim of this review is to analyze the existing clinical data with the major focus on the potential of SGLT-2i in modulating or preventing fluid retention in patients at risk or active symptomatic HFrEF. Although edema/congestion is associated with poor HF outcomes, clinical diagnosis of edema is often limited to subjective patient symptoms and clinical signs from physical exam. Objective diagnostic imaging, laboratory tools and algorithms for assessment and early identification of edema are limited [8,9,51,56,57,59–67]. Limitations in the quantitative assessment of edema/congestion have hampered the evaluation of direct SGLT-2i edema-related outcomes in clinical studies and clinical trials.

2. Impact of SGLT-2i on Diuretic, Natriuretic and Renal Hemodynamic Outcomes in HFrEF: Focus on Edema/Congestion

The exact mechanism(s) by which SGLT-2i exert beneficial effects on HFrEF outcomes has yet to be elucidated. Currently there are numerous theories and hypothesized mechanisms focusing on cardioprotective benefits of SGLT-2i [15–17,37–48,68]. However, these theories when applied solely, are insufficient to explain the reduction of HHF rate and mortality by SGLT-2i-based therapies in patients with HFrEF.

HF decompensation events related to edema/congestion are the primary cause of the HHF and re-hospitalization. SGLT-2i may reduce HHF rate and benefit patients with HFrEF by concomitant beneficial modulation of pathologically deregulated mechanisms causing an imbalance of salt-water homeostasis manifesting as clinically evident edema/congestion. The mechanisms contributing to edema/congestion attenuation in HFrEF by treatment with SGLT-2i [15–17,37–48,68,69] are summarized on Figure 1.

2.1. Impact of SGLT-2i on Natriuresis and Osmotic Diuresis

SGLT-2i may benefit patients with HFrEF by promotion of natriuresis-suppression of sodium reabsorption in the kidney, which is pathologically increased in HF causing deregulation of salt-water homeostasis manifesting as clinically evident edema, and associated diuresis leading to decongestion.

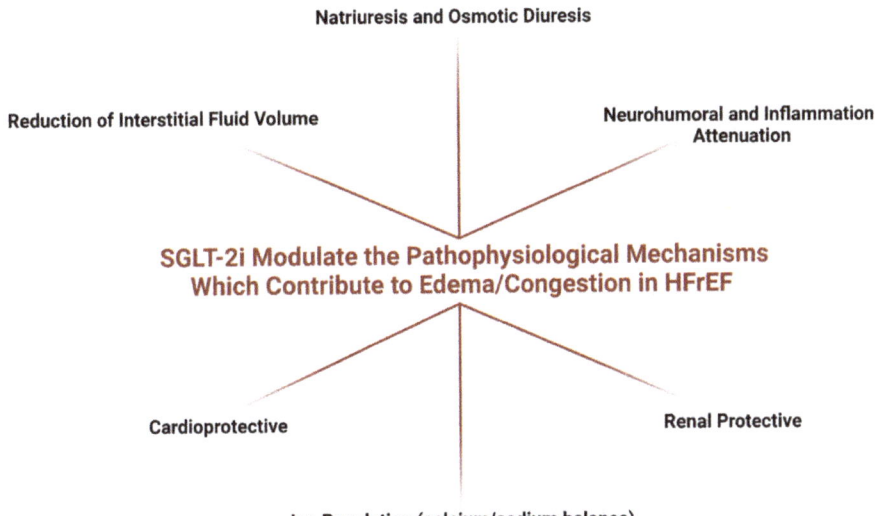

Figure 1. Summary of Mechanisms Contributing to Outcomes of SGLT-2i on Edema/Congestion in HFrEF [15–17,37–48,68,69].

Blockade of the SGLT-2 in the proximal convoluted tubule inhibits the reabsorption of 30–50% of filtered glucose. This effect is accompanied by a significant increase in urinary sodium excretion, leading to a potent combined osmotic diuretic and natriuretic effect and an ensuing favorable reduction in plasma volume, blood pressure, and interstitial fluid volume [28,29,70]. Treatment with dapagliflozin has been associated with a reduction in mean 24-h blood pressure measurements, as well as a greater reduction in body weight and plasma volume compared to hydrochlorothiazide [71]. The beneficial impact of SGLT-2i on these parameters can be attributed to the immediate diuretic action and fluid loss that occurs because of increased urinary sodium and glucose excretion. Prolonged inhibition of SGLT-2 also favorably affects sodium excretion while concurrent activation of compensatory mechanisms, such as increased renin and vasopressin secretion, restores extracellular volume homeostasis, thereby preventing the deleterious effects of excessive diuresis or dehydration [72,73].

The impressive benefits of SGLT-2i on HF outcomes may not be explained by their diuretic effects alone, since other diuretics have not been associated with reduction in HHF and death [44,74]. In fact, prolonged use of loop diuretics in the setting of acute decompensated HF has been linked to worsening outcomes and increased mortality. This is most likely due to the risk of hypotension, electrolyte imbalance, and reduced renal perfusion if inadequately titrated. Reduced arterial filling can further activate RAAS, leading to greater sodium and water retention which can worsen peripheral and pulmonary edema [39,75]. In contrast, treatment with SGLT-2i may control electrolyte balance and renal perfusion that delay or prevent renal hyperfiltration.

2.2. SGLT-2i Reduced Pathological HF-Related Intestinal Fluid Volume Rather Than Blood Plasma Volume

The DAPA-HF trial showed that treatment with dapagliflozin was associated with a larger increase in electrolyte free water clearance compared to a traditional loop diuretic. A mathematical integrated cardiorenal modeling analysis showed that SGLT-2i may generate Na^+-free water clearance and its diuretic mechanism is distinct from other Na^+-driven diuretic classes. Therefore, it was hypothesized that SGLT-2i reduces pathological HF interstitial fluid volume to a greater extent than blood plasma volume [39,76], which is in contrast to other diuretics. This difference may be mediated by peripheral sequestration of osmotically inactive sodium. It has been shown that sodium can be stored in the skin and other tissues, likely by binding with negatively charged proteoglycans [17]. When excess water relative to sodium is removed and sodium concentration within the interstitial compartment rises, peripheral tissues can sequester sodium [39]. This peripheral sequestration of sodium reduces the water volume needed to maintain the equilibrium of sodium concentration between the interstitial and intravascular compartments. This coupled with low cardiac output associated with HFrEF leads to a maladaptive neurohumoral response. If SGLT-2i relieves fluid accumulation in HF by reducing congestion in the interstitial space, arterial filling and organ perfusion may remain intact. Therefore, SGLT-2i may more efficiently impact HF edema/congestion without the deleterious effects from other types of diuretics.

2.3. Impact of SGLT-2i on Renal Function

Renal and cardiovascular hemodynamics are highly interdependent. In primary cardiovascular dysfunction, the heart is unable to adequately pump blood into the systemic circulation, causing prerenal hypoperfusion [77]. The reduced total renal blood flow and glomerular filtration rate (GFR) contribute to increased sodium retention and to edema formation in patients with congestive HF [8,78–80]. Beneficial renal hemodynamic effects of SGLT-2i observed in clinical trials in patients with and without diabetes likely support glycemic-independent nature of such improvement.

SGLT-2i can potentially mitigate the fluid retention that occurs as a result of inadequate renal blood flow. Treatment with SGLT-2i directly affects the physiology of tubuloglomerular feedback. Blockade of SGLT-2-mediated reabsorption of sodium and glucose leads to increased sodium delivery to the distal tubule [81]. Increased sodium concentration activates the juxtaglomerular apparatus and subsequent vasoconstriction of the afferent arteriole. This lowers glomerular hydrostatic pressure and decreases the GFR. Lowering the GFR at the start of treatment with SGLT-2i (GFR normalizes soon after) delays the onset of glomerular hyperfiltration that progressively leads to diabetic nephropathy. Several cardiovascular outcome trials, such as CREDENCE and DAPA-HF, reported a significant reduction in the rate of hyperfiltration at the onset of treatment as well as a long-term reduction in the overall decline of GFR [20,24,81].

Also, it was proposed that SGLT-2i could protect against renal failure by attenuating latent renal congestion by diminishing excessive sodium and water from the interstitial space of the kidney parenchyma. This mechanism might be beneficial even at asymptomatic HF [82].

2.4. Effects of SGLT-2i on Neurohumoral Activation

The pathophysiology of HFrEF involves prolonged activation of the SNS and classical RAAS, compromised angiotensin converting enzyme 2-angiotensin (1–7) axis of RAAS, and impairment of NP system and nitric oxide (NO) pathway associated with accumulation of sodium and body fluid, blood pressure and cardiac remodeling [13,65,83–90]. Reduced cardiac output causes persistent sympathetic activation and a maladaptive cycle that perpetuates fluid retention and edema. There exists evidence to suggest that SGLT-2i may modulate this deleterious sympathetic response. Several clinical trials have shown that treatment with SGLT-2i was not associated with a reflex increase in heart rate in response to blood pressure reduction [48]. This can be considered a marker of sympathetic suppression. Similar findings have been shown in experimental animal studies. Dampening of neurohormonal activation was seen in a group of empagliflozin-treated, nondiabetic pigs with HF. This group had lower plasma levels of norepinephrine catabolites [91].

The diuretic, natriuretic and cardiac hemodynamic outcomes of SGLT-2i associated with reduced congestion in HFrEF patients with and without T2DM might potentially lead to classical RAAS overactivation. However, the data on association between chronic treatment with SGLT-2i and classical RAAS systemic and renal activation are complicated and mostly limited to the patients with T2DM and translational models of T2DM [92].

3. Overview of SGLT-2i Treatment Outcomes Contributing to Edema/Congestion Modulation in HFrEF-Related Clinical Trials

The overall results of the randomized clinical trials strongly support a role for SGLT-2i in the treatment of HFrEF patients independently of their glycemic status and might suggest its effects on maintaining normal fluid homeostasis. Results of HF-associated clinical trials demonstrated benefits on cardiovascular outcomes, renal function, and plasma ANP/BNP and NT-pro-BNP levels with a significant reduction in mortality and HHF and overall quality of life.

3.1. Impact of SGLT-2i on Death and Hospitalization Rates

Reductions in premature mortality and HHF rates are the primarily endpoints in the HFrEF-associated clinical trials. In randomized controlled trials, SGLT-2i added to guideline-directed pharmacological therapy reduced HHF or cardiovascular-related mortality in HFrEF. As HF-related edema is strongly associated with HHF and mortality [5–7,49–52,54,57–60,93–95] a potential SGLT-2i impact on edema attenuation may contribute to the reduction in HHF and premature mortality. The major outcome measures in primary HFrEF clinical trials are summarized in Table 1.

SGLT-2i have become the subject of investigation in several cardiovascular outcome trials within the past six years. Trial data assessing cardiovascular risk in patients with T2DM treated with SGLT-2i has shown possible off target benefits for cardiovascular disease and HF. The EMPA-REG OUTCOME trial demonstrated a significant reduction in the rate of major adverse cardiac events (MACE) in patients with T2DM and established atherosclerotic cardiovascular disease (ASCVD) treated with empagliflozin [18]. The CANVAS trial yielded similar results in the same target population of patient with T2DM and ASCVD treated with canagliflozin [19]. These trials, as well as DECLARE-TIMI and CREDENCE, also demonstrated a significant reduction in the rate HHF [18–20,97]. However, these studies primarily included diabetic patients without evidence of pre-existing HF at baseline. The DAPA-HF (Dapagliflozin and Prevention of Adverse outcome in Heart Failure) trial was a cardiovascular outcome trial designed to assess the effect of SGLT-2i in patients with pre-existing HFrEF, with or without T2DM. The primary outcome of a composite of a first episode of worsening HF (HHF or an urgent visit resulting in IV therapy for HF) or cardiovascular death occurred in 16.3% of patients in the dapagliflozin group versus 21.2% in the placebo group [24]. This finding was significant across all prespecified subgroups, including those with and without T2DM. In this trial, patients experienced less symptoms of HF in the dapagliflozin arm compared to conventional therapy. This was evidenced by improvement in the Kansas City Cardiomyopathy Questionnaire (KCCQ) score. This finding was also homogenous across prespecified subgroups. The EMPEROR-Reduced trial (assessing outcome of empagliflozin in HFrEF) evaluated the same target population as DAPA-HF, however it included patients with markedly reduced EF and elevated NPs [27]. The primary outcome was a composite of HHF or cardiovascular death. The overall combined risk was 25% lower in the empagliflozin group than in the placebo group [27]. Patients in the empagliflozin group were also more likely to experience an improvement in NYHA functional class compared to the placebo group. In the pilot EMPA-RESPONSE-AHF, treatment with empagliflozin reduced a combined endpoint of worsening HF, HHF or death for 60 days in patients with acute HF [29]. Dapagliflozin reduced the risk of total (first and repeat) HHF and cardiovascular death [98]. A post hoc analysis of DAPA-HF showed that in patients with dapagliflozin reduced the risk of sudden death when added to conventional therapy [99]. Dapagliflozin reduced the risk of worsening HF, cardiovascular death, and all-cause death irrespective of sex [100]. Thus, data from the multiple clinical trials show that in HFrEF SGLT-2i improves cardiovascular outcomes with a significant reduction in mortality and HHF regardless of T2DM status [14,18–35,47,97]. A meta-analysis investigating the overall effect of SGLT-2i on cardiovascular outcomes in patients with HF concluded that they significantly reduced the risk of cardiovascular death and HHF by 23%. SGLT-2i were robustly effective in HFrEF subgroup regardless of T2DM and tended to be effective in HFpEF [101].

Table 1. SGLT-2i treatment outcome in primary HFrEF clinical trials.

HF Clinical Trial	Study Population Inclusion Criteria	Major Outcome Measures	Summary
DAPA-HF Dapagliflozin: 10 mg or 5 mg tablets given once daily/up to 27.8 months. McMurray et al., 2019 [24]	• HFrEF (LVEF ≤ 40%), with/without T2DM. • Sample size—4744 • Male/female, ≥18 years • Symptomatic HFrEF (NYHA functional class II–IV), for ≥2 months • LVEF ≤ 40% • Elevated NT-proBNP Patients should receive background OMT for HFrEF according to locally recognized guidelines • eGFR ≥ 30 mL/min/1.73 m² at enrolment	Dapagliflozin vs. pacebo groups: • Composite of a first episode of worsening HF (hospitalization or an urgent visit resulting in IV therapy for HF) or CV death-event rate of 16.3% vs. 21.2%; • Composite of HHF or CV death-lower; (HR = 0.75, 0.65–0.85) • Total number of hospitalizations for HF and CV death-fewer (16.1% vs. 20.9%)	Dapagliflozin reduced HHF and CV death
EMPEROR-REDUCED Empagliflozin: 10 mg/once daily/up to 1040 days Packer et al., 2020 [27]	• Chronic HFrEF (LVEF ≤ 40%), irrespective of diabetes status. • Sample size—3730 • Male/female, ≥18 years • EF ≥ 36% to ≤40%: NT-proBNP ≥ 500 pg/mL or patients without AF and NT-proBNP ≥ 5000 pg/mL for patients with AF • EF ≥ 31% to ≤35%: NT-proBNP ≥1000 pg/mL for patients without AF and NT-proBNP ≥ 2000 pg/mL for patients with AF • EF ≤ 30%: NT-proBNP ≥ 600 pg/mL for patients without AF and NT-proBNP ≥ 1200 pg/mL for patients with AF • EF ≤ 40% and hospitalization for HF in the past 12 months: NT-proBNP ≥ 600 pg/mL for patients without AF and NT-proBNP ≥ 1200 pg/mL for patients with AF	Empagliflozin vs. placebo group: • Reduced hospitalization for worsening HF or CV death; • Overall combined risk was 25% lower in the empagliflozin group • The occurrence of all adjudicated hospitalizations for HF (first and recurrent events)—31% lower; Rate of decline in the eGFR was slower	Empagliflozin reduced HHF and CV death; preserved renal function

Table 1. *Cont.*

HF Clinical Trial	Study Population Inclusion Criteria	Major Outcome Measures	Summary
EMPA-TROPISM Empagliflozin: 10mg/once daily/6 months Santos-Gallegos et al., 2021 [96]	<ul><li>HFrEF</li><li>Sample Size—84</li><li>Male/female, ≥18 years</li><li>Diagnosis of Heart failure (NYHA II to III)</li><li>LVEF < 50% on echocardiography</li><li>cMRI in the previous 6 months</li><li>Have stable symptoms and therapy for HF within the last 3 months.</li></ul>	Empagliflozin vs. placebo group from baseline to 6 months: <ul><li>LV end-systolic volume: 26.6 mL vs. −0.5 mL ($p < 0.001$);</li><li>LV end-diastolic volume: 25.1 vs. −1.5 mL ($p < 0.001$);</li><li>LVEF: 6.0% vs. −0.1% ($p < 0.001$);</li><li>LV mass: −17.8 g/m² vs. 4.1 g/m² ($p < 0.001$);</li><li>Peak VO2: 1.1 mL/kg/min vs. −0.5 mL/kg/min ($p = 0.017$);</li><li>6-min walk test: 82 vs. −35 min ($p < 0.001$).</li></ul>	Empagliflozin improved cardiac function (suggesting cardiac pressure overload improvement) and patient exercise capacity
EMPA-RESPONSE-AHF Empagliflozin: 10 mg/daily/30 days Damman et al., 2020 [29]	<ul><li>Acute HF; Congestive HF with decompensation</li><li>Sample size—80</li><li>Male/female, ≥18 years</li><li>Hospitalized for AHF:<ul><li>Dyspnea at rest</li><li>Signs of congestion, such as edema, rales, and/or congestion on chest radiograph</li><li>BNP ≥ 350 pg/mL or NT-proBNP ≥ 1400 pg/mL (Patients with AF: BNP ≥ 500 pg/mL or NT-proBNP ≥ 2000 pg/mL)</li></ul></li><li>Treated with loop diuretics</li><li>Able to be randomized within 24 h</li><li>Able and willing to provide freely given written informed consent</li><li>eGFR (CKD-EPI) ≥ 30 mL/min/1.73 m²</li></ul>	Empagliflozin vs. placebo group: <ul><li>No difference was observed in VAS dyspnea score, diuretic response, length of stay, or change in NT-proBNP;</li><li>Reduced a combined endpoint of in-hospital worsening HF, rehospitalization for HF or death at 60 days compared with placebo [4 (10%) vs. 13 (33%); $p = 0.014$];</li><li>Urinary output significantly greater [difference 3449 (95% confidence interval 578–6321) mL; $p < 0.01$];</li><li>No adverse effects on blood pressure or renal function.</li></ul>	Empagliflozin reduced HHF; acute setting and small sample size limited results

Dapagliflozin and Prevention of Adverse-outcomes in Heart Failure (DAPA-HF); Empagliflozin Outcome in Chronic Heart Failure with Reduced Ejection Fraction (EMPEROR-REDUCED); Are the "Cardiac Benefits" of Empagliflozin Independent of Its Hypoglycemic Activity? (EMPA-TROPISM); Effects of Empagliflozin on Clinical Outcomes in Patients with Acute Decompensated HF (EMPA-RESPONSE-AHF); Type 2 diabetes mellitus (T2DM); Atherosclerotic cardiovascular disease (ASCVD); Myocardial infarction (MI); Cardiovascular (CV); CV disease (CVD); Hospitalization for heart failure (HHF); Heart failure (HF); Left ventricular ejection fraction (LVEF); Heart failure with reduced ejection fraction (HFrEF); Left ventricular (LV); Estimated glomerular filtration rate (eGFR); Chronic kidney disease (CKD); End-stage renal disease (ESRD); Hazard ratio (HR); Atrial fibrillation (AF).

In summary, randomized clinical trials support the hypothesis that SGLT-2i provides cardiovascular benefits and a reduction in HHF rates via an unknown mechanism in addition to those affecting blood glucose regulation and might suggest that SGLT-2i benefits patients with HFrEF with or without T2DM in part through attenuation of edema/congestion.

3.2. Impact of SGLT-2i on Cardiac Remodeling and Metabolism

The EMPA-TROPISM double-blind, placebo-controlled clinical trial evaluated the effects of empagliflozin on cardiac remodeling in nondiabetic patients with HFrEF [96]. Treatment with empagliflozin was associated with significant reductions in LV end systolic volume and end diastolic volume as well as increased EF and decreased LV mass [96].

A secondary analysis of the comparative cardiac MRI data at baseline and after 6 months of nondiabetic HFrEF patients enrolled in the EMPA-TROPISM clinical trial revealed that empagliflozin significantly improved adiposity (epicardial adipose tissue), interstitial myocardial fibrosis, aortic stiffness [102].

MRI-determined LV end-systolic volume and LV end-diastolic volume index were significantly reduced in another randomized, double-blind, placebo-controlled trial (SUGAR-DM-HF) with HFrEF patients (NYHA functional class II to IV) with prediabetes/diabetes treated with empagliflozin [103].

The EMPA-VISION clinical trial (double-blind, randomized, placebo-controlled) was designed to assess the effects of empagliflozin treatment on cardiac energy metabolism in HFrEF patients with or without T2DM using longitudinal MRI [104]. Additional studies are underway to explore the potential metabolic alterations from SGLT-2i therapy for HFrEF. Important to note, cardiac cachexia and sarcopenia which result from a negative metabolic state of advanced HFrEF, may be an additional source of extracellular water via hydrolysis (See 3.6 for Impacts of SGLT-2i on Fluid Retention).

3.3. Impact of SGLT-2i on Plasma Biomarkers

Plasma levels of ANP/BNP and their NT-pro-forms are strongly associated with HFrEF decompensation related to clinical symptoms from fluid and salt retention and play crucial role in the clinical assessment of decompensation in patients with HF [5,6,105–107].

The impact of the SGLT-2i on a broad range of plasma biomarkers in clinical and pre-clinical HFrEF was comprehensively reviewed [108]. Here, we briefly summarize the influence of SGLT-2i on plasma levels of NPs and inflammatory markers that might indicate congestion status in patients with HFrEF in randomized clinical trials.

In the DEFINE-HF clinical trial, HFrEF patients (NYHA functional class II–III, eGFR $\geq$ 30 mL/min/1.73 m^2, and elevated NT-proBNP) receiving dapagliflozin over 12 weeks did not show difference n mean NT-proBNP, however, there were increases in the proportion of patients with clinically meaningful improvements in KCCQ score or NPs [25]. In DAPA-HF trial treatment of HFrEF patients (NYHA functional class II–IV, increased NT-pro-BNP) with dapagliflozin for 8 months caused significant reduction in NT-proBNP levels (by 300 pg/mL) vs. placebo, which was consistent with a reduction of the risk of HF progression, death and improved HF symptoms [109]. In the EMPEROR-Reduced trial (HFrEF patients with elevated levels of BNP), patients treated with empagliflozin experienced greater reductions in NT-proBNP concentrations compared to placebo. There was also a reduced risk of adverse HF outcomes regardless of baseline NT-proBNP levels [27]. Treatment with empagliflozin significantly reduced plasma ANP/BNP levels when assessed after 1, 3, 6 and 12 months vs. baseline in small randomized study of Japanese patients with chronic HFrEF and T2DM [110]. It is important to note that assessments of the NT-pro-BNP level may be affected by chronic kidney dysfunction (eGFR $\leq$ 60 mL/min/1.73 m^2) [84,111,112], and increased body mass index [88,112].

Chronic sustained inflammation promotes pathological cardiac remodeling, LV dysfunction, pleural/pulmonary/systemic edema in HFrEF [113–115]. Therefore, inflammatory plasma biomarkers might indirectly reflect the congestion status in HFrEF patients. Proteomic analysis revealed that treatment of nondiabetic HFrEF patients with empagliflozin vs. placebo (EMPA-TROPISM clinical trial) was associated with a significant reduction in inflammatory biomarkers [102]. Therapy with SLT-2i decreased plasma levels of inflammatory markers such as tumor necrosis factor-1, fibronectin, and matrix metalloproteinase 7 in patients randomized to canagliflozin vs. glimepiride [116]. These results suggest that SGLT-2i contributes to the suppression of inflammation-related molecular processes and may attenuate associated endothelial dysfunction as supported by preclinical studies [117–119], and therefore prevent vascular leakage which contributes to edema/congestion.

3.4. Impact of SGLT-2i on Renal Function

Chronic renal dysfunction (eGFR ≤ 60 mL/min/1.73 m^2) accelerates HFrEF decompensation and mortality [120–122]. The DAPA-HF trial assessed the safety and efficacy of dapagliflozin in patients with HFrEF with or without T2DM. Treatment with dapagliflozin slowed the rate of decline in eGFR. The benefits of dapagliflozin on morbidity and mortality were not affected by baseline kidney function [123]. The rate of decline in eGFR was slower in the empagliflozin group than in the placebo group in the EMPEROR-Reduced trial [27].

The experimental trials with canagliflozin (CREDENCE) and prespecified subgroup meta-analyses from DAPA-HF (dapagliflozin) and EMPEROR-Reduced (empagliflozin) have demonstrated that SGLT-2i has beneficial effects on renal outcomes in patients with HFrEF regardless of T2DM and chronic kidney disease (CKD) status [32,41,84,85]. Treatment with canagliflozin was associated with 30% reduction in the primary composite outcome of end-stage kidney disease (dialysis, transplantation, or sustained eGFR of <15 mL/min/1.73 m^2) [20]. A secondary composite outcome of ESRD, doubling of serum creatinine, and renal death was reduced by 34% [20]. These improved renal outcomes were observed in addition to improved cardiovascular outcomes. Treatment with canagliflozin was associated with a 20% decrease in the risk of myocardial infarction (MI), stroke, and cardiovascular death. HHF was reduced by 39% [20]. These findings were observed in conjunction with only a slight reduction in Hemoglobin A1c, which suggests that the mechanisms of the observed benefit are independent of the glucose lowering effect of SGLT-2i.

3.5. Impact of SGLT-2i on Functional Status and Quality of Life

In many clinical trials (DEFINE-HF, DAPA-HF, EMPEROR-REDUCED, EMPA-TROPISM, and SOLOIST-WHF), HFrEF patients treated with SGLT-2i experienced reduced clinical symptoms of HF compared to patients treated with only conventional therapy, as was evidenced by improvement in the KCCQ score from baseline [124]. The EMPA-TROPISM clinical trial evaluated the effects of empagliflozin on functional capacity, and quality of life nondiabetic patients with HFrEF [96]. HFrEF patient functional status was significantly improved in the empagliflozin sub-group vs. placebo group, evidenced by enhanced oxygen consumption and improvement in a 6-min walk test. Patients in the empagliflozin treatment subgroup also reported a lower symptom burden and improved quality of life (21 +/− 18 vs. 2 +/− 15; $p < 0.001$) on the KCCQ [96]. A secondary analysis of the EMPEROR-Reduced trial found that empagliflozin significantly improved patient health status as assessed by the KCCQ-CSS by 1.5 to 2.0 points. Empagliflozin led to more 5-point, 10-point, and 15-point improvements in and fewer deteriorations in KCCQ-CSS at 3 months compared to placebo [125]. The improved functional status assessed by KCCQ was also reported for HFrEF patients treated with dapagliflozin vs. placebo in DEFINE-HF [25] and DAPA-HF trials [30,109]. Treatment of HFrEF patients with dapagliflozin improved clinical symptoms, physical function, and health-related quality of life regardless of sex [100]. Using a new type of study design, the CHIEF-HF trail (randomized, double-blind, controlled), focused on patient-centered outcomes and conducted in a completely remote fashion, showed canagliflozin significantly improved patient symptom burden after 12 weeks of treatment (KCCQ Total Symptom Score improvement by 4.3 points), regardless of EF or T2DM status [126]. Collectively, these data emphasize substantial benefits of SGLT-2i in improvement of HF symptoms, function and quality of life in HFrEF patients.

3.6. Direct Impact of SGLT-2i on Fluid Retention

One method commonly used to quantify the extent of peripheral edema is fluid weight gain. Several of the HF-associated clinical trials reported an overall decrease in weight and waist circumference in the patients treated with an SGLT-2i [106]. Meta-analysis of eight randomized-controlled trials (a combined cohort of 5233 HF patients without T2DM) reported 20% relative risk reduction in cardiovascular and HHF, associated with a reduction in body weight (-1.21 kg, $p < 0.001$), body mass index (-0.47 kg/m^2, $p < 0.001$) in patients treated with SGLT-2i vs. those without treatment [127]. The post-hoc analysis of the SONAR trial (patients with T2DM and CKD), show that six-weeks treatment SGLT-2i added to an endothelin receptor antagonist decreased body weight, a surrogate for fluid retention [128].

Since major HF symptoms are associated with fluid retention and vascular congestion, SGLT-2i must significantly improve the volume status of patients with HF. An ongoing clinical trial called EMPULSE is currently investigating the effects of empagliflozin on all-cause mortality and HHF for acute HF with signs of dyspnea, fluid overload, and elevated NPs [107]. This trial will be assessing the clinical benefit and safety of empagliflozin in this population. The results will shed light on whether SGLT-2i provides any benefits in patients with acute symptomatic HF.

4. Discussion

Two independent clinical trials, DAPA-HF and EMPEROR-Reduced, showed that SGLT-2i (dapagliflozin and empagliflozin), reduce HHF and all-cause cardiovascular death, and improved renal outcomes in HFrEF patients with or without diabetes independently from co-administration of OMT. These significant benefits have been associated with improving functional status and quality of life. The pathophysiologic mechanisms and molecular pathways underlying the benefits of SGLT-2i in HFrEF are complex and remain incompletely understood.

The HHF and re-hospitalization rates reflect HF decompensation events related to clinical symptoms caused by edema/congestion. Thus, reducing HHF/re-hospitalization is directly related to the suppression/prevention of edema/congestion exacerbation. In patients with HFrEF, edema/congestion develops, as a pathophysiologic outcome, under control of interdependent functional crosstalk between dynamic cardiac function and remodeling, chronic inflammation, endothelial dysfunction, changes in peripheral vasculature system, and pathological neurohormonal activation of SNS-RAAS and impairment of NPs and NO-related mechanisms. Comorbidities with renal or pulmonary abnormalities aggravate these pathologies. Treatment of HFrEF patients (with or without T2DM) with SGLT-2i leads to diuresis/natriuresis stimulation (reduced volume overload), improvement of overall cardiac function (improved cardiac output), and reduction (significant or mild) of NP plasma levels. The impact of the SGLT-2i on the classical RAAS overactivation and impairment of NP/NO mechanisms in HFrEF remains to be determined.

In contrast with other diuretics, treatment with SGLT-2i likely controls electrolyte balance and renal perfusion. A mathematic integrated cardiorenal modeling analysis of the DAPA-HF clinical trial predicts that SGLT-2i relives HF-related edema/congestion by reducing pathologically elevated interstitial fluid volume without significantly reducing blood plasma volume (i.e., normalizing blood volume homeostasis—or reducing volume overload stress on the heart). The ability of SGLT-2i to suppress chronic inflammation and, eventually, attenuate endothelial dysfunction suggests that SGLT-2i may control/prevent fluid leakage from the vascular compartment to the interstitial space and prevent edema development. The summary of SGLT-2i outcomes in HFrEF associated with edema/congestion repressing shown in the Figure 2.

The prevention and detection of pathological fluid is important for HF outcomes. SGLT-2i appear to prevent and delay HF progression, but additional research is needed and ongoing.

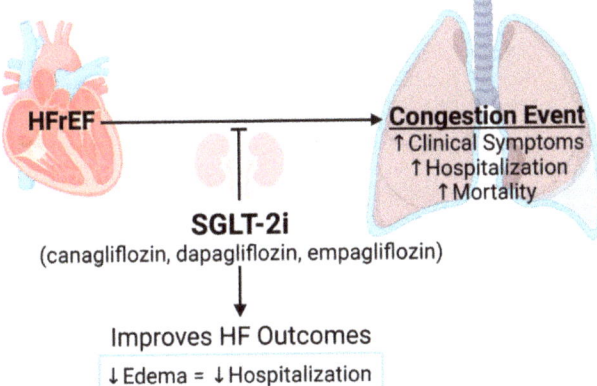

Figure 2. Schematic presentation of SGLT-2i Contribution to Attenuation of Edema/Congestion in HFrEF. Created with BioRender.com.

5. Conclusions

Late stage HF is characterized by the generation of edema/congestion leading to clinical symptoms and hospitalization. Clinical HFrEF studies summarized in this review suggest that SGLT-2i treatment may attenuate the pathological salt-water retention; however, additional studies should be designed to investigate HFrEF edema/congestion as a primary outcome.

Author Contributions: Conceptualization and methodology, I.P.G.; validation: R.D.S. and G.L.R.; investigation: M.H., R.D.S., M.E.M. and I.P.G.; writing—original draft preparation, M.H., M.E.M. and I.P.G.; writing—review and editing, R.D.S., G.L.R. and I.P.G.; formatting for publication, R.D.S.; supervision, I.P.G. All authors have read and agreed to the published version of the manuscript.

Funding: Supported by research funds from the University of Arizona, College of Medicine-Phoenix.

Conflicts of Interest: The authors declare no conflict of interest.

Abbreviations

AF	Atrial Fibrillation
ANP/NT-proANP	Atrial natriuretic peptide/N-terminal-proANP
ASCVD	Atherosclerotic cardiovascular disease
BNP/NT-proBNP	Brain/B-type natriuretic peptide/N-terminal-proBNP
CKD	Chronic kidney disease
CSS	Clinical summary score
CV	Cardiovascular
EF	Ejection fraction
eGFR	Estimated glomerular filtration rate
ESRD	End-stage renal disease
HF	Heart failure
HFrEF	Heart failure with reduced ejection fraction
HFpEF	Heart failure with preserved ejection fraction
HHF	Hospitalization due to heart failure
HR	Hazard ratio
KCCQ	Kansas City Cardiomyopathy Questionnaire
LVEF	Left ventricular ejection fraction
MACE	Major adverse cardiac events
NO	Nitric oxide
NPs	Natriuretic peptides
NYHA	New York Heart Association

OMT	Optimal medical therapy
RAAS	Renin-angiotensin-aldosterone system
SGLT-2i	Sodium-glucose cotransporter-2 inhibitors
SNS	Sympathetic nervous system
T2DM/T1DM	Type 2/Type 1 diabetes mellitus

References

1. McDonagh, T.A.; Metra, M.; Adamo, M.; Gardner, R.S.; Baumbach, A.; Bohm, M.; Burri, H.; Butler, J.; Celutkiene, J.; Chioncel, O.; et al. 2021 Esc Guidelines for the Diagnosis and Treatment of Acute and Chronic Heart Failure. *Eur. Heart J.* **2021**, *42*, 3599–3726. [CrossRef] [PubMed]
2. Bozkurt, B.; Coats, A.J.; Tsutsui, H.; Abdelhamid, M.; Adamopoulos, S.; Albert, N.; Anker, S.D.; Atherton, J.; Bohm, M.; Butler, J.; et al. Universal Definition and Classification of Heart Failure: A Report of the Heart Failure Society of America, Heart Failure Association of the European Society of Cardiology, Japanese Heart Failure Society and Writing Committee of the Universal Definition of Heart Failure. *J. Card. Fail.* **2021**, *27*, 387–413. [CrossRef]
3. Bozkurt, B.; Coats, A.J.S.; Tsutsui, H.; Abdelhamid, C.M.; Adamopoulos, S.; Albert, N.; Anker, S.D.; Atherton, J.; Bohm, M.; Butler, J.; et al. Universal Definition and Classification of Heart Failure: A Report of the Heart Failure Society of America, Heart Failure Association of the European Society of Cardiology, Japanese Heart Failure Society and Writing Committee of the Universal Definition of Heart Failure: Endorsed by the Canadian Heart Failure Society, Heart Failure Association of India, Cardiac Society of Australia and New Zealand, and Chinese Heart Failure Association. *Eur. J. Heart Fail.* **2021**, *23*, 352–380. [CrossRef]
4. Weber, K.T. Aldosterone in Congestive Heart Failure. *N. Engl. J. Med.* **2001**, *345*, 1689–1697. [CrossRef] [PubMed]
5. Ware, L.B.; Matthay, M.A. Clinical Practice. Acute Pulmonary Edema. *N. Engl. J. Med.* **2005**, *353*, 2788–2796. [CrossRef] [PubMed]
6. Writing Committee Members; Yancy, C.W.; Jessup, M.; Bozkurt, B.; Butler, J.; Casey, D.E., Jr.; Drazner, M.H.; Fonarow, G.C.; Geraci, S.A.; Horwich, T.; et al. 2013 Accf/Aha Guideline for the Management of Heart Failure: A Report of the American College of Cardiology Foundation/American Heart Association Task Force on Practice Guidelines. *Circulation* **2013**, *128*, e240–e327. [CrossRef]
7. Clark, A.L.; Cleland, J.G. Causes and Treatment of Oedema in Patients with Heart Failure. *Nat. Rev. Cardiol.* **2013**, *10*, 156–170. [CrossRef]
8. Parrinello, G.; Greene, S.J.; Torres, D.; Alderman, M.; Bonventre, J.V.; Di Pasquale, P.; Gargani, L.; Nohria, A.; Fonarow, G.C.; Vaduganathan, M.; et al. Water and Sodium in Heart Failure: A Spotlight on Congestion. *Heart Fail. Rev.* **2015**, *20*, 13–24. [CrossRef]
9. Miller, W.L. Fluid Volume Overload and Congestion in Heart Failure: Time to Reconsider Pathophysiology and How Volume Is Assessed. *Circ. Heart Fail.* **2016**, *9*, e002922. [CrossRef]
10. Lam, C.S.P.; Yancy, C. Universal Definition and Classification of Heart Failure: Is It Universal? Does It Define Heart Failure? *J. Card. Fail.* **2021**, *27*, 509–511. [CrossRef]
11. Hunt, S.A.; Baker, D.W.; Chin, M.H.; Cinquegrani, M.P.; Feldman, A.M.; Francis, G.S.; Ganiats, T.G.; Goldstein, S.; Gregoratos, G.; Jessup, M.L.; et al. Guidelines for the Evaluation and Management of Chronic Heart Failure in the Adult: Executive Summary a Report of the American College of Cardiology/American Heart Association Task Force on Practice Guidelines (Committee to Revise the 1995 Guidelines for the Evaluation and Management of Heart Failure): Developed in Collaboration with the International Society for Heart and Lung Transplantation; Endorsed by the Heart Failure Society of America. *Circulation* **2001**, *104*, 2996–3007. [CrossRef] [PubMed]
12. Dzau, V.J.; Colucci, W.S.; Hollenberg, N.K.; Williams, G.H. Relation of the Renin-Angiotensin-Aldosterone System to Clinical State in Congestive Heart Failure. *Circulation* **1981**, *63*, 645–651. [CrossRef] [PubMed]
13. Sullivan, R.D.; Mehta, R.M.; Tripathi, R.; Reed, G.L.; Gladysheva, I.P. Renin Activity in Heart Failure with Reduced Systolic Function-New Insights. *Int. J. Mol. Sci.* **2019**, *20*, 3182. [CrossRef] [PubMed]
14. Lam, C.S.P.; Chandramouli, C.; Ahooja, V.; Verma, S. Sglt-2 Inhibitors in Heart Failure: Current Management, Unmet Needs, and Therapeutic Prospects. *J. Am. Heart Assoc.* **2019**, *8*, e013389. [CrossRef]
15. Correale, M.; Petroni, R.; Coiro, S.; Antohi, E.L.; Monitillo, F.; Leone, M.; Triggiani, M.; Ishihara, S.; Dungen, H.D.; Sarwar, C.M.S.; et al. Paradigm Shift in Heart Failure Treatment: Are Cardiologists Ready to Use Gliflozins? *Heart Fail. Rev.* **2021**, 1–17. [CrossRef]
16. Lytvyn, Y.; Bjornstad, P.; Udell, J.A.; Lovshin, J.A.; Cherney, D.Z.I. Sodium Glucose Cotransporter-2 Inhibition in Heart Failure: Potential Mechanisms, Clinical Applications, and Summary of Clinical Trials. *Circulation* **2017**, *136*, 1643–1658. [CrossRef]
17. Wojcik, C.; Warden, B.A. Mechanisms and Evidence for Heart Failure Benefits from Sglt2 Inhibitors. *Curr. Cardiol. Rep.* **2019**, *21*, 130. [CrossRef]
18. Zinman, B.; Wanner, C.; Lachin, J.M.; Fitchett, D.; Bluhmki, E.; Hantel, S.; Mattheus, M.; Devins, T.; Johansen, O.E.; Woerle, H.J.; et al. Empagliflozin, Cardiovascular Outcomes, and Mortality in Type 2 Diabetes. *N. Engl. J. Med.* **2015**, *373*, 2117–2128. [CrossRef]
19. Neal, B.; Perkovic, V.; Matthews, D.R. Canagliflozin and Cardiovascular and Renal Events in Type 2 Diabetes. *N. Engl. J. Med.* **2017**, *377*, 2099. [CrossRef]
20. Perkovic, V.; Jardine, M.J.; Neal, B.; Bompoint, S.; Heerspink, H.J.L.; Charytan, D.M.; Edwards, R.; Agarwal, R.; Bakris, G.; Bull, S.; et al. Canagliflozin and Renal Outcomes in Type 2 Diabetes and Nephropathy. *N. Engl. J. Med.* **2019**, *380*, 2295–2306. [CrossRef]

21. Solomon, S.D.; McMurray, J.J.V.; Anand, I.S.; Ge, J.; Lam, C.S.P.; Maggioni, A.P.; Martinez, F.; Packer, M.; Pfeffer, M.A.; Pieske, B.; et al. Committees. Angiotensin-Neprilysin Inhibition in Heart Failure with Preserved Ejection Fraction. *N. Engl. J. Med.* **2019**, *381*, 1609–1620. [CrossRef] [PubMed]
22. McMurray, J.J.V.; DeMets, D.L.; Inzucchi, S.E.; Kober, L.; Kosiborod, M.N.; Langkilde, A.M.; Martinez, F.A.; Bengtsson, O.; Ponikowski, P.; Sabatine, M.S.; et al. A Trial to Evaluate the Effect of the Sodium-Glucose Co-Transporter 2 Inhibitor Dapagliflozin on Morbidity and Mortality in Patients with Heart Failure and Reduced Left Ventricular Ejection Fraction (Dapa-Hf). *Eur. J. Heart Fail.* **2019**, *21*, 665–675. [CrossRef] [PubMed]
23. McMurray, J.J.V.; DeMets, D.L.; Inzucchi, S.E.; Kober, L.; Kosiborod, M.N.; Langkilde, A.M.; Martinez, F.A.; Bengtsson, O.; Ponikowski, P.; Sabatine, M.S.; et al. The Dapagliflozin and Prevention of Adverse-Outcomes in Heart Failure (Dapa-Hf) Trial: Baseline Characteristics. *Eur. J. Heart Fail.* **2019**, *21*, 1402–1411. [CrossRef] [PubMed]
24. McMurray, J.J.V.; Solomon, S.D.; Inzucchi, S.E.; Kober, L.; Kosiborod, M.N.; Martinez, F.A.; Ponikowski, P.; Sabatine, M.S.; Anand, I.S.; Belohlavek, J.; et al. Dapagliflozin in Patients with Heart Failure and Reduced Ejection Fraction. *N. Engl. J. Med.* **2019**, *381*, 1995–2008. [CrossRef] [PubMed]
25. Nassif, M.E.; Windsor, S.L.; Tang, F.; Khariton, Y.; Husain, M.; Inzucchi, S.E.; McGuire, D.K.; Pitt, B.; Scirica, B.M.; Austin, B.; et al. Dapagliflozin Effects on Biomarkers, Symptoms, and Functional Status in Patients with Heart Failure with Reduced Ejection Fraction: The Define-Hf Trial. *Circulation* **2019**, *140*, 1463–1476. [CrossRef] [PubMed]
26. Jensen, J.; Omar, M.; Kistorp, C.; Poulsen, M.K.; Tuxen, C.; Gustafsson, I.; Kober, L.; Gustafsson, F.; Fosbol, E.; Bruun, N.E.; et al. Empagliflozin in Heart Failure Patients with Reduced Ejection Fraction: A Randomized Clinical Trial (Empire Hf). *Trials* **2019**, *20*, 374. [CrossRef] [PubMed]
27. Packer, M.; Anker, S.D.; Butler, J.; Filippatos, G.; Pocock, S.J.; Carson, P.; Januzzi, J.; Verma, S.; Tsutsui, H.; Brueckmann, M.; et al. Cardiovascular and Renal Outcomes with Empagliflozin in Heart Failure. *N. Engl. J. Med.* **2020**, *383*, 1413–1424. [CrossRef]
28. Zannad, F.; Ferreira, J.P.; Pocock, S.J.; Anker, S.D.; Butler, J.; Filippatos, G.; Brueckmann, M.; Ofstad, A.P.; Pfarr, E.; Jamal, W.; et al. Sglt2 Inhibitors in Patients with Heart Failure with Reduced Ejection Fraction: A Meta-Analysis of the Emperor-Reduced and Dapa-Hf Trials. *Lancet* **2020**, *396*, 819–829. [CrossRef]
29. Damman, K.; Beusekamp, J.C.; Boorsma, E.M.; Swart, H.P.; Smilde, T.D.J.; Elvan, A.; van Eck, J.W.M.; Heerspink, H.J.L.; Voors, A.A. Randomized, Double-Blind, Placebo-Controlled, Multicentre Pilot Study on the Effects of Empagliflozin on Clinical Outcomes in Patients with Acute Decompensated Heart Failure (Empa-Response-Ahf). *Eur. J. Heart Fail.* **2020**, *22*, 713–722. [CrossRef]
30. Kosiborod, M.N.; Jhund, P.S.; Docherty, K.F.; Diez, M.; Petrie, M.C.; Verma, S.; Nicolau, J.C.; Merkely, B.; Kitakaze, M.; DeMets, D.L.; et al. Effects of Dapagliflozin on Symptoms, Function, and Quality of Life in Patients with Heart Failure and Reduced Ejection Fraction: Results from the Dapa-Hf Trial. *Circulation* **2020**, *141*, 90–99. [CrossRef]
31. Solomon, S.D.; Jhund, P.S.; Claggett, B.L.; Dewan, P.; Kober, L.; Kosiborod, M.N.; Martinez, F.A.; Ponikowski, P.; Sabatine, M.S.; Inzucchi, S.E.; et al. Effect of Dapagliflozin in Patients with Hfref Treated with Sacubitril/Valsartan: The Dapa-Hf Trial. *JACC Heart Fail.* **2020**, *8*, 811–818. [CrossRef] [PubMed]
32. Docherty, K.F.; Jhund, P.S.; Inzucchi, S.E.; Kober, L.; Kosiborod, M.N.; Martinez, F.A.; Ponikowski, P.; DeMets, D.L.; Sabatine, M.S.; Bengtsson, O.; et al. Effects of Dapagliflozin in Dapa-Hf According to Background Heart Failure Therapy. *Eur. Heart J.* **2020**, *41*, 2379–2392. [CrossRef] [PubMed]
33. Martinez, F.A.; Serenelli, M.; Nicolau, J.C.; Petrie, M.C.; Chiang, C.E.; Tereshchenko, S.; Solomon, S.D.; Inzucchi, S.E.; Kober, L.; Kosiborod, M.N.; et al. Efficacy and Safety of Dapagliflozin in Heart Failure with Reduced Ejection Fraction According to Age: Insights from Dapa-Hf. *Circulation* **2020**, *141*, 100–111. [CrossRef] [PubMed]
34. Serenelli, M.; Bohm, M.; Inzucchi, S.E.; Kober, L.; Kosiborod, M.N.; Martinez, F.A.; Ponikowski, P.; Sabatine, M.S.; Solomon, S.D.; DeMets, D.L.; et al. Effect of Dapagliflozin According to Baseline Systolic Blood Pressure in the Dapagliflozin and Prevention of Adverse Outcomes in Heart Failure Trial (Dapa-Hf). *Eur. Heart J.* **2020**, *41*, 3402–3418. [CrossRef] [PubMed]
35. Jackson, A.M.; Dewan, P.; Anand, I.S.; Belohlavek, J.; Bengtsson, O.; de Boer, R.A.; Bohm, M.; Boulton, D.W.; Chopra, V.K.; DeMets, D.L.; et al. Dapagliflozin and Diuretic Use in Patients with Heart Failure and Reduced Ejection Fraction in Dapa-Hf. *Circulation* **2020**, *142*, 1040–1054. [CrossRef]
36. Packer, M. Are the Benefits of Sglt2 Inhibitors in Heart Failure and a Reduced Ejection Fraction Influenced by Background Therapy? Expectations and Realities of a New Standard of Care. *Eur. Heart J.* **2020**, *41*, 2393–2396. [CrossRef]
37. McMurray, J. Empa-Reg—The "Diuretic Hypothesis. *J. Diabetes Complicat.* **2016**, *30*, 3–4. [CrossRef]
38. Rahman, A.; Hitomi, H.; Nishiyama, A. Cardioprotective Effects of Sglt2 Inhibitors Are Possibly Associated with Normalization of the Circadian Rhythm of Blood Pressure. *Hypertens Res.* **2017**, *40*, 535–540. [CrossRef]
39. Hallow, K.M.; Helmlinger, G.; Greasley, P.J.; McMurray, J.J.V.; Boulton, D.W. Why Do Sglt2 Inhibitors Reduce Heart Failure Hospitalization? A Differential Volume Regulation Hypothesis. *Diabetes Obes. Metab.* **2018**, *20*, 479–487. [CrossRef]
40. Bertero, E.; Prates Roma, L.; Ameri, P.; Maack, C. Cardiac Effects of Sglt2 Inhibitors: The Sodium Hypothesis. *Cardiovasc. Res.* **2018**, *114*, 12–18. [CrossRef]
41. Bell, R.M.; Yellon, D.M. Sglt2 Inhibitors: Hypotheses on the Mechanism of Cardiovascular Protection. *Lancet Diabetes Endocrinol.* **2018**, *6*, 435–437. [CrossRef]
42. Verma, S.; Rawat, S.; Ho, K.L.; Wagg, C.S.; Zhang, L.; Teoh, H.; Dyck, J.E.; Uddin, G.M.; Oudit, G.Y.; Mayoux, E.; et al. Empagliflozin Increases Cardiac Energy Production in Diabetes: Novel Translational Insights into the Heart Failure Benefits of Sglt2 Inhibitors. *JACC Basic Transl. Sci.* **2018**, *3*, 575–587. [CrossRef] [PubMed]

43. Yoshihara, F.; Imazu, M.; Hamasaki, T.; Anzai, T.; Yasuda, S.; Ito, S.; Yamamoto, H.; Hashimura, K.; Yasumura, Y.; Mori, K.; et al. An Exploratory Study of Dapagliflozin for the Attenuation of Albuminuria in Patients with Heart Failure and Type 2 Diabetes Mellitus (Dapper). *Cardiovasc. Drugs Ther.* **2018**, *32*, 183–190. [CrossRef] [PubMed]
44. Lopaschuk, G.D.; Verma, S. Mechanisms of Cardiovascular Benefits of Sodium Glucose Co-Transporter 2 (Sglt2) Inhibitors: A State-of-the-Art Review. *JACC Basic Transl. Sci.* **2020**, *5*, 632–644. [CrossRef] [PubMed]
45. Nightingale, B. A Review of the Proposed Mechanistic Actions of Sodium Glucose Cotransporter-2 Inhibitors in the Treatment of Heart Failure. *Cardiol. Res.* **2021**, *12*, 60–66. [CrossRef]
46. Packer, M. Differential Pathophysiological Mechanisms in Heart Failure with a Reduced or Preserved Ejection Fraction in Diabetes. *JACC Heart Fail.* **2021**, *9*, 535–549. [CrossRef]
47. Gupta, M.; Rao, S.; Manek, G.; Fonarow, G.C.; Ghosh, R.K. The Role of Dapagliflozin in the Management of Heart Failure: An Update on the Emerging Evidence. *Ther. Clin. Risk Manag.* **2021**, *17*, 823–830. [CrossRef]
48. Fathi, A.; Vickneson, K.; Singh, J.S. Sglt2-Inhibitors; More Than Just Glycosuria and Diuresis. *Heart Fail. Rev.* **2021**, *26*, 623–642. [CrossRef]
49. Metra, M.; O'Connor, C.M.; Davison, B.A.; Cleland, J.G.; Ponikowski, P.; Teerlink, J.R.; Voors, A.A.; Givertz, M.M.; Mansoor, G.A.; Bloomfield, D.M.; et al. Early Dyspnoea Relief in Acute Heart Failure: Prevalence, Association with Mortality, and Effect of Rolofylline in the Protect Study. *Eur. Heart J.* **2011**, *32*, 1519–1534. [CrossRef]
50. Mentz, R.J.; Stevens, S.R.; DeVore, A.D.; Lala, A.; Vader, J.M.; AbouEzzeddine, O.F.; Khazanie, P.; Redfield, M.M.; Stevenson, L.W.; O'Connor, C.M.; et al. Decongestion Strategies and Renin-Angiotensin-Aldosterone System Activation in Acute Heart Failure. *JACC Heart Fail.* **2015**, *3*, 97–107. [CrossRef]
51. Pellicori, P.; Kaur, K.; Clark, A.L. Fluid Management in Patients with Chronic Heart Failure. *Card. Fail. Rev.* **2015**, *1*, 90–95. [CrossRef] [PubMed]
52. Melenovsky, V.; Andersen, M.J.; Andress, K.; Reddy, Y.N.; Borlaug, B.A. Lung Congestion in Chronic Heart Failure: Haemodynamic, Clinical, and Prognostic Implications. *Eur. J. Heart Fail.* **2015**, *17*, 1161–1171. [CrossRef] [PubMed]
53. Chioncel, O.; Mebazaa, A.; Harjola, V.P.; Coats, A.J.; Piepoli, M.F.; Crespo-Leiro, M.G.; Laroche, C.; Seferovic, P.M.; Anker, S.D.; Ferrari, R.; et al. Clinical Phenotypes and Outcome of Patients Hospitalized for Acute Heart Failure: The Esc Heart Failure Long-Term Registry. *Eur. J. Heart Fail.* **2017**, *19*, 1242–1254. [CrossRef] [PubMed]
54. Aimo, A.; Vergaro, G.; Giannoni, A.; Emdin, M. Wet Is Bad: Residual Congestion Predicts Worse Prognosis in Acute Heart Failure. *Int. J. Cardiol.* **2018**, *258*, 201–202. [CrossRef]
55. Selvaraj, S.; Claggett, B.; Pozzi, A.; McMurray, J.J.V.; Jhund, P.S.; Packer, M.; Desai, A.S.; Lewis, E.F.; Vaduganathan, M.; Lefkowitz, M.P.; et al. Prognostic Implications of Congestion on Physical Examination among Contemporary Patients with Heart Failure and Reduced Ejection Fraction: Paradigm-Hf. *Circulation* **2019**, *140*, 1369–1379. [CrossRef]
56. Pellicori, P.; Khan, M.J.I.; Graham, F.J.; Cleland, J.G.F. New Perspectives and Future Directions in the Treatment of Heart Failure. *Heart Fail. Rev.* **2020**, *25*, 147–159. [CrossRef] [PubMed]
57. Palazzuoli, A.; Evangelista, I.; Nuti, R. Congestion Occurrence and Evaluation in Acute Heart Failure Scenario: Time to Reconsider Different Pathways of Volume Overload. *Heart Fail. Rev.* **2020**, *25*, 119–131. [CrossRef]
58. DeFilippis, E.M.; Van Spall, H.G.C. Improving Health-Related Quality of Life for Women with Acute Heart Failure: Chronically Undertreated. *JACC Heart Fail.* **2021**, *9*, 346–348. [CrossRef]
59. Lombardi, C.M.; Cimino, G.; Pellicori, P.; Bonelli, A.; Inciardi, R.M.; Pagnesi, M.; Tomasoni, D.; Ravera, A.; Adamo, M.; Carubelli, V.; et al. Congestion in Patients with Advanced Heart Failure: Assessment and Treatment. *Heart Fail. Clin.* **2021**, *17*, 575–586. [CrossRef]
60. Gheorghiade, M.; Filippatos, G.; De Luca, L.; Burnett, J. Congestion in Acute Heart Failure Syndromes: An Essential Target of Evaluation and Treatment. *Am. J. Med.* **2006**, *119*, S3–S10. [CrossRef]
61. Pang, P.S.; Cleland, J.G.; Teerlink, J.R.; Collins, S.P.; Lindsell, C.J.; Sopko, G.; Peacock, W.F.; Fonarow, G.C.; Aldeen, A.Z.; Kirk, J.D.; et al. A Proposal to Standardize Dyspnoea Measurement in Clinical Trials of Acute Heart Failure Syndromes: The Need for a Uniform Approach. *Eur. Heart J.* **2008**, *29*, 816–824. [CrossRef] [PubMed]
62. Gheorghiade, M.; Follath, F.; Ponikowski, P.; Barsuk, J.H.; Blair, J.E.; Cleland, J.G.; Dickstein, K.; Drazner, M.H.; Fonarow, G.C.; Jaarsma, T.; et al. Assessing and Grading Congestion in Acute Heart Failure: A Scientific Statement from the Acute Heart Failure Committee of the Heart Failure Association of the European Society of Cardiology and Endorsed by the European Society of Intensive Care Medicine. *Eur. J. Heart Fail.* **2010**, *12*, 423–433. [CrossRef] [PubMed]
63. Girerd, N.; Seronde, M.F.; Coiro, S.; Chouihed, T.; Bilbault, P.; Braun, F.; Kenizou, D.; Maillier, B.; Nazeyrollas, P.; Roul, G.; et al. Integrative Assessment of Congestion in Heart Failure Throughout the Patient Journey. *JACC Heart Fail.* **2018**, *6*, 273–285. [CrossRef] [PubMed]
64. Sullivan, R.D.; Mehta, R.M.; Tripathi, R.; Gladysheva, I.P.; Reed, G.L. Normalizing Plasma Renin Activity in Experimental Dilated Cardiomyopathy: Effects on Edema, Cachexia, and Survival. *Int. J. Mol. Sci.* **2019**, *20*, 3886. [CrossRef] [PubMed]
65. Tripathi, R.; Sullivan, R.D.; Fan, T.M.; Mehta, R.M.; Gladysheva, I.P.; Reed, G.L. A Low-Sodium Diet Boosts Ang (1-7) Production and No-Cgmp Bioavailability to Reduce Edema and Enhance Survival in Experimental Heart Failure. *Int. J. Mol. Sci.* **2021**, *22*, 4035. [CrossRef]
66. Pirrotta, F.; Mazza, B.; Gennari, L.; Palazzuoli, A. Pulmonary Congestion Assessment in Heart Failure: Traditional and New Tools. *Diagnostics* **2021**, *11*, 1306. [CrossRef]

67. Reed, G.L.; Gladysheva, I.P.; Sullivan, R.D.; Mehta, R.M. Method of Personalized Treatment for Cardiomyopathy and Heart Failure and Associated Diseases by Measuring Edema and Cachexia/Sarcopenia. U.S. Patent 17/313,904, 6 May 2021. Available online: https://www.freepatentsonline.com/y2021/0263120.html (accessed on 26 February 2022).
68. Takeuchi, T.; Dohi, K.; Omori, T.; Moriwaki, K.; Sato, Y.; Nakamori, S.; Fujimoto, N.; Fujii, E.; Yamada, N.; Ito, M. Diuretic Effects of Sodium-Glucose Cotransporter 2 Inhibitor in Patients with Type 2 Diabetes Mellitus and Heart Failure. *Int. J. Cardiol.* **2015**, *201*, 1–3. [CrossRef]
69. Lee, H.C.; Shiou, Y.L.; Jhuo, S.J.; Chang, C.Y.; Liu, P.L.; Jhuang, W.J.; Dai, Z.K.; Chen, W.Y.; Chen, Y.F.; Lee, A.S. The Sodium-Glucose Co-Transporter 2 Inhibitor Empagliflozin Attenuates Cardiac Fibrosis and Improves Ventricular Hemodynamics in Hypertensive Heart Failure Rats. *Cardiovasc. Diabetol.* **2019**, *18*, 45. [CrossRef]
70. Packer, M. Activation and Inhibition of Sodium-Hydrogen Exchanger Is a Mechanism That Links the Pathophysiology and Treatment of Diabetes Mellitus with That of Heart Failure. *Circulation* **2017**, *136*, 1548–1559. [CrossRef]
71. Lambers Heerspink, H.J.; de Zeeuw, D.; Wie, L.; Leslie, B.; List, J. Dapagliflozin a Glucose-Regulating Drug with Diuretic Properties in Subjects with Type 2 Diabetes. *Diabetes Obes. Metab.* **2013**, *15*, 853–862. [CrossRef]
72. Eickhoff, M.K.; Dekkers, C.C.J.; Kramers, B.J.; Laverman, G.D.; Frimodt-Moller, M.; Jorgensen, N.R.; Faber, J.; Danser, A.H.J.; Gansevoort, R.T.; Rossing, P.; et al. Effects of Dapagliflozin on Volume Status When Added to Renin-Angiotensin System Inhibitors. *J. Clin. Med.* **2019**, *8*, 779. [CrossRef] [PubMed]
73. Masuda, T.; Muto, S.; Fukuda, K.; Watanabe, M.; Ohara, K.; Koepsell, H.; Vallon, V.; Nagata, D. Osmotic Diuresis by Sglt2 Inhibition Stimulates Vasopressin-Induced Water Reabsorption to Maintain Body Fluid Volume. *Physiol. Rep.* **2020**, *8*, e14360. [CrossRef] [PubMed]
74. Marx, N.; McGuire, D.K. Sodium-Glucose Cotransporter-2 Inhibition for the Reduction of Cardiovascular Events in High-Risk Patients with Diabetes Mellitus. *Eur. Heart J.* **2016**, *37*, 3192–3200. [CrossRef] [PubMed]
75. Rossignol, P.; Hernandez, A.F.; Solomon, S.D.; Zannad, F. Heart Failure Drug Treatment. *Lancet* **2019**, *393*, 1034–1044. [CrossRef]
76. Yu, H.; Basu, S.; Hallow, K.M. Cardiac and Renal Function Interactions in Heart Failure with Reduced Ejection Fraction: A Mathematical Modeling Analysis. *PLoS Comput. Biol.* **2020**, *16*, e1008074. [CrossRef] [PubMed]
77. Rangaswami, J.; Bhalla, V.; Blair, J.E.A.; Chang, T.I.; Costa, S.; Lentine, K.L.; Lerma, E.V.; Mezue, K.; Molitch, M.; Mullens, W.; et al. Cardiorenal Syndrome: Classification, Pathophysiology, Diagnosis, and Treatment Strategies: A Scientific Statement from the American Heart Association. *Circulation* **2019**, *139*, e840–e878. [CrossRef] [PubMed]
78. Merrill, A.J. Edema and Decreased Renal Blood Flow in Patients with Chronic Congestive Heart Failure: Evidence of "Forward Failure" as the Primary Cause of Edema. *J. Clin. Invest.* **1946**, *25*, 389–400. [CrossRef]
79. Kilcoyne, M.M.; Schmidt, D.H.; Cannon, P.J. Intrarenal Blood Flow in Congestive Heart Failure. *Circulation* **1973**, *47*, 786–797. [CrossRef]
80. Verbrugge, F.H.; Guazzi, M.; Testani, J.M.; Borlaug, B.A. Altered Hemodynamics and End-Organ Damage in Heart Failure: Impact on the Lung and Kidney. *Circulation* **2020**, *142*, 998–1012. [CrossRef]
81. Nespoux, J.; Vallon, V. Renal Effects of Sglt2 Inhibitors: An Update. *Curr. Opin. Nephrol. Hypertens.* **2020**, *29*, 190–198. [CrossRef]
82. Kuriyama, S. A Potential Mechanism of Cardio-Renal Protection with Sodium-Glucose Cotransporter 2 Inhibitors: Amelioration of Renal Congestion. *Kidney Blood Press. Res.* **2019**, *44*, 449–456. [CrossRef] [PubMed]
83. Cotton, J.M.; Kearney, M.T.; Shah, A.M. Nitric Oxide and Myocardial Function in Heart Failure: Friend or Foe? *Heart* **2002**, *88*, 564–566. [CrossRef] [PubMed]
84. Ibebuogu, U.N.; Gladysheva, I.P.; Houng, A.K.; Reed, G.L. Decompensated Heart Failure Is Associated with Reduced Corin Levels and Decreased Cleavage of Pro-Atrial Natriuretic Peptide. *Circ. Heart Fail.* **2011**, *4*, 114–120. [CrossRef] [PubMed]
85. Dries, D.L. Process Matters: Emerging Concepts Underlying Impaired Natriuretic Peptide System Function in Heart Failure. *Circ. Heart Fail.* **2011**, *4*, 107–110. [CrossRef] [PubMed]
86. Sayer, G.; Bhat, G. The Renin-Angiotensin-Aldosterone System and Heart Failure. *Cardiol. Clin.* **2014**, *32*, 21–32. [CrossRef]
87. Volpe, M.; Carnovali, M.; Mastromarino, V. The Natriuretic Peptides System in the Pathophysiology of Heart Failure: From Molecular Basis to Treatment. *Clin. Sci.* **2016**, *130*, 57–77. [CrossRef]
88. Zaidi, S.S.; Ward, R.D.; Ramanathan, K.; Yu, X.; Gladysheva, I.P.; Reed, G.L. Possible Enzymatic Downregulation of the Natriuretic Peptide System in Patients with Reduced Systolic Function and Heart Failure: A Pilot Study. *BioMed Res. Int.* **2018**, *2018*, 7279036. [CrossRef]
89. Tripathi, R.; Wang, D.; Sullivan, R.; Fan, T.H.; Gladysheva, I.P.; Reed, G.L. Depressed Corin Levels Indicate Early Systolic Dysfunction before Increases of Atrial Natriuretic Peptide/B-Type Natriuretic Peptide and Heart Failure Development. *Hypertension* **2016**, *67*, 362–367. [CrossRef]
90. Tripathi, R.; Sullivan, R.; Fan, T.M.; Wang, D.; Sun, Y.; Reed, G.L.; Gladysheva, I.P. Enhanced Heart Failure, Mortality and Renin Activation in Female Mice with Experimental Dilated Cardiomyopathy. *PLoS ONE* **2017**, *12*, e0189315. [CrossRef]
91. Santos-Gallego, C.G.; Requena-Ibanez, J.A.; San Antonio, R.; Ishikawa, K.; Watanabe, S.; Picatoste, B.; Flores, E.; Garcia-Ropero, A.; Sanz, J.; Hajjar, R.J.; et al. Empagliflozin Ameliorates Adverse Left Ventricular Remodeling in Nondiabetic Heart Failure by Enhancing Myocardial Energetics. *J. Am. Coll. Cardiol.* **2019**, *73*, 1931–1944. [CrossRef]
92. Ansary, T.M.; Nakano, D.; Nishiyama, A. Diuretic Effects of Sodium Glucose Cotransporter 2 Inhibitors and Their Influence on the Renin-Angiotensin System. *Int. J. Mol. Sci.* **2019**, *20*, 629. [CrossRef] [PubMed]

93. Maggioni, A.P.; Dahlstrom, U.; Filippatos, G.; Chioncel, O.; Leiro, M.C.; Drozdz, J.; Fruhwald, F.; Gullestad, L.; Logeart, D.; Metra, M.; et al. Eurobservational Research Programme: The Heart Failure Pilot Survey (Esc-Hf Pilot). *Eur. J. Heart Fail.* **2010**, *12*, 1076–1084. [CrossRef] [PubMed]
94. Rubio-Gracia, J.; Demissei, B.G.; Ter Maaten, J.M.; Cleland, J.G.; O'Connor, C.M.; Metra, M.; Ponikowski, P.; Teerlink, J.R.; Cotter, G.; Davison, B.A.; et al. Prevalence, Predictors and Clinical Outcome of Residual Congestion in Acute Decompensated Heart Failure. *Int. J. Cardiol.* **2018**, *258*, 185–191. [CrossRef] [PubMed]
95. Yancy, C.W.; Jessup, M.; Bozkurt, B.; Butler, J.; Casey, D.E., Jr.; Drazner, M.H.; Fonarow, G.C.; Geraci, S.A.; Horwich, T.; Januzzi, J.L.; et al. 2013 Accf/Aha Guideline for the Management of Heart Failure: A Report of the American College of Cardiology Foundation/American Heart Association Task Force on Practice Guidelines. *J. Am. Coll. Cardiol.* **2013**, *62*, e147–e239. [CrossRef]
96. Santos-Gallego, C.G.; Vargas-Delgado, A.P.; Requena-Ibanez, J.A.; Garcia-Ropero, A.; Mancini, D.; Pinney, S.; Macaluso, F.; Sartori, S.; Roque, M.; Sabatel-Perez, F.; et al. Randomized Trial of Empagliflozin in Nondiabetic Patients with Heart Failure and Reduced Ejection Fraction. *J. Am. Coll. Cardiol.* **2021**, *77*, 243–255. [CrossRef]
97. Wiviott, S.D.; Raz, I.; Sabatine, M.S. Dapagliflozin and Cardiovascular Outcomes in Type 2 Diabetes. Reply. *N. Engl. J. Med.* **2019**, *380*, 1881–1882. [CrossRef]
98. Jhund, P.S.; Ponikowski, P.; Docherty, K.F.; Gasparyan, S.B.; Bohm, M.; Chiang, C.E.; Desai, A.S.; Howlett, J.; Kitakaze, M.; Petrie, M.C.; et al. Dapagliflozin and Recurrent Heart Failure Hospitalizations in Heart Failure with Reduced Ejection Fraction: An Analysis of Dapa-Hf. *Circulation* **2021**, *143*, 1962–1972. [CrossRef]
99. Curtain, J.P.; Docherty, K.F.; Jhund, P.S.; Petrie, M.C.; Inzucchi, S.E.; Kober, L.; Kosiborod, M.N.; Martinez, F.A.; Ponikowski, P.; Sabatine, M.S.; et al. Effect of Dapagliflozin on Ventricular Arrhythmias, Resuscitated Cardiac Arrest, or Sudden Death in Dapa-Hf. *Eur. Heart J.* **2021**, *42*, 3727–3738. [CrossRef]
100. Butt, J.H.; Docherty, K.F.; Petrie, M.C.; Schou, M.; Kosiborod, M.N.; O'Meara, E.; Katova, T.; Ljungman, C.E.A.; Diez, M.; Ogunniyi, M.O.; et al. Efficacy and Safety of Dapagliflozin in Men and Women with Heart Failure with Reduced Ejection Fraction: A Prespecified Analysis of the Dapagliflozin and Prevention of Adverse Outcomes in Heart Failure Trial. *JAMA Cardiol.* **2021**, *6*, 678–689. [CrossRef]
101. Lu, Y.; Li, F.; Fan, Y.; Yang, Y.; Chen, M.; Xi, J. Effect of Sglt-2 Inhibitors on Cardiovascular Outcomes in Heart Failure Patients: A Meta-Analysis of Randomized Controlled Trials. *Eur. J. Intern. Med.* **2021**, *87*, 20–28. [CrossRef]
102. Requena-Ibanez, J.A.; Santos-Gallego, C.G.; Rodriguez-Cordero, A.; Vargas-Delgado, A.P.; Mancini, D.; Sartori, S.; Atallah-Lajam, F.; Giannarelli, C.; Macaluso, F.; Lala, A.; et al. Mechanistic Insights of Empagliflozin in Nondiabetic Patients with Hfref: From the Empa-Tropism Study. *JACC Heart Fail.* **2021**, *9*, 578–589. [CrossRef] [PubMed]
103. Lee, M.M.Y.; Brooksbank, K.J.M.; Wetherall, K.; Mangion, K.; Roditi, G.; Campbell, R.T.; Berry, C.; Chong, V.; Coyle, L.; Docherty, K.F.; et al. Effect of Empagliflozin on Left Ventricular Volumes in Patients with Type 2 Diabetes, or Prediabetes, and Heart Failure with Reduced Ejection Fraction (Sugar-Dm-Hf). *Circulation* **2021**, *143*, 516–525. [CrossRef] [PubMed]
104. Hundertmark, M.J.; Agbaje, O.F.; Coleman, R.; George, J.T.; Grempler, R.; Holman, R.R.; Lamlum, H.; Lee, J.; Milton, J.E.; Niessen, H.G.; et al. Design and Rationale of the Empa-Vision Trial: Investigating the Metabolic Effects of Empagliflozin in Patients with Heart Failure. *ESC Heart Fail.* **2021**, *8*, 2580–2590. [CrossRef] [PubMed]
105. Tanajak, P.; Sa-Nguanmoo, P.; Sivasinprasasn, S.; Thummasorn, S.; Siri-Angkul, N.; Chattipakorn, S.C.; Chattipakorn, N. Cardioprotection of Dapagliflozin and Vildagliptin in Rats with Cardiac Ischemia-Reperfusion Injury. *J. Endocrinol.* **2018**, *236*, 69–84. [CrossRef] [PubMed]
106. Lee, P.C.; Ganguly, S.; Goh, S.Y. Weight Loss Associated with Sodium-Glucose Cotransporter-2 Inhibition: A Review of Evidence and Underlying Mechanisms. *Obes. Rev.* **2018**, *19*, 1630–1641. [CrossRef]
107. Tromp, J.; Ponikowski, P.; Salsali, A.; Angermann, C.E.; Biegus, J.; Blatchford, J.; Collins, S.P.; Ferreira, J.P.; Grauer, C.; Kosiborod, M.; et al. Sodium-Glucose Co-Transporter 2 Inhibition in Patients Hospitalized for Acute Decompensated Heart Failure: Rationale for and Design of the Empulse Trial. *Eur. J. Heart Fail.* **2021**, *23*, 826–834. [CrossRef]
108. Ibrahim, N.E.; Januzzi, J.L. Sodium-Glucose Co-Transporter 2 Inhibitors and Insights from Biomarker Measurement in Heart Failure Patients. *Clin. Chem.* **2021**, *67*, 79–86. [CrossRef]
109. Butt, J.H.; Adamson, C.; Docherty, K.F.; de Boer, R.A.; Petrie, M.C.; Inzucchi, S.E.; Kosiborod, M.N.; Maria Langkilde, A.; Lindholm, D.; Martinez, F.A.; et al. Efficacy and Safety of Dapagliflozin in Heart Failure with Reduced Ejection Fraction According to N-Terminal Pro-B-Type Natriuretic Peptide: Insights from the Dapa-Hf Trial. *Circ. Heart Fail.* **2021**, *14*, 1305–1318. [CrossRef]
110. Sezai, A.; Sekino, H.; Unosawa, S.; Taoka, M.; Osaka, S.; Tanaka, M. Canagliflozin for Japanese Patients with Chronic Heart Failure and Type Ii Diabetes. *Cardiovasc. Diabetol.* **2019**, *18*, 76. [CrossRef]
111. Takase, H.; Dohi, Y. Kidney Function Crucially Affects B-Type Natriuretic Peptide (Bnp), N-Terminal Probnp and Their Relationship. *Eur. J. Clin. Investig.* **2014**, *44*, 303–308. [CrossRef]
112. Bhatt, A.S.; Cooper, L.B.; Ambrosy, A.P.; Clare, R.M.; Coles, A.; Joyce, E.; Krishnamoorthy, A.; Butler, J.; Felker, G.M.; Ezekowitz, J.A.; et al. Interaction of Body Mass Index on the Association between N-Terminal-Pro-B-Type Natriuretic Peptide and Morbidity and Mortality in Patients with Acute Heart Failure: Findings from Ascend-Hf (Acute Study of Clinical Effectiveness of Nesiritide in Decompensated Heart Failure). *J. Am. Heart Assoc.* **2018**, *7*, e006740. [CrossRef] [PubMed]
113. Wiig, H. Pathophysiology of Tissue Fluid Accumulation in Inflammation. *J. Physiol.* **2011**, *589*, 2945–2953. [CrossRef] [PubMed]
114. Van Linthout, S.; Tschope, C. Inflammation - Cause or Consequence of Heart Failure or Both? *Curr. Heart Fail. Rep.* **2017**, *14*, 251–265. [CrossRef] [PubMed]

115. Murphy, S.P.; Kakkar, R.; McCarthy, C.P.; Januzzi, J.L., Jr. Inflammation in Heart Failure: Jacc State-of-the-Art Review. *J. Am. Coll. Cardiol.* **2020**, *75*, 1324–1340. [CrossRef] [PubMed]
116. Heerspink, H.J.L.; Perco, P.; Mulder, S.; Leierer, J.; Hansen, M.K.; Heinzel, A.; Mayer, G. Canagliflozin Reduces Inflammation and Fibrosis Biomarkers: A Potential Mechanism of Action for Beneficial Effects of Sglt2 Inhibitors in Diabetic Kidney Disease. *Diabetologia* **2019**, *62*, 1154–1166. [CrossRef]
117. Alshnbari, A.S.; Millar, S.A.; O'Sullivan, S.E.; Idris, I. Effect of Sodium-Glucose Cotransporter-2 Inhibitors on Endothelial Function: A Systematic Review of Preclinical Studies. *Diabetes Ther.* **2020**, *11*, 1947–1963. [CrossRef]
118. Ugusman, A.; Kumar, J.; Aminuddin, A. Endothelial Function and Dysfunction: Impact of Sodium-Glucose Cotransporter 2 Inhibitors. *Pharmacol. Ther.* **2021**, *224*, 107832. [CrossRef]
119. Dyck, J.R.B.; Sossalla, S.; Hamdani, N.; Coronel, R.; Weber, N.C.; Light, P.E.; Zuurbier, C.J. Cardiac Mechanisms of the Beneficial Effects of Sglt2 Inhibitors in Heart Failure: Evidence for Potential Off-Target Effects. *J. Mol. Cell. Cardiol.* **2022**, *167*, 17–31. [CrossRef]
120. Schefold, J.C.; Filippatos, G.; Hasenfuss, G.; Anker, S.D.; von Haehling, S. Heart Failure and Kidney Dysfunction: Epidemiology, Mechanisms and Management. *Nat. Rev. Nephrol.* **2016**, *12*, 610–623. [CrossRef]
121. Damman, K.; Masson, S.; Lucci, D.; Gorini, M.; Urso, R.; Maggioni, A.P.; Tavazzi, L.; Tarantini, L.; Tognoni, G.; Voors, A.; et al. Progression of Renal Impairment and Chronic Kidney Disease in Chronic Heart Failure: An Analysis from Gissi-Hf. *J. Card Fail.* **2017**, *23*, 2–9. [CrossRef]
122. Adamska-Welnicka, A.; Welnicki, M.; Mamcarz, A.; Gellert, R. Chronic Kidney Disease and Heart Failure-Everyday Diagnostic Challenges. *Diagnostics* **2021**, *11*, 2164. [CrossRef] [PubMed]
123. Jhund, P.S.; Solomon, S.D.; Docherty, K.F.; Heerspink, H.J.L.; Anand, I.S.; Bohm, M.; Chopra, V.; de Boer, R.A.; Desai, A.S.; Ge, J.; et al. Efficacy of Dapagliflozin on Renal Function and Outcomes in Patients with Heart Failure with Reduced Ejection Fraction: Results of Dapa-Hf. *Circulation* **2021**, *143*, 298–309. [CrossRef] [PubMed]
124. Green, C.P.; Porter, C.B.; Bresnahan, D.R.; Spertus, J.A. Development and Evaluation of the Kansas City Cardiomyopathy Questionnaire: A New Health Status Measure for Heart Failure. *J. Am. Coll. Cardiol.* **2000**, *35*, 1245–1255. [CrossRef]
125. Butler, J.; Anker, S.D.; Filippatos, G.; Khan, M.S.; Ferreira, J.P.; Pocock, S.J.; Giannetti, N.; Januzzi, J.L.; Pina, I.L.; Lam, C.S.P.; et al. Empagliflozin and Health-Related Quality of Life Outcomes in Patients with Heart Failure with Reduced Ejection Fraction: The Emperor-Reduced Trial. *Eur. Heart J.* **2021**, *42*, 1203–1212. [CrossRef]
126. Spertus, J.A.; Birmingham, M.C.; Nassif, M.; Damaraju, C.V.; Abbate, A.; Butler, J.; Lanfear, D.E.; Lingvay, I.; Kosiborod, M.N.; Januzzi, J.L. The Sglt2 Inhibitor Canagliflozin in Heart Failure: The Chief-Hf Remote, Patient-Centered Randomized Trial. *Nat. Med.* **2022**, 1–5. [CrossRef]
127. Teo, Y.H.; Teo, Y.N.; Syn, N.L.; Kow, C.S.; Yoong, C.S.Y.; Tan, B.Y.Q.; Yeo, T.C.; Lee, C.H.; Lin, W.; Sia, C.H. Effects of Sodium/Glucose Cotransporter 2 (Sglt2) Inhibitors on Cardiovascular and Metabolic Outcomes in Patients without Diabetes Mellitus: A Systematic Review and Meta-Analysis of Randomized-Controlled Trials. *J. Am. Heart Assoc.* **2021**, *10*, e019463. [CrossRef]
128. Heerspink, H.J.L.; Kohan, D.E.; de Zeeuw, D. New Insights from Sonar Indicate Adding Sodium Glucose Co-Transporter 2 Inhibitors to an Endothelin Receptor Antagonist Mitigates Fluid Retention and Enhances Albuminuria Reduction. *Kidney Int.* **2021**, *99*, 346–349. [CrossRef]

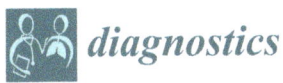

Article

A Multivariate Model to Predict Chronic Heart Failure after Acute ST-Segment Elevation Myocardial Infarction: Preliminary Study

Valentin Elievich Oleynikov, Elena Vladimirovna Averyanova, Anastasia Aleksandrovna Oreshkina, Nadezhda Valerievna Burko *, Yulia Andreevna Barmenkova, Alena Vladimirovna Golubeva and Vera Aleksandrovna Galimskaya

Department of Therapy, Medical Institute, Penza State University, 440026 Penza, Russia;
v.oleynikof@gmail.com (V.E.O.); averyanova-elena90@bk.ru (E.V.A.); anast.oreschckina@yandex.ru (A.A.O.);
yulenka.gsk@gmail.com (Y.A.B.); fialmy@mail.ru (A.V.G.); vera-budanova@mail.ru (V.A.G.)
* Correspondence: hopeful.n@mail.ru; Tel.: +7-9869366220

Abstract: A multivariate model for predicting the risk of decompensated chronic heart failure (CHF) within 48 weeks after ST-segment elevation myocardial infarction (STEMI) has been developed and tested. Methods. The study included 173 patients with acute STEMI aged 51.4 (95% confidence interval (CI): 42–61) years. Two-dimensional (2D) speckle-tracking echocardiography (STE) has been performed on the 7th–9th days, and at the 12th, 24th, and 48th weeks after the index event with the analysis of volumetric parameters and values for global longitudinal strain (GLS), global circumferential strain (GCS), and global radial strain (GRS). A 24-h ECG monitoring (24 h ECG) of the electrocardiogram (ECG) to assess heart rate turbulence (HRT) has been performed on the 7th–9th days of STEMI. The study involved two stages of implementation. At the first stage, a multivariate model to assess the risk of CHF progression within 48 weeks after STEMI has been built on the basis of examination and follow-up data for 113 patients (group M). At the second stage, the performance of the model has been assessed based on a 48-week follow-up of 60 patients (group T). Results. A multivariate regression model for CHF progression in STEMI patients has been created based on the results of the first stage. It included the following parameters: HRT, left ventricular (LV) end-systolic dimension (ESD), and GLS. The contribution of each factor for the relative risk (RR) of decompensated CHF has been found: 3.92 (95% CI: 1.66–9.25) ($p = 0.0018$) for HRT; 1.04 (95% CI: 1.015–1.07) ($p = 0.0027$) for ESD; 0.9 (95% CI: 0.815–0.98) ($p = 0.028$) for GLS. The diagnostic efficiency of the proposed model has been evaluated at the second stage. It appeared to have a high specificity of 83.3%, a sensitivity of 95.8%, and a diagnostic accuracy of 93.3%. Conclusion. The developed model for predicting CHF progression within 48 weeks after STEMI has a high diagnostic efficiency and can be used in early stages of myocardial infarction to stratify the risk of patients.

Keywords: myocardial infarction; chronic heart failure; heart rate variability; 2D echocardiography; 24-h ECG monitoring

Citation: Oleynikov, V.E.; Averyanova, E.V.; Oreshkina, A.A.; Burko, N.V.; Barmenkova, Y.A.; Golubeva, A.V.; Galimskaya, V.A. A Multivariate Model to Predict Chronic Heart Failure after Acute ST-Segment Elevation Myocardial Infarction: Preliminary Study. *Diagnostics* 2021, 11, 1925. https://doi.org/10.3390/diagnostics11101925

Academic Editor: Gino Seravalle Seravalle

Received: 19 August 2021
Accepted: 4 October 2021
Published: 18 October 2021

Publisher's Note: MDPI stays neutral with regard to jurisdictional claims in published maps and institutional affiliations.

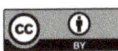

Copyright: © 2021 by the authors. Licensee MDPI, Basel, Switzerland. This article is an open access article distributed under the terms and conditions of the Creative Commons Attribution (CC BY) license (https://creativecommons.org/licenses/by/4.0/).

1. Introduction

Chronic heart failure (CHF) has become a major public health problem of the 21st century, significantly reducing the life potential of the population worldwide. Major causes of CHF are arterial hypertension and coronary heart disease [1,2]. A combination of both diseases occurs in more than half of patients [2,3].

Annual costs of treating CHF patients grow progressively due to an increase in the life expectancy of patients [4,5]. According to a large-scale meta-analysis [5], a five-year life expectancy in patients with CHF has increased by 59.7% as compared to the 1970s. Improvement of the quality of care and expanding the range of drugs after severe cardiovascular events help to maintain the quality of life of patients at an acceptable level for a long period of time. However, the financial aspect of this issue is rather burdensome [4–6].

Nowadays, patients with acute ST-segment elevation myocardial infarction (STEMI) receive high-quality treatment due to the achievements of interventional cardiology and drugs that are able to restore and "revive" hibernating cardiomyocytes in the infarct zone. Thus, the prognosis of patients after myocardial infarction has significantly improved in the era of pharmacoinvasive therapy [7,8]. According to the French Registry of Acute ST-Elevation or Non-ST-Elevation Myocardial Infarction [7], a six-month mortality rate in patients after STEMI decreased from 17.2% in 1995 to 6.9% in 2010, and 5.3% in 2015.

Due to the increase in the survival rate of patients with myocardial infarction, the prediction and prevention of CHF decompensation are the key tasks for the cardiological community [9].

Currently, there are some urgent problems, dealing with the introduction of the possibilities of laboratory and instrumental diagnostic methods to predict the risk of developing CHF decompensation, and how to reduce the risk of re-hospitalization of patients. To predict a high risk of CHF in early stages of STEMI is essential for personalized anti-remodeling therapy, reliable recommendations for therapeutic rehabilitation, and timely cardiac surgery.

The aim of this study was to create a model for reliable risk prediction of CHF progression after acute STEMI during a 48-week follow-up using a combination of echocardiography (EchoCG) and 24 h ECG monitoring.

2. Materials and Methods

A total of 1256 STEMI patients were examined in the Emergency Cardiology Department of the Regional Clinical Hospital n. a. N.N. Burdenko (Penza, Russia). According to evaluated inclusion/exclusion criteria, a total of 173 STEMI patients were enrolled in the study. The study protocol and informed consent were approved by the Local Ethics Committee at Penza State University.

The study included patients having met the following criteria: aged 35–65 years; acute STEMI of any localization, confirmed by laboratory and instrumental methods (increased troponin levels, ECG data, coronary angiography (CA), EchoCG). The main exclusion criteria were as follows: repeated and recurrent myocardial infarction; stenosis of more than 30% of the left coronary artery; stenosis of more than 50% of other coronary arteries, except for an infarct-related one; NYHA class II-IV of CHF; non-sinus rhythm; severe concomitant diseases.

The average age of the patients was 51.4 (95% CI: 42–61) years, men prevailed—152 patients (87.8%). Two-dimensional EchoCG has been performed on the 7th–9th days, and at the 12th, 24th, and 48th weeks after STEMI using a MyLab90 ultrasound scanner (Esaote, Genoa, Italy) with analysis of generally accepted volumetric parameters. The ejection fraction (EF) has been calculated using a modified Simpson method. The end-diastolic volume index (EDVI) and the end-systolic volume index (ESVI) have been determined by indexing to body surface area (BSA). Speckle-tracking EchoCG has been performed using Esaote XStrain™ software. The values for global longitudinal strain (GLS), global circumferential strain (GCS), and global radial strain (GRS) have been estimated [10].

A 12-lead 24-h ECG monitoring has been carried out using Holter Analysis-Astrocard complex devices (Meditek Ltd., Moscow, Russia) on the 7th–9th days of STEMI. Episodes of ischemia, arrhythmias have been assessed: ventricular and supraventricular extrasystoles, running of stable and unstable tachycardias, paroxysms of atrial fibrillation and flutter, ventricular fibrillation, conduction disturbances—sinoatrial and atrioventricular blockades. An analysis of heart rate turbulence (HRT) has been performed on the basis of the 24-h ECG. The deviation of at least one of two parameters has been taken as pathological HRT: turbulence onset (TO) <0%), and turbulence slope (TS) >2.5 ms/RR). Heart rate variability (HRV) has been assessed by temporal (SDNN—standard deviation of the average values of RR-intervals; SDNNi—mean value of standard deviations of RR intervals for a 5-min recording; SDANN—standard deviation of the average values of sinus RR intervals for 5 min), and spectral characteristics (TotP—total spectrum power; LfP—low-frequency component of the spectrum; HfP—high-frequency component of the spectrum; L/H—vagosympathetic balance index) [11].

The level of brain natriuretic peptide (BNP) has been determined on the 7th–9th days after STEMI. A six-minute walk test has been performed to determine NYHA class of CHF starting from the 12th week of the postinfarction period.

The progression of CHF in the postinfarction period has been considered to be the endpoint, determined by the development of one of the following events [12,13]: hospitalization of the patient due to decompensation of CHF; decrease in EF compared to baseline values with the patient's transition from the group with preserved EF (HFpEF) to the group with mid-range (HFmrEF) or reduced (HFrEF) ejection fraction, or from HFmrEF to HFrEF group; a six-minute walk test results corresponding to NYHA class II-IV of CHF.

The STEMI patients have been receiving treatment in accordance with the ESC Clinical Practice Guidelines [14]. Percutaneous coronary intervention (PCI) with stenting (100%) has been carried out in all patients on the first day of STEMI. Twenty (33.3%) patients have undergone pharmacoinvasive reperfusion—systemic thrombolytic therapy (TT) and PCI.

The study involved two stages of implementation. At the first stage, a multivariate model for assessing the risk of CHF progression within 48 weeks after STEMI has been built on the basis of examination and follow-up data for 113 patients (group "M"). At the second stage, the sensitivity and specificity of the multivariate model for the risk of CHF decompensation has been tested based on a 48-week follow-up of 60 patients (group "T").

Statistical data processing has been performed using the licensed version of STATISTICA 13.0 program (StatSoft, Inc., OC, OK, USA). All values of quantitative traits are given with the 95% confidence interval (CI). The McNemar criterion has been used when comparing qualitative characteristics for paired samples, and χ^2 test has been used for independent samples. To determine the influence of the parameters on the endpoint development, and to estimate the relative risk (RR) and 95% CI, the method of univariate analysis by applying logistic regression has been used. The value of $p < 0.05$ was taken as a threshold of statistical significance. To include the indicators in a multivariate model using the Cox multiple linear regression, the absence of a correlation between thereof should be a prerequisite. To assess the information content and adequacy of the logistic model, the coefficients of sensitivity and specificity have been determined. Sensitivity (Se) is the ability of a diagnostic method to give a reliable result, and specificity (Sp) is the ability of a diagnostic method not to provide false positive results in the absence of a disease [15].

3. Results

According to the results of the first stage of the study [16], the endpoints had been achieved in 26 (23%) patients of group "M". Nine (35%) patients were hospitalized due to decompensation of CHF; NYHA class III of CHF was estimated in 2 (7.7%) patients according to a six-minute walk test; a decrease in EF was determined in 19 (73%) patients with the transition from HFpEF: to HFmrEF—in 11 (58%), to HFrEF—in 4 (21%), from HFmrEF to HFrEF—in 4 (21%) patients.

The following factors for CHF progression have been established according to the univariate regression analysis of data from 113 STEMI patients: pathological values of TO and HRT, BNP level, ESD, GLS, GCS, and GRS values obtained on the 7th–9th days of STEMI (Table 1). The EF has shown no diagnostic significance in detecting CHF progression.

Considering correlations between given parameters and using a stepwise variable selection method, a multivariate regression model for CHF progression in STEMI patients has been created. It includes HRT, ESD, and GLS values, and has the form of the formula:

$$h = h_0(t) \cdot \exp(1.366539 \cdot X_1 + 0.043323 \cdot X_2 - 0.108260 \cdot X_3) \qquad (1)$$

where: X_1 is equal to 1.0 with pathological HRT on the 7th–9th days of STEMI, and it is equal to 0 with normal HRT; X_2—ESD, mm; X_3—GLS, %; $h_0(t)$—baseline risk of 0.018611 at the 6th week, 0.100065 at the 12th week, 0.108673 at the 16th week, 0.181305 at the 24th week, and 0.212152 at the 48th week. The risk of predicting CHF has been calculated at the 6th, 12th, 16th, 24th, and 48th weeks of the postinfarction period. We have concluded that if the value of h was higher than 1.0, CHF progression was predicted; if the value of h was less than 1.0, there was a stable course of the postinfarction period.

Table 1. Parameters correlating with CHF progression within 48 weeks after STEMI.

Variable	Univariate Analysis		Multivariate Analysis	
	RR (95% CI)	p	RR (95% CI)	p
Pathological TO	2.75 (1.191–6.326)	0.018	-	-
Pathological HRT	2.64 (1.17–5.92)	0.019	3.92 (1.66–9.25)	0.0018
SDANN	0.98 (0.97–1.0)	0.11	-	-
HfP	1.0 (0.99–1.01)	0.22	-	-
BNP	1.001 (1.0001–1.0002)	0.023	-	-
ESD	1.04 (1.01–1.07)	0.0022	1.04 (1.015–1.07)	0.0027
GLS	0.89 (0.82–0.98)	0.017	0.9 (0.815–0.98)	0.028
GCS	0.92 (0.86–0.98)	0.01	-	-
GRS	0.95 (0.92–0.99)	0.012	-	-

Note: BNP—brain natriuretic peptide; HfP—high-frequency component of the spectrum; SDANN—standard deviation of the average values of sinus RR intervals for 5 min; TO—turbulence onset; ESD—end-systolic dimension; RR—relative risk; HRT—heart rate turbulence. The values are given with 95% CI.

The analysis of variance (ANOVA) has shown that the present model of differentiation of patients by the nature of the postinfarction period has a high information content: the Wilk's Lambda = 0.83243, F (3109) = 7.3139 (p = 0.00016).

At the second stage, the performance of the developed multivariate model has been tested in group "T" (60 patients). Table 2 shows comparative characteristics of groups "M" and "T". There were no significant differences in age, a number of concomitant conditions, and localization of the infarction area in the groups. However, the patients with burdened heredity for cardiovascular diseases were found more frequently in group "T".

Table 2. Drug therapy in group "M" and group "T".

Group of Drugs	Group "M" (n = 113)			Group "T" (n = 60)			p 1–4	p 2–5	p 3–6
	7th–9th Day	12th Week	48th Week	7th–9th Day	12th Week	48th Week			
	1	2	3	4	5	6			
Beta-blockers	86 (76%)	81 (73%)	74 (65%)	48 (80%)	40 (67%)	36 (60%)	0.56	0.494	0.476
ACE inhibitors/ARBs	93 (82%)	87 (77%)	61 (70%)	53 (88%)	44 (73%)	39 (65%)	0.299	0.594	0.163
Diuretics	21 (19%)	17 (15%)	15 (13%)	9 (15%)	7 (12%)	7 (12%)	0.554	0.541	0.763
Calcium channel blockers	10 (8.8%)	13 (12%)	8 (7.1%)	4 (6.7%)	5 (8.3%)	4 (6.7%)	0.617	0.516	0.919
Class III antiarrhythmic agents	6 (5.3%)	2 (1.8%)	3 (2.7%)	3 (5%)	1 (1.7%)	1 (1.7%)	0.931	0.961	0.681

Note: ARBs—angiotensin II receptor blockers, ACE inhibitors—angiotensin-converting enzyme inhibitors.

CHF progression was recorded in 12 (20%) patients of group "T" over the 48-week follow-up. One (8.3%) patient was hospitalized due to CHF decompensation; NYHA class III of CHF was estimated in 2 (16.7%) patients according to the six-minute walk test; a ecrease in EF was determined in 9 (75%) patients: with the transition from HFpEF to HFmrEF—in 3 (25%), and from HFmrEF to HFrEF—in 6 (50%) patients.

Sensitivity, specificity, and diagnostic accuracy of the method have been determined to assess the adequacy of the presented logistic regression individual risk model for predicting CHF.

Table 3 shows the results of testing a multivariate model for predicting CHF progression in patients of group "T" (n = 60) within 48 weeks after STEMI.

Table 3. Test results of a model for predicting CHF progression in patients of group "T" (n = 60) within 48 weeks after STEMI.

Period after STEMI	12th Week	24th Week	48th Week
True positive, n	1	6	10
False positive, n	4	2	2
False negative, n	2	3	2
True negative, n	53	49	46
Sensitivity, %	33.3%	66.7%	83.3%
Specificity, %	93%	96.1%	95.8%
Diagnostic accuracy, %	90%	91.7%	93.3%

The diagnostic model is characterized by low sensitivity with a high level of specificity and diagnostic accuracy at the 12th week. However, sensitivity of the model has increased to 83.3% by the 48th week at the later stages of the postinfarction period. Thus, the individual risk model for predicting CHF after STEMI has acceptable sensitivity, high specificity, and diagnostic accuracy and can be used in early stages of STEMI (on the 7th–9th days) to identify patients with a high risk of CHF decompensation.

4. Discussion

Late and/or unsuccessful pharmacoinvasive revascularization, large-size myocardial infarction, life-threatening arrhythmias, old and senile age, lack of previous drug therapy of cardiovascular diseases, type 2 diabetes, and comorbidity are known as factors to be associated with a high risk of CHF progression [4,5,12,17]. Various combinations thereof affect the risk of developing CHF in different ways, which, however, requires proof in appropriate multivariate models.

BNP is one of the most common CHF indicators [12,18]. According to some researches [19], such biomarkers as N-terminal pro-brain natriuretic peptide (NT-proBNP), pentraxin-related protein (PTX-3) and, to a lesser extent, stimulating growth factor 2 (ST2), have demonstrated their prognostic significance in diagnosis of cardiovascular complications with a sensitivity of 78.79% and a specificity of 86.67% (area under the curve, AUC 0.73). The current study has also established the role of BNP in long-term prognosis in STEMI patients, but this parameter has not been included in the multivariate model.

Investigation of cardiac biomechanics is essential in assessing the function of the entire cardiovascular system in patients with myocardial infarction, since this group of patients has a high risk of CHF progression due to left ventricular (LV) pathological remodeling. As LV EF is the most studied, the expediency of its monitoring in CHF is beyond doubt, since reduced ejection fraction is associated with an unsatisfactory prognosis, poor quality of life of patients, increased mortality and hospitalization rates [4,5,12,20]. A decrease in LV EF during dynamic follow-up is a direct indicator of CHF progression. Despite that a decrease in EF with the transition of a patient from HFpEF to HFmrEF or HFrEF, and from HFmrEF to HFrEF in the post-infarction period, has been regarded as one of the manifestations of CHF progression in the current study, the initial values of the LV EF on the 7th–9th days of STEMI did not demonstrate diagnostic significance in detecting CHF progression in the postinfarction period.

Many researchers have found that HRV is a valid factor for a high risk of mortality and CHF progression [11,21]. Low values of parameters for HRV spectral analysis (HfP) and temporal analysis (SDAAN) are associated with an increase in the probability of CHF decompensation.

HRT is an appropriate technique for stratification of CHF risk in postinfarction patients [11]. A group of researchers led by Cygankiewicz [22] have established a correlation between HRT, EF, and class of CHF. In the current study, it has been revealed that pathological values of TO and impaired HRT on the 7th–9th days of STEMI were independent factors of CHF decompensation.

Another urgent problem is the risk stratification of life-threatening rhythm disturbances in CHF patients who have had myocardial infarction. Due to the lack of an accurate system for determining the risk of sudden death in such patients, implantation of a cardioverter defibrillator is not always properly performed [23–25]. Some researchers believe that a deeper investigation of the global strain characteristics would help unify the selection of patients [26,27]. Special attention is paid to the GLS parameter, since it has been established to be an indicator of an unfavorable course of CHF, and is associated with a decrease in the functional status of patients and an increase in the volume of the LV [28,29]. In the current study, low values of three parameters (GLS, GCS, and GRS) have been independently associated with CHF progression within the next 48 weeks after STEMI.

An integrated approach is essential to apply for assessing the risk of CHF progression. Determination of individual parameters does not reflect a complex clinical and functional picture and cannot be used in patients after STEMI. The best way to assess the risk of developing decompensated CHF is a combination of several parameters reflecting the condition of the cardiovascular system as a whole.

According to the Meta-Analysis Global Group in Chronic Heart Failure (MAGGIC) research, a risk score for prediction of mortality in CHF has been constructed from 13 patient characteristics: age, EF, NYHA class, serum creatinine, diabetes, systolic blood pressure, body mass index, heart failure duration, current smoker, chronic obstructive pulmonary disease, gender, not prescribed a beta-blocker, and not prescribed an ACE inhibitor or ARBs. The difference between the model-predicted and the observed 3-year mortality in the six risk groups varied between 5% and −12% [30]. An addition of BNP or NT-proBNP to the model has significantly increased the predictive significance of the MAGGIC risk score [31].

Other researchers [32] have proposed the BARDICHE-index to assess the risk of hospitalization and mortality in patients with CHF based on body mass index, age, resting systolic blood pressure, dyspnea, NT-proBNP, glomerular filtration rate, resting heart rate, and exercise performance using the six-minute walk test. Outcome has been predicted independently of EF and gender.

As there are no available publications describing the calculation of the risk of CHF progression based on a combined assessment of volumetric and strain characteristics of the LV myocardium together with determination of autonomic rhythm regulation, the approach to risk stratification of STEMI patients is to improve the diagnostic accuracy of prediction. A multivariate diagnostic model for predicting CHF progression within 48 weeks after STEMI has been created and successfully tested. Its high specificity, diagnostic accuracy and sensitivity have been proved in the current study.

5. Conclusions

The proposed multivariate model for predicting CHF decompensation within 48 weeks after myocardial infarction, which includes such parameters as heart rate turbulence, left ventricular end-systolic dimension, and global longitudinal strain, has an adequate specificity of 83.3%, a high sensitivity of 95.8%, and a diagnostic accuracy of 93.3%. This technique can be used in the early stages of myocardial infarction to identify patients with a high risk of heart failure progression within the next 48-weeks of postinfarction period.

6. Study Limitations

The present study included young and middle-aged patients predominantly (35–65 years old) with primary STEMI with hemodynamically significant stenosis of exclusively infarct-related coronary artery, without a history of CHF. These strict inclusion criteria have been driven by the attempt to exclude the influence of other factors that could lead to myocardial remodeling before the index event (STEMI) and affect the baseline values of the volumetric and deformation characteristics of the myocardium. For this reason, the number of the study participants was relatively small. The authors consider the present study a preliminary one in the process of searching and refining the combination of predictors of the development and progression of CHF after STEMI.

Author Contributions: Conceptualization, V.E.O. and V.A.G.; methodology, E.V.A.; software, A.A.O.; validation, V.A.G., Y.A.B. and A.V.G.; formal analysis, Y.A.B.; investigation, E.V.A. and A.V.G.; resources, V.E.O.; data curation, V.A.G.; writing—original draft preparation, E.V.A.; writing—review and editing, N.V.B.; visualization, A.A.O.; supervision, N.V.B.; project administration, V.E.O.; funding acquisition, V.E.O. All authors have read and agreed to the published version of the manuscript.

Funding: The work was carried out with financial support: a grant from the President of the Russian Federation for the government support of the young Russian scientists—Candidates and Doctors of sciences.

Institutional Review Board Statement: The study was conducted according to the guidelines of the Declaration of Helsinki, and approved by the Local Ethics Committee of the Penza State University (protocol code 253 and date of approval—28 September 2014).

Informed Consent Statement: Informed consent was obtained from all subjects involved in the study.

Data Availability Statement: The data presented in this study are available on request from the corresponding author. The data are not publicly available due to ethical reasons.

Conflicts of Interest: The authors declare no conflict of interest.

References

1. Dunlay, S.M.; Roger, V.L.; Redfield, M.M. Epidemiology of heart failure with preserved ejection fraction. *Nat. Rev. Cardiol.* **2017**, *14*, 591–602. [CrossRef] [PubMed]
2. Ziaeian, B.; Fonarow, B.Z.G.C. Epidemiology and aetiology of heart failure. *Nat. Rev. Cardiol.* **2016**, *13*, 368–378. [CrossRef] [PubMed]
3. Yancy, C.W.; Jessup, M.; Bozkurt, B.; Butler, J.; Casey, D.; Colvin, M.M.; Drazner, M.H.; Filippatos, G.S.; Fonarow, G.C.; Givertz, M.M.; et al. 2017 ACC/AHA/HFSA focused update of the 2013 ACCF/AHA guideline for the management of heart failure: A Report of the American College of Cardiology/American Heart Association Task Force on Clinical Practice Guidelines and the Heart Failure Society of America. *Circulation* **2017**, *136*, e137–e161. [CrossRef]
4. Yang, X.; Lupón, J.; Vidán, M.T.; Ferguson, C.; Gastelurrutia, P.; Newton, P.J.; Macdonald, P.S.; Bueno, H.; Bayés-Genís, A.; Woo, J.; et al. Impact of frailty on mortality and hospitalization in chronic heart failure: A systematic review and meta-analysis. *J. Am. Heart Assoc.* **2018**, *7*, e008251. [CrossRef] [PubMed]
5. Jones, N.; Roalfe, A.K.; Adoki, I.; Hobbs, F.R.; Taylor, C.J. Survival of patients with chronic heart failure in the community: A systematic review and meta-analysis. *Eur. J. Heart Fail.* **2019**, *21*, 1306–1325. [CrossRef] [PubMed]
6. Yu, D.S.F.; Li, P.W.C.; Yue, S.C.S.; Wong, J.; Yan, B.; Tsang, K.K.; Choi, K.C.; Doris, Y.S.F. The effects and cost-effectiveness of an empowerment-based self-care programme in patients with chronic heart failure: A study protocol. *J. Adv. Nurs.* **2019**, *75*, 3740–3748. [CrossRef] [PubMed]
7. Puymirat, E.; Simon, T.; Cayla, G.; Cottin, Y.; Elbaz, M.; Coste, P.; Lemesle, G.; Motreff, P.; Popovic, B.; Khalife, K.; et al. Acute Myocardial Infarction. *Circulation* **2017**, *136*, 1908–1919. [CrossRef] [PubMed]
8. Johansson, S.; Rosengren, A.; Young, K.; Jennings, E. Mortality and morbidity trends after the first year in survivors of acute myocardial infarction: A systematic review. *BMC Cardiovasc. Disord.* **2017**, *17*, 1–8. [CrossRef] [PubMed]
9. Bahit, M.C.; Kochar, A.; Granger, C.B. Post-myocardial infarction heart failure. *JACC Heart Fail.* **2018**, *6*, 179–186. [CrossRef] [PubMed]
10. Mitchell, C.; Rahko, P.S.; Blauwet, L.A.; Canaday, B.; Finstuen, J.A.; Foster, M.C.; Horton, K.; Ogunyankin, K.O.; Palma, R.A.; Velazquez, E.J. Guidelines for performing a comprehensive transthoracic echocardiographic examination in adults: Recommendations from the American Society of Echocardiography. *J. Am. Soc. Echocardiogr.* **2019**, *32*, 1–64. [CrossRef]
11. Steinberg, J.S.; Varma, N.; Cygankiewicz, I.; Aziz, P.; Balsam, P.; Baranchuk, A.; Cantillon, D.J.; Dilaveris, P.; Dubner, S.J.; El-Sherif, N.; et al. 2017 ISHNE-HRS expert consensus statement on ambulatory ECG and external cardiac monitoring/telemetry. *Heart Rhythm.* **2017**, *14*, e55–e96. [CrossRef]
12. Ponikowski, P.; Voors, A.A.; Anker, S.D.; Bueno, H.; Cleland, J.G.F.; Coats, A.J.S.; Falk, V.; González-Juanatey, J.R.; Harjola, V.-P.; A Jankowska, E.; et al. 2016 ESC Guidelines for the diagnosis and treatment of acute and chronic heart failure. *Eur. Heart J.* **2016**, *37*, 2129–2200. [CrossRef] [PubMed]

13. Mareev, V.Y.; Medical Scientific and Educational Centre of Moscow State University; Fomin, I.V.; Ageev, F.T.; Begrambekova, Y.L.; Vasyuk, Y.; Garganeeva, A.A.; Gendlin, G.E.; Glezer, M.G.; Gote, S.V.; et al. Russian Heart Failure Society, Russian Society of Cardiology. Russian Scientific Medical Society of Internal Medicine Guidelines for Heart failure: Chronic (CHF) and acute decompensated (ADHF). Diagnosis, prevention and treatment. *Kardiologiia* **2018**, *17*, 1–164. [CrossRef]
14. Arslan, F.; Bongartz, L.; Berg, J.M.T.; Jukema, J.W.; Appelman, Y.; Liem, A.H.; De Winter, R.J.; Hof, A.W.J.V.; Damman, P. 2017 ESC guidelines for the management of acute myocardial infarction in patients presenting with ST-segment elevation: Comments from the Dutch ACS working group. *Neth. Heart J.* **2018**, *26*, 417–421. [CrossRef] [PubMed]
15. Lang, T.A. *How to Describe Statistics in Medicine. Guide for Authors, Editors and Reviewers*, 2nd ed.; Leonova, V.P., Ed.; Prakticheskaya Meditsina: Moskva, Russia, 2016; p. 480. (In Russian)
16. Oleynikov, V.E.; Dushina, E.V.; Golubeva, A.V.; Barmenkova, J.A. Early predictors of heart failure progression in patients after myocardial infarction. *Kardiologiia* **2020**, *60*, 84–93. [CrossRef]
17. Ouwerkerk, W.; Voors, A.A.; Zwinderman, A.H. Factors influencing the predictive power of models for predicting mortality and/or heart failure hospitalization in patients with heart failure. *JACC Heart Fail.* **2014**, *2*, 429–436. [CrossRef]
18. Fazlinezhad, A.; Rezaeian, M.K.; Yousefzadeh, H.; Ghaffarzadegan, K.; Khajedaluee, M. Plasma Brain Natriuretic Peptide (BNP) as an indicator of left ventricular function, early outcome and mechanical complications after acute myocardial infarction. *Clin. Med. Insights Cardiol.* **2011**, *5*, CMC-S7189. [CrossRef]
19. Khamitova, A.F.; Lakman, I.A.; Akhmetvaleev, R.R.; Tulbaev, E.L.; Gareeva, D.F.; Zagidullin, S.Z.; Zagidullin, N.S. Multifactor predictive model in patients with myocardial infarction based on modern biomarkers. *Kardiologiia* **2020**, *60*, 14–20. [CrossRef]
20. Murphy, S.P.; Ibrahim, N.E.; Januzzi, J.L. Heart Failure with Reduced Ejection Fraction. *JAMA* **2020**, *324*, 488–504. [CrossRef]
21. La Rovere, M.T.; Pinna, G.D.; Maestri, R.; Barlera, S.; Bernardinangeli, M.; Veniani, M.; Nicolosi, G.L.; Marchioli, M.; Tavazzi, L.; GISSI-HF Investigators. Autonomic markers and cardiovascular and arrhythmic events in heart failure patients: Still a place in prognostication? Data from the GISSI-HF trial. *Eur. J. Heart Fail.* **2012**, *14*, 1410–1419. [CrossRef] [PubMed]
22. Cygankiewicz, I. Heart Rate Turbulence. *Prog. Cardiovasc. Dis.* **2013**, *56*, 160–171. [CrossRef]
23. Priori, S.G.; Blomström-Lundqvist, C.; Mazzanti, A.; Blom, N.; Borggrefe, M.; Camm, J.; Elliott, P.; Fitzsimons, D.; Hatala, R.; Hindricks, G.; et al. 2015 ESC Guidelines for the management of patients with ventricular arrhythmias and the prevention of sudden cardiac death. *Europace* **2015**, *17*, 1601–1687. [CrossRef] [PubMed]
24. Gasparyan, A.Z.; Shlevkov, N.B.; Skvortsov, A.A. Possibilities of modern biomarkers for assessing the risk of developing ventricular tachyarrhythmias and sudden cardiac death in patients with chronic heart failure. *Kardiologiia* **2020**, *60*, 101–108. [CrossRef]
25. Haugaa, K.H.; Dan, G.-A.; Iliodromitis, K.; Lenarczyk, R.; Marinskis, G.; Osca, J.; Scherr, D.; Dagres, N. Management of patients with ventricular arrhythmias and prevention of sudden cardiac death—translating guidelines into practice: Results of the European Heart Rhythm Association survey. *Europace* **2018**, *20*, f249–f253. [CrossRef] [PubMed]
26. Dandel, M.; Javier, M.F.D.M.; Delmo, E.M.J.; Loebe, M.; Hetzer, R. Weaning from ventricular assist device support after recovery from left ventricular failure with or without secondary right ventricular failure. *Cardiovasc. Diagn. Ther.* **2021**, *11*, 226–242. [CrossRef]
27. Haugaa, K.; Grenne, B.L.; Eek, C.H.; Ersbøll, M.; Valeur, N.; Svendsen, J.H.; Florian, A.; Sjøli, B.; Brunvand, H.; Køber, L.; et al. Strain Echocardiography Improves Risk Prediction of Ventricular Arrhythmias After Myocardial Infarction. *JACC Cardiovasc. Imaging* **2013**, *6*, 841–850. [CrossRef]
28. Stanton, T.; Leano, R.; Marwick, T.H. Prediction of all-cause mortality from global longitudinal speckle strain: Comparison with ejection fraction and wall motion scoring. *Circulation. Cardiovasc. Imaging* **2009**, *2*, 356–364. [CrossRef]
29. Zhang, K.W.; French, B.; Khan, A.M.; Plappert, T.; Fang, J.C.; Sweitzer, N.K.; Borlaug, B.A.; Chirinos, J.A.; Sutton, M.S.J.; Cappola, T.P.; et al. Strain Improves Risk Prediction Beyond Ejection Fraction in Chronic Systolic Heart Failure. *J. Am. Heart Assoc.* **2014**, *3*, e000550. [CrossRef]
30. Sartipy, U.; Dahlström, U.; Edner, M.; Lund, L.H. Predicting survival in heart failure: Validation of the MAGGIC heart failure risk score in 51 043 patients from the Swedish Heart Failure Registry. *Eur. J. Heart Fail.* **2013**, *16*, 173–179. [CrossRef]
31. Khanam, S.S.; Choi, E.; Son, J.-W.; Lee, J.-W.; Youn, Y.J.; Yoon, J.; Lee, S.-H.; Kim, J.-Y.; Ahn, S.G.; Ahn, M.-S.; et al. Validation of the MAGGIC (Meta-Analysis Global Group in Chronic Heart Failure) heart failure risk score and the effect of adding natriuretic peptide for predicting mortality after discharge in hospitalized patients with heart failure. *PLoS ONE* **2018**, *13*, e0206380. [CrossRef] [PubMed]
32. Uszko-Lencer, N.H.; Frankenstein, L.; Spruit, M.A.; Maeder, M.T.; Gutmann, M.; Muzzarelli, S.; Osswald, S.; Pfisterer, M.E.; Zugck, C.; Brunner-La Rocca, H.P.; et al. Predicting hospitalization and mortality in patients with heart failure: The BARDICHE-index. *Int. J. Cardiol.* **2017**, *227*, 901–907. [CrossRef]

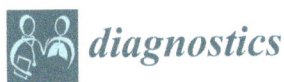

Article

Long-Term Effects of Angiotensin Receptor–Neprilysin Inhibitors on Myocardial Function in Chronic Heart Failure Patients with Reduced Ejection Fraction

Gregor Poglajen [1,2,*], Ajda Anžič-Drofenik [1], Gregor Zemljič [1], Sabina Frljak [1], Andraž Cerar [1], Renata Okrajšek [1], Miran Šebeštjen [1,2] and Bojan Vrtovec [1,2]

1 Advanced Heart Failure and Transplantation Center, Department of Cardiology, University Medical Center Ljubljana, 1000 Ljubljana, Slovenia; ajda.drofenik@gmail.com (A.A.-D.); gregor.zemljic@kclj.si (G.Z.); sabina.frljak@kclj.si (S.F.); andraz.cerar@kclj.si (A.C.); renata.okrajsek@kclj.si (R.O.); miran.sebestjen@kclj.si (M.Š.); bojan.vrtovec@kclj.si (B.V.)
2 Department of Internal Medicine, Faculty of Medicine, University of Ljubljana, 1000 Ljubljana, Slovenia
* Correspondence: gregor.poglajen@kclj.si

Received: 1 June 2020; Accepted: 27 July 2020; Published: 28 July 2020

Abstract: Background. We sought to evaluate the long-term effects of angiotensin receptor blocker–neprilysin inhibitor (ARNI) therapy on reverse remodeling of the failing myocardium in HFrEF patients. Methods. We performed a prospective non-randomized longitudinal study on 228 HFrEF patients treated with ARNI at our center. Prior to ARNI introduction all patients received stable doses of ACEI/ARB for at least six months. Clinical, biochemical and echocardiography data were obtained at ARNI introduction and 12-month follow-up. Results At follow-up, we found significant improvements in LVEF (29.7% ± 8% vs. 36.5% ± 9%; $p < 0.001$), LVOT-VTI (14.8 ± 4.2 cm vs. 17.2 ± 4.2 cm; $p < 0.001$), TAPSE (1.7 ± 0.5 cm vs. 2.1 ± 0.6 cm; $p < 0.001$) and LV-EDD (6.5 ± 0.8 cm vs. 6.3 ± 0.9 cm; $p = 0.001$). NT-proBNP serum levels also decreased significantly (1324 (605, 3281) pg/mL vs. 792 (329, 2022) pg/mL; $p = 0.001$). A total of 102 (45%) of patients responded favorably to ARNI (ΔLVEF < +5%; Group A) and 126 (55%) patients achieved ΔLVEF ≥ +5% (Group B). The two groups differed significantly in age, heart failure etiology, baseline LVEF and baseline NT-proBNP. On multivariable analysis, nonischemic heart failure, LVEF < 30% and NT-proBNP < 1500 pg/mL emerged as independent correlates of favorable response to ARNI therapy. Conclusion. ARNI therapy appears to improve echocardiographic parameters of left and right ventricular function in HFrEF patients above the effect of pre-existing optimal medical management. These effects may be particularly pronounced in patients with nonischemic heart failure, LVEF < 30% and lower degree of neurohumoral activation.

Keywords: angiotensin receptor–neprilysin inhibitor; echocardiography; HFrEF

1. Introduction

With the publication of paradigm-HF trial (prospective comparison of ARNI with ACEI to determine impact on global mortality in heart failure) in 2014 [1] angiotensin receptor blocker–neprilysin inhibitors (ARNI) became a new promising class of drugs for the treatment of patients with heart failure with reduced ejection fraction (HFrEF). The study demonstrated that in HFrEF patient treatment with ARNI, compared to angiotensin converting enzyme inhibitor (ACEI) enalapril, resulted in significant benefits considering heart failure hospitalizations and cardiovascular (CV) and all-cause mortality [1]. Subsequent transition and pioneer-HF trials further demonstrated comparable safety and superior efficacy of ARNI over ACEI also in HFrEF patients with more advanced stages of the disease, largely establishing ARNI as an evolving first-line treatment approach in this patient population [2,3]. However, despite these encouraging findings, the underlying mechanisms still remain incompletely understood.

Studies of guidelines-based optimal heart failure medical therapy using angiotensin converting enzyme inhibitors (ACEI), angiotensin II receptor blockers (ARB), beta receptor blocking agents (β-blockers) and mineralocorticoid receptor antagonists (MRA) have demonstrated that improved clinical outcomes of HFrEF patients were associated with the reverse remodeling of the failing myocardium [4] which largely predicated on the inhibition of renin–angiotensin–aldosterone axis. Available data have suggested that in this patient cohort superior clinical response to ARNI over ACEI stems from a dual inhibition of renin–angiotensin–aldosterone axis and neprilysin, the latter resulting in an increased bioactivity of natriuretic and other vasoactive peptides [5]. However, until recently the association between ARNI-associated dual inhibition and myocardial reverse remodeling in HFrEF patients remained unexplored.

The recently published prove-HF trial confirmed the association of reverse remodeling and neurohumoral modulation in HFrEF patients treated with ARNI, demonstrating a significant correlation between changes in serum NT-proBNP and parameters of left ventricular volume and function in these patients [6]. While the results of several other small-scale reports are in line with prove-HF data [7–9], it is important to emphasize that the vast majority of presently available clinical data focus solely on the short-term effects of ARNI on left ventricular structure and function. In contrast, currently there are very few data on the long-term effects of ARNI therapy on myocardial reverse remodeling. What is more, no study to date addressed the effects of ARNI on the right ventricular function in HFrEF patients. This is relevant as in this patient cohort right ventricular dysfunction has been established as an important determinant of symptomatic limitations, cardiovascular outcomes and survival [10].

The aim of our study was therefore to evaluate the long-term effects of ARNI therapy on ventricular reverse remodeling in a HFrEF patient population.

2. Materials and Methods

2.1. Study Population

We performed a single-center open-label prospective non-randomized longitudinal study to explore the effects of ARNI on the ventricular reverse remodeling in HFrEF patients (Figure 1). The study protocol was approved by the National medical ethics committee (decision document 0120–355/2017/6). All patients with HFrEF of ischemic and non-ischemic etiology that were treated at our center between years 2016 and 2019 were considered for the participation in the study. The inclusion criteria for the participation in the study were: patient age > 18 years, guideline-based heart failure medical management (OMT) for at least 6 months, established left ventricular systolic dysfunction (LVEF < 40%) and an established diagnosis of nonischemic dilated cardiomyopathy (DCMP) (as per European Society of Cardiology position statement [11]) or an established diagnosis of ischemic heart failure (ICM) without a possibility of percutaneous or surgical revascularization [12]. Exclusion criteria were as follows: patients with established heart failure with preserved ejection fraction (HFpEF), any hospitalization for severe worsening of heart failure (worsening heart failure requiring inotropic support) or acute myocardial infarction within 6 months before study enrollment, cardiac resynchronization therapy within 6 months before enrollment, patients with significant improvement of LVEF (ΔLVEF > +5% in 6 months prior to enrollment) on current optimal heart failure therapy and patients currently participating in other interventional studies. Of 322 assessed patients 26 did not meet the inclusion/exclusion criteria and 33 patients declined to participate in the study. Upon follow-up evaluation additional 35 patients were excluded due to the incomplete clinical, biochemical or echocardiographic data. Ultimately, 228 patients were included in the final data analysis. Informed consent was obtained from all patients before they were enrolled in the study.

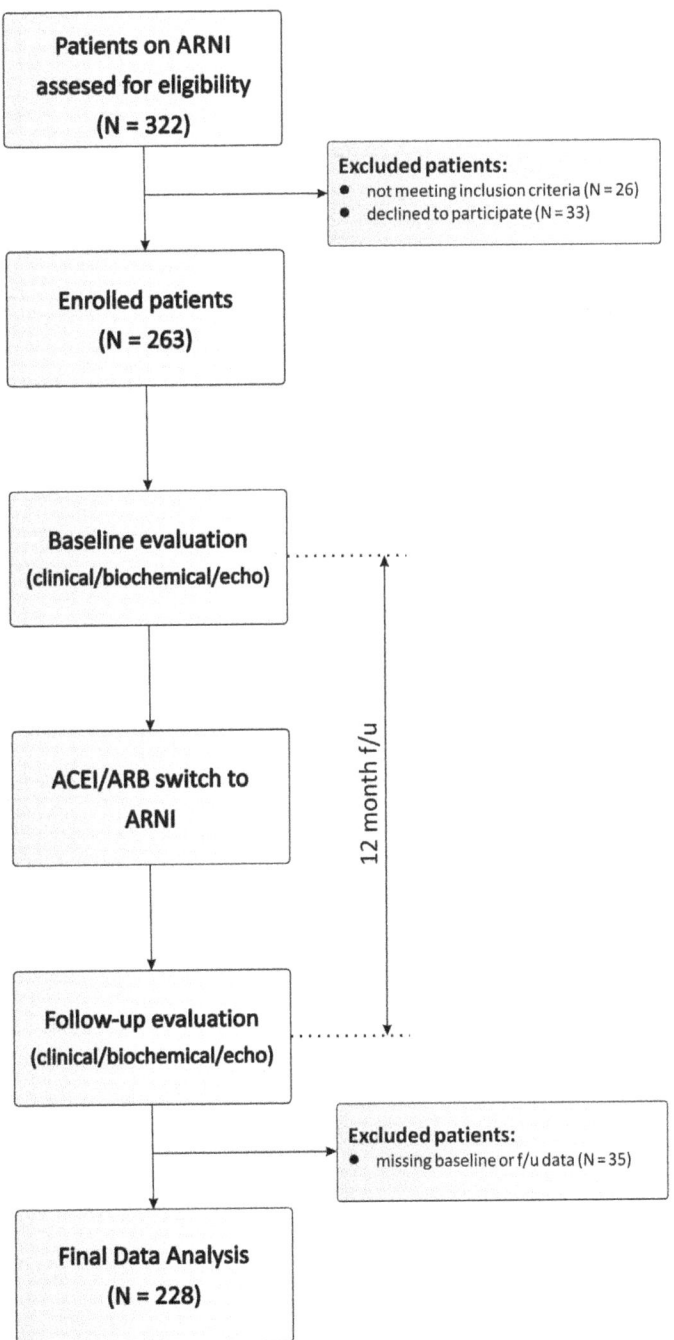

Figure 1. Study consort diagram.

2.2. Study Design

At enrollment, all patients were started on a sacubitril/valsartan dose per our institution's protocol (Figure 1): if the patients were on an ACEI or ARB dose of at least 50% of target dose, they were started on an ARNI dose of 49/51 mg q12. Patients on an ACEI or ARB dose of less than 50% of target dose or with a history of hypotension (systolic blood pressure < 90 mmHg), liver or kidney insufficiency were initiated on an ARNI dose of 24/26 mg q12. ARNI uptitration was performed on weekly intervals if tolerated by the patient. During the study period patients maintained the doses of β-blockers and MRAs. Clinical, biochemical and echocardiographic data were collected at baseline and 12-month follow-up. Favorable response to ARNI therapy was defined as an increase in left ventricular ejection fraction (LVEF) ≥5% at 12-month follow-up [4].

2.3. Laboratory Tests

Laboratory tests (biochemistry, CBC, renal function tests and liver function test) were collected at baseline and at 12-month follow-up. All samples were collected in accordance with the institutional protocols and delivered to the institutional laboratory that was blinded to patient clinical data for the analysis.

2.4. NT-proBNP Measurement

Blood sample was collected at baseline and at 12-month follow-up. EDTA-coated, aprotinin-containing test tubes were used. Immediately after the blood sample was obtained, it was placed on ice (for up to 4 h) and centrifuged at 4500 rpm for 15 min at 0 °C. After centrifugation, the serum was extracted from the test tube and stored separately (at −80 °C). All NT-proBNP assays were done using a standard commercial kit (Roche Diagnostics, Rotkreuz, Switzerland) at a hospital's central independent laboratory which was blinded to the patients' clinical status and medication data.

2.5. Echocardiography

Transthoracic echocardiography was performed at baseline and 12 months according to American Society of Echocardiography (ASE) and European Association of Cardiovascular Imaging (EACVI) recommendations [13]. A cardiac ultrasound system (GE Vivid E9, Vingmed ultrasound, Horten, Norway) was used for imaging. All images were stored and analyzed at the end of the follow-up by an independent echocardiographer who was blinded to the patients' therapeutic status and the timing of the recordings. Left ventricular function was assessed by left ventricular ejection fraction that was determined based on Simpson's biplane rule. Right ventricular function was assessed by tricuspid annular plane systolic excursion (TAPSE).

2.6. Study End Points

The primary end point was a change in LVEF between baseline and 12-month follow-up. Secondary end points were the changes in TAPSE, left ventricular outflow tract velocity–time integral (LVOT VTI) and left ventricular end-diastolic diameter (LVEDD) between baseline and 12-month follow-up. In exploratory data analysis, we aimed to identify predictors of favorable response to ARNI therapy.

2.7. Statistical Methods and Analysis

Categorical variables are presented as count (percent) and were compared using a chi-squared test or nonparametric Fischer exact test. Continuous variables are reported either as mean (±SD) or median (IQR). Continuous variables were compared using Student's t-test, ANOVA or Mann–Whitney nonparametric test. Pearson correlation model was used to assess the potential correlation between two continuous variables. Shapiro–Wilk test was used to test for the normality of data distribution. Statistical significance was assumed for p-values of <0.05. All statistical analyses were performed with SPSS version 20.0 (IBM, Chicago, IL, USA).

3. Results

3.1. Patient Characteristics

Baseline patient characteristics are outlined in Table 1. Majority of the patients included in our analysis were male with non-ischemic heart failure. Roughly half of the patients had a history of hypertension and hyperlipidemia and about a quarter of the patients had type 2 diabetes. The average LVEF and LVEDD were 30% and 6.5 cm, respectively. End-organ function was not significantly affected in any of the patients and no relevant biochemical abnormalities were registered. The baseline median (IQR) value of serum NT-proBNP was 1324 (605, 3281) pg/mL. At enrollment, all patients had been receiving maximal tolerated doses of optimal medical therapy. All patients received ACEI/ARB and β-blockers and 69% of patients also received MRAs. On average patient achieved 70% of recommended target dose of ACEI/ARB, 63% of recommended target dose of β-blockers and 95% of recommended target dose of MRA. While ACEI or ARB was switched for ARNI at enrollment, the doses of β-blockers and MRAs were not altered during the study period. The diuretic therapy was adjusted per discretion of the treating cardiologist. The average duration between baseline and follow-up visit in our patient cohort was 377 days.

Table 1. Baseline patient characteristics.

Variable	Baseline (N = 228)	Follow-Up (N = 228)	p
Age, y	57 ± 11		/
Male gender (%)	189 (83)		/
Ischemic heart failure (%)	82 (36)		/
Sodium, mmol/L	140 ± 2	141 ± 3	0.78
Potassium, mmol/L	4.7 ± 0.5	4.8 ± 0.4	0.45
Creatinine, μmol/L	95 ± 34	97 ± 38	0.48
Bilirubin, μmol/L	17 ± 13	16 ± 10	0.28
NT-proBNP, pg/mL (IQR)	1324 (605, 3281)	792 (329, 2022)	0.001
Comorbidities			
Hypertension (%)	123 (54)		/
Diabetes (%)	52 (23)		/
Hyperlipidemia (%)	129 (57)		/
Chronic kidney disease (%)	56 (24)		/
Atrial fibrillation (%)	67 (29)		/
Baseline medical therapy			
ACEI/ARB (%)	228 (100)	0	/
% of target dose	70	0	/
ARNI (%)	0	228 (100)	/
% of target dose	0	69	/
Beta blockers (%)	228 (100)	228 (100)	/
% of target dose	63	63	/
MRA (%)	157 (69)	157 (69)	/
% of target dose	100	100	/
Digoxin (%)	23 (10)	27 (12)	0.58
ICD/CRT (%)	64 (28)	64 (28)	/

Legend: ACEI—angiotensin converting enzyme inhibitor; ARB—angiotensin receptor blocker; ARNI—angiotensin receptor blocker/neprilysin inhibitor; ICD—implantable cardioverter defibrillator; CRT—cardiac resynchronization therapy.

3.2. Effects of ARNI on Ventricular Reverse Remodeling

The effects of ARNI on the left and right ventricular reverse remodeling are outlined in Figure 2. Our results suggest that when in HFrEF patients ACEI or ARB therapy is switched to ARNI, this is associated with an additional improvement of left ventricular structure and function as we observed a significant increase in LVEF (29.7% ± 8% at baseline vs. 36.5% ± 9% at follow-up; $p < 0.001$) and LVOT VTI (14.8 ± 4.2 cm vs. 17.2 ± 4.2 cm; $p < 0.001$). At the same time, a decrease in LVEDD (6.5 ± 0.8 cm vs. 6.3 ± 0.9 cm; $p = 0.001$) was noted. Importantly, our data also showed that in this patient cohort ARNI therapy was associated with a significant improvement in right ventricular function as TAPSE changed from 1.7 ± 0.5 cm at baseline to 2.1 ± 0.6 cm ($p < 0.001$) at 12-month follow-up.

3.3. The Association of Neurohumoral Modulation and Reverse Remodeling

Our data also confirmed the beneficial effects of ARNI on neurohumoral modulation as NT-proBNP serum levels decreased significantly between baseline and 12-month follow-up (1324 (605, 3281) pg/mL vs. 792 (329, 2022) pg/mL; $p = 0.001$). However, we did not find a correlation between changes in NT-proBNP serum levels and LVEF (Pearson's $r^2 = 0.01$) or TAPSE (Pearson's $r^2 = 0.003$).

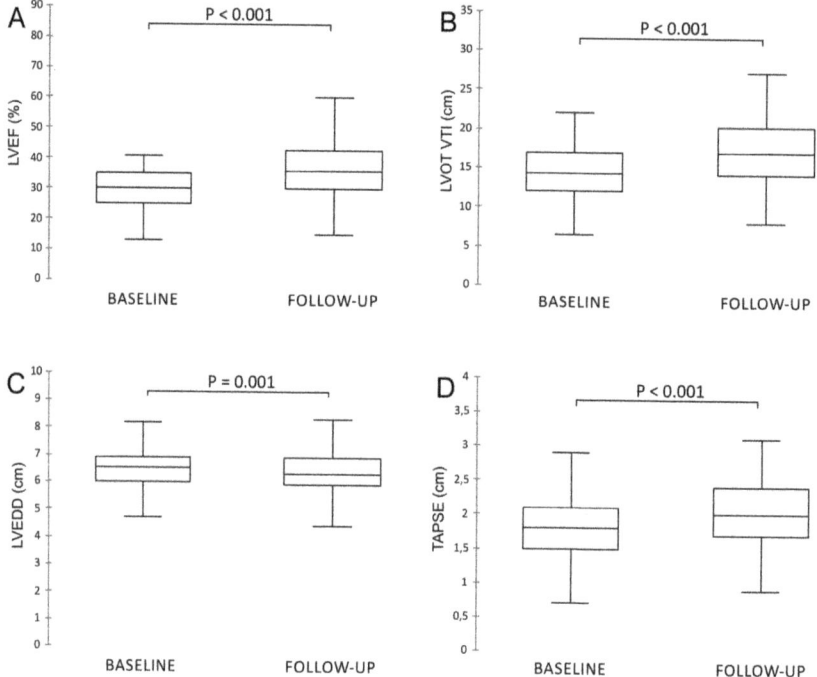

Figure 2. Compared to baseline, angiotensin receptor blocker–neprilysin inhibitor (ARNI) therapy showed significant improvement in (**A**) left ventricular systolic dysfunction (LVEF), (**B**) left ventricular outflow tract velocity–time integral (LVOT VTI) and (**C**) left ventricular end-diastolic diameter (LVEDD) and (**D**) tricuspid annular plane systolic excursion (TAPSE) at 12-month follow-up.

3.4. Response to ARNI and Reverse Remodeling

We further stratified patients according to the magnitude of the response to ARNI therapy (Table 2). We compared patients, in whom LVEF increased less than 5% in the 12-month follow-up period (Group A; $N = 102$, 45%) to patients, in whom an increase in LVEF of 5% or more was observed (Group B; $N = 126$, 55%). In Group A 50% of patients displayed a less than 5% increase of LVEF, in 6% of patients LVEF remained unchanged and in 44% of patients LVEF decreased. In the latter subgroup the mean decrease of LVEF was −4.6%. Comparing the two groups, we found significant differences in age (60 ± 10 years in Group A vs. 55 ± 11 years in Group B; $p = 0.005$), heart failure etiology (ischemic: 48% vs. 28%; $p = 0.002$), baseline LVEF (33% ± 7% vs. 27% ± 8%; $p < 0.001$) and baseline NT-proBNP 1612 (709, 3573) pg/mL vs. 1112 (513, 3027) pg/mL; $p = 0.03$). Our data also showed that more patients in Group A received low dose of ARNI (22% vs. 12%; $p = 0.03$), while there were no differences regarding the intermediate (38% vs. 39%; $p = 0.94$) and high (40% vs. 49%; $p = 0.47$) ARNI doses between the two groups. On multivariable analysis, nonischemic heart failure, baseline LVEF < 30% and baseline NT-proBNP serum levels less than 1500 pg/mL emerged as independent predictors of favorable response to ARNI therapy (Table 3).

Table 2. Baseline characteristics of patients according to the response to ARNI therapy.

Variable	Group A (N = 102)	Group B (N = 126)	p
Age, y	60 ± 10	55 ± 11	0.005
Male gender (%)	84 (82)	106 (84)	0.97
Ischemic heart failure (%)	49 (48)	35 (28)	0.002
Creatinine, μmol/L	100 ± 39	95 ± 37	0.39
Bilirubin, μmol/L	16 ± 8	15 ± 12	0.74
NT-proBNP, pg/mL (IQR)	1612 (709, 3573)	1112 (513, 3027)	0.03
LVEF (%)	33 ± 7	27 ± 8	<0.001
LVEDD, cm	6.5 ± 0.9	6.5 ± 0.7	0.75
TAPSE, cm	1.7 ± 0.5	1.7 ± 0.4	0.78
Comorbidities			
Hypertension (%)	59 (58)	63 (50)	0.20
Diabetes (%)	27 (26)	26 (21)	0.41
Hyperlipidemia (%)	62 (61)	67 (53)	0.19
Chronic kidney disease (%)	24 (23)	32 (25)	0.89
Atrial fibrillation (%)	32 (31)	35 (28)	0.76
Baseline medical therapy			
ACEI/ARB (%)	102 (100)	126 (100)	/
Beta blockers (%)	102 (100)	126 (100)	/
MRA (%)	85 (83)	93 (74)	0.86
Digoxin (%)	12 (12)	11 (9)	0.53
ICD/CRT (%)	34 (33)	29 (23)	0.10
ARNI dose			
Low dose (%)	22 (22)	15 (12)	0.03
Intermediate dose (%)	39 (38)	49 (39)	0.94
High dose (%)	41 (40)	62 (49)	0.47

Table 3. Multivariable analysis of predictors of response to ARNI therapy.

Variable	B	p	95% Confidence Interval	
			Lower Bound	Upper Bound
Age > 60 years	−0.129	0.713	0.443	1.745
Ischemic heart failure	−0.699	0.044	0.252	0.981
LVEF > 30%	−1.711	0.001	0.087	0.374
NT-proBNP > 1500 pg/mL	−0.813	0.035	0.208	0.945
Low-dose ARNI therapy	−0.588	0.232	0.212	1.456

Evaluation of the response to ARNI therapy according to the ARNI dose (Figure 3) showed that the low dose of ARNI was associated with lower increases in LVEF (+3.8% ± 7.2%) and TAPSE (−0.1 ± 0.7 cm) than intermediate (LVEF: +8.2% ± 11.1%; TAPSE +0.5 ± 0.6 cm) or high doses of ARNI (LVEF: +8.7% ± 9.8%; TAPSE +0.4 ± 0.7 cm).

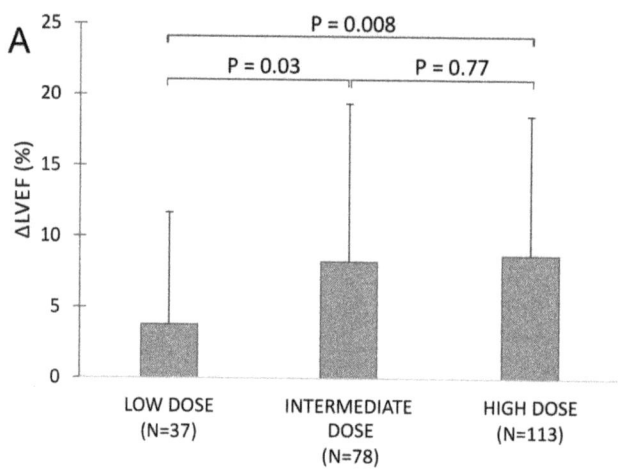

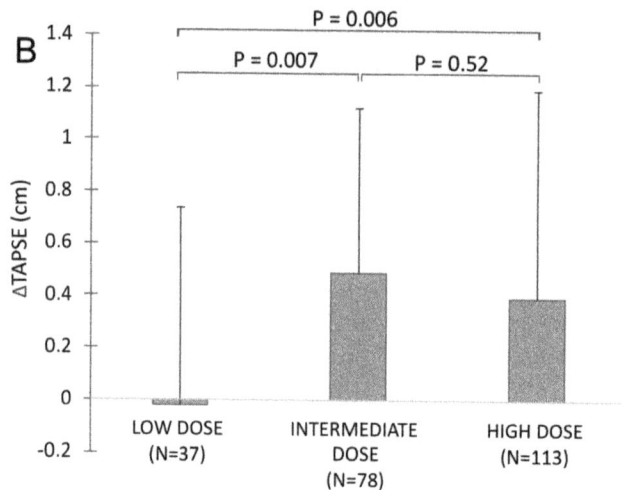

Figure 3. Effect of ARNI dose on (**A**) LVEF and on (**B**) TAPSE.

4. Discussion

The current analysis suggests that in HFrEF patients previously treated with maximal tolerated doses of guideline-based medical therapy a switch to ARNI-based medical regimen may further promote reverse remodeling of the failing myocardium and that this response is likely dose-dependent. Our data additionally suggest that these beneficial effects are particularly pronounced in patients with non-ischemic heart failure, with lower baseline LVEF and with less prominent baseline neurohumoral activation.

In the past 20 years, four major drug classes (ACEI, ARB, β-blockers and MRAs) were introduced for the treatment of HFrEF. Inhibiting the renin–angiotensin–aldosterone axis they have significantly improved the morbidity and mortality of these patients [14–17]. Importantly, the beneficial effects of these medical therapies were repeatedly associated with their potential to promote myocardial reverse remodeling manifested mainly by the reduction of left ventricular size and improvement of its function [18]. While paradigm-HF and pioneer-HF data clearly demonstrated superior clinical efficacy of ARNI therapy compared to ACEI in terms of reduced heart failure-associated hospital admissions, cardiovascular and all-cause mortality, until recently the association between these clinical effects and reverse remodeling of the failing myocardium remained unexplored [1,2]. Basing largely on the small patient cohorts and short-term follow-up recently published data support the association between ARNI and left ventricular reverse remodeling as these studies consistently showed an improvement in left ventricular ejection fraction (ΔLVEF +4–5%) and a decrease in left ventricular size (ΔLVEDD—6% or ΔLVEDV—8–10%) after three months of ARNI therapy [7–9]. A large prove-HF trial corroborated these initial findings and further established long-term beneficial effects of ARNI therapy on left ventricular reverse remodeling as significant improvements in left ventricular ejection fraction (ΔLVEF +9.4%) and size (ΔLVEDV–14%) were established 12 months after the initiation of ARNI therapy [6]. Apart from prove-HF trial our study is the only prospective study to date evaluating long-term effects of ARNI therapy on myocardial reverse remodeling in HFrEF patient population. Our results are in line with the prove-HF data as we have also established comparable long-term improvements in left ventricular size (ΔLVEDD–4% and function (ΔLVEF +6.8%) in HFrEF patients receiving ARNI therapy. Taken together, these data show that in the HFrEF patient population ARNI therapy may lead to early and, importantly, lasting improvement in myocardial reverse remodeling.

While emerging data suggest a significant benefit of ARNI therapy on left ventricular reverse remodeling there are currently almost no data available on the effects of ARNI on right ventricular function in HFrEF patient population. Bayard et al. failed to establish any benefit of ARNI therapy on right ventricular function in 52 patients with HFrEF as no changes in TAPSE were observed throughout the study period (3 months) [9]. Contrary to these conclusions our data suggest that ARNI therapy may be associated with an improvement of right ventricular function as TAPSE improved significantly after 12 months of ARNI therapy in our patient cohort. This differences in results could partly be attributed to the differences in sample size as the study of Bayard et al. was likely underpowered to adequately evaluate the effects of ARNI therapy on TAPSE. Additionally, prove-HF trial, while not specifically evaluating right ventricular function, indirectly supports our results as it demonstrated positive effects of ARNI therapy on left ventricular diastolic function showing a significant decrease in left atrial volume index and left ventricular end-diastolic filling pressure (E/e') at 12-month follow-up [6]. These observations were further supported by Mullens et al. demonstrating that ARNI therapy may result in a prolonged left ventricular diastolic filling time and in a significant reduction in number of patients demonstrating restrictive mitral filling pattern [8]. Collectively, these results may suggest that ARNI therapy could reduce right ventricular afterload indirectly through the improvement of left ventricular diastolic function. This in combination with the effects of ARNI-induced dual neurohumoral blockade on intravascular volume reduction (right ventricular preload reduction) and anti-inflammatory and anti-fibrotic effects that ARNI therapy exerts on the failing myocardium may explain an improved right ventricular systolic function, established in our trial [19]. This could also translate into clinical relevance as right ventricular dysfunction has been established as an important determinant of symptomatic limitations, cardiovascular outcomes and survival in HFrEF and HFpEF patients alike [10].

In accordance with previously published literature [1,2,19] our data also confirmed the beneficial effects of ARNI on neurohumoral modulation as NT-proBNP serum levels decreased significantly between baseline and 12-month follow-up, supporting the dual neurohumoral blockade as a primary pathophysiological mechanism of ARNI therapy. However, we have failed to establish a correlation between changes in NT-proBNP serum levels and changes in left ventricular ejection fraction or TAPSE, respectively. This finding contrasts the conclusion of prove-HF trial, where a weak, but significant correlation was established between reduction in NT-proBNP and improvements in markers of left ventricular structure and function [6]. Several explanations may be offered to justify this discrepancy: (1) whereas the correlation between changes NT-proBNP concentrations and markers of left structure and function were the primary end-point of prove-HF, this was a subject of exploratory analysis in our trial; (2) the population in the prove-HF trial was more than three times the size of the population included in our analysis; and (3) our patient cohort was roughly 10 years younger, had higher prevalence of male patients, much higher baseline NT-proBNP serum levels and significantly higher percentage of patients treated with MRAs. Any of these differences could confound a potential association between changes in serum NT-proBNP and changes in structure and function of left or right ventricle in our patient cohort.

Considering the response to ARNI therapy our data suggest that patients with non-ischemic heart failure, patients with left ventricular ejection fraction less than 30% and with less pronounced neurohumoral activation may display particularly good response to ARNI therapy. In terms of left ventricular ejection fraction and neurohumoral activation these results are supported by paradigm-HF data that showed better clinical response to ARNI therapy in patients with lower left ventricular ejection fraction and with NT-proBNP levels below the median value [1]. While this may seem counterintuitive, these findings may be explained by an elegant study of Gremmler et al. who showed that in stable/compensated HFrEF patients NT-proBNP serum levels appear to be highest with LVEF between 30–40% (around 2000 pg/mL). In patients with LVEF between 15% to 30%, NT-proBNP serum levels decreased to around 1500 pg/mL [20]. While pathophysiological background of this remains inadequately explained it is speculated that HFrEF patients with LVEF between 30 and 40% may develop higher wall tension in the failing myocardium, so the stimulus for natriuretic peptide excretion could be more pronounced in this patient cohort. Similarly, in the field of cardiac resynchronization therapy (CRT) REVERSE study investigators showed that patients with left ventricular ejection fraction < 30% displayed significant improvements in clinical response to CRT as well as in echocardiographic parameters of left ventricular reverse remodeling that may be even more pronounced than in patients with left ventricular ejection fraction > 30% [21]. Our data also suggest better response to ARNI therapy in patients with non-ischemic heart failure as left ventricular ejection fraction improved for +9.4% in patients with non-ischemic heart failure and for +4.5% in patients with ischemic heart failure. This may seem intuitive as impaired coronary perfusion may significantly diminish the capacity of the failing myocardium to recover its structure and/or function. Nevertheless, paradigm-HF sub-analysis demonstrated similar clinical benefits in patients with ischemic and non-ischemic heart failure receiving ARNI therapy [22]. It can be argued that a relative increase in left ventricular ejection fraction of +4.9% in favor of patient with non-ischemic heart failure seen in our data are likely not sufficient to translate to meaningful differences in clinical outcomes between patients with ischemic and non-ischemic heart failure.

Finally, in our patient cohort a dose-dependent effect of ARNI therapy was noted as an increase in left ventricular ejection fraction and TAPSE was significantly lower in patients receiving low dose of ARNI than in patients receiving intermediate or high doses of ARNI. We did not observe any differences in response to ARNI between the groups of patients receiving intermediate or high ARNI doses. These observations are in line with the data from Mullens et al. who also demonstrated dose-dependent effect of ARNI therapy [8]. Importantly, a similar dose-dependent effect has been noted for most the heart failure therapies to date [18,23], again stressing the importance of heart failure therapy titration in HFrEF patient population. Interestingly, in prove-HF trial this dose-dependent effect was blunted, likely due to the fact that 67% of the prove-HF patient population reached the high ARNI dose and most the remaining 33% of patients reached the intermediate dose of ARNI [6].

Our study has several limitations that must be acknowledged. First is its single-group, open-label design. However, this study design may be justified due to a widespread bioavailability of ARNI, its class I clinical practice guideline recommendation and proven superiority over ACEI/ARB in most the HFrEF patients. Second, compared to some recently published heart failure trials, there may be an underrepresentation of the female gender in our study. Third, the size of our study sample—despite being second only to prove-HF considering the studies analyzing echocardiographic response to ARNI therapy—is still relatively small. Therefore, our study was likely not sufficiently powered for some performed analyses, such as a correlation between changes in serum NT-proBNP and left ventricular ejection fraction or TAPSE. Fourth, while many more informative and intricate echocardiographic parameters could be assessed, we chose only the most robust and easily accessible ones for our analysis in order to make our conclusions applicable not only to the tertiary centers with access to the advanced imaging technology, but also to the general cardiology practices. We acknowledge that adding other echocardiographic parameters to the analysis may add novel insights into the reverse-remodeling in the HFrEF patient population and fully support the verification of our preliminary data in such a trial.

5. Conclusions

ARNI therapy appears to promote long-term reverse remodeling of both left and right ventricle in HFrEF patient populations, above and beyond the effect of pre-existing optimal medical management. These effects may be particularly pronounced in patients with nonischemic heart failure, LVEF < 30% and lower degree of neurohumoral activation.

Author Contributions: G.P.: Conceptualization, study design, investigation, writing—original draft preparation; A.A.-D.: Data curation, data analysis, writing—original draft preparation; G.Z.: Investigation; S.F.: Investigation; Writing—review and editing; A.C.: Methodology; R.O.: Investigation; M.Š.: Investigation; B.V.: Investigation, Supervision, Writing—review and editing. All authors have read and agreed to the published version of the manuscript.

Funding: This research received no external funding.

Conflicts of Interest: The authors declare no conflict of interest.

References

1. McMurray, J.J.; Packer, M.; Desai, A.S.; Gong, J.; Lefkowitz, M.P.; Rizkala, A.R.; Rouleau, J.L.; Shi, V.C.; Solomon, S.D.; Swedberg, K.; et al. Angiotensin-Neprilysin Inhibition versus Enalapril in Heart Failure. *N. Engl. J. Med.* **2014**, *371*, 993–1004. [CrossRef] [PubMed]
2. Devore, A.D.; Braunwald, E.; Morrow, D.A.; Duffy, C.I.; Ambrosy, A.P.; Chakraborty, H.; McCague, K.; Rocha, R.; Velazquez, E.J. Initiation of Angiotensin-Neprilysin Inhibition After Acute Decompensated Heart Failure: Secondary Analysis of the Open-label Extension of the PIONEER-HF Trial. *JAMA Cardiol.* **2020**, *5*, 202–207. [CrossRef] [PubMed]
3. Wachter, R.; Senni, M.; Belohlavek, J.; Straburzynska-Migaj, E.; Witte, K.K.; Kobalava, Z.; Fonseca, C.; Goncalvesova, E.; Cavusoglu, Y.; Fernandez, A.; et al. Initiation of sacubitril/valsartan in haemodynamically stabilised heart failure patients in hospital or early after discharge: Primary results of the randomised TRANSITION study. *Eur. J. Heart Fail.* **2019**, *21*, 998–1007. [CrossRef] [PubMed]
4. Kramer, D.G.; Trikalinos, T.A.; Kent, D.M.; Antonopoulos, G.V.; Konstam, M.A.; Udelson, J.E. Quantitative Evaluation of Drug or Device Effects on Ventricular Remodeling as Predictors of Therapeutic Effects on Mortality in Patients With Heart Failure and Reduced Ejection Fraction. *J. Am. Coll. Cardiol.* **2010**, *56*, 392–406. [CrossRef]
5. Mangiafico, S.; Costello-Boerrigter, L.C.; Andersen, I.A.; Cataliotti, A.; Burnett, J.C. Neutral endopeptidase inhibition and the natriuretic peptide system: An evolving strategy in cardiovascular therapeutics. *Eur. Heart J.* **2012**, *34*, 886–893. [CrossRef]
6. Januzzi, J.L.; Prescott, M.F.; Butler, J.; Felker, G.M.; Maisel, A.S.; McCague, K.; Camacho, A.; Piña, I.L.; Rocha, R.A.; Shah, A.M.; et al. Association of Change in N-Terminal Pro-B-Type Natriuretic Peptide Following Initiation of Sacubitril-Valsartan Treatment With Cardiac Structure and Function in Patients With Heart Failure With Reduced Ejection Fraction. *JAMA* **2019**, *322*, 1–11. [CrossRef]
7. Almufleh, A.; Marbach, J.; Chih, S.; Stadnick, E.; Davies, R.; Liu, P.; Mielniczuk, L. Ejection fraction improvement and reverse remodeling achieved with Sacubitril/Valsartan in heart failure with reduced ejection fraction patients. *Am. J. Cardiovasc. Dis.* **2017**, *7*, 108–113.
8. Martens, P.; Beliën, H.; Dupont, M.; Vandervoort, P.; Mullens, W. The reverse remodeling response to sacubitril/valsartan therapy in heart failure with reduced ejection fraction. *Cardiovasc. Ther.* **2018**, *36*, e12435. [CrossRef]
9. Bayard, G.; Da Costa, A.; Pierrard, R.; Roméyer-Bouchard, C.; Guichard, J.B.; Isaaz, K. Impact of sacubitril/valsartan on echo parameters in heart failure patients with reduced ejection fraction a prospective evaluation. *IJC Heart Vasc.* **2019**, *25*, 100418. [CrossRef]

10. Raina, A.; Meeran, T. Right Ventricular Dysfunction and Its Contribution to Morbidity and Mortality in Left Ventricular Heart Failure. *Curr. Heart Fail. Rep.* **2018**, *15*, 94–105. [CrossRef]
11. Elliott, P.; Andersson, B.; Arbustini, E.; Bilinska, Z.; Cecchi, F.; Charron, P.; Dubourg, O.; Kühl, U.; Maisch, B.; McKenna, W.J.; et al. Classification of the cardiomyopathies. *Kardiol. Pol.* **2008**, *66*, 270–276. [CrossRef] [PubMed]
12. Ponikowski, P.; Voors, A.A.; Anker, S.D.; Bueno, H.; Cleland, J.G.F.; Coats, A.J.S.; Falk, V.; González-Juanatey, J.R.; Harjola, V.-P.; Jankowska, E.A.; et al. 2016 ESC Guidelines for the diagnosis and treatment of acute and chronic heart failure. *Eur. J. Heart Fail.* **2016**, *18*, 891–975. [CrossRef] [PubMed]
13. Lang, R.M.; Badano, L.P.; Mor-Avi, V.; Afilalo, J.; Armstrong, A.; Ernande, L.; Flachskampf, F.A.; Foster, E.; Goldstein, S.A.; Kuznetsova, T.; et al. Recommendations for Cardiac Chamber Quantification by Echocardiography in Adults: An Update from the American Society of Echocardiography and the European Association of Cardiovascular Imaging. *Eur. Heart J. Cardiovasc. Imaging.* **2015**, *16*, 233–271. [CrossRef] [PubMed]
14. The Consensus Trial Study Group. Effects of Enalapril on Mortality in Severe Congestive Heart Failure. *N. Engl. J. Med.* **1987**, *316*, 1429–1435. [CrossRef]
15. SOLVD Investigators. Effect of Enalapril on Survival in Patients with Reduced Left Ventricular Ejection Fractions and Congestive Heart Failure. *N. Engl. J. Med.* **1991**, *325*, 293–302. [CrossRef]
16. CIBIS-II Investigators. The Cardiac Insufficiency Bisoprolol Study II (CIBIS-II): A randomised trial. *Lancet* **1999**, *353*, 9–13. [CrossRef] [PubMed]
17. Pitt, B.; Zannad, F.; Remme, W.J.; Cody, R.; Castaigne, A.; Perez, A.; Palensky, J.; Wittes, J. The Effect of Spironolactone on Morbidity and Mortality in Patients with Severe Heart Failure. *N. Engl. J. Med.* **1999**, *341*, 709–717. [CrossRef]
18. Nijst, P.; Martens, P.; Mullens, W. Heart Failure with Myocardial Recovery—The Patient Whose Heart Failure Has Improved: What Next? *Prog. Cardiovasc. Dis.* **2017**, *60*, 226–236. [CrossRef]
19. D'Elia, E.; Iacovoni, A.; Vaduganathan, M.; Lorini, F.L.; Perlini, S.; Senni, M. Neprilysin inhibition in heart failure: Mechanisms and substrates beyond modulating natriuretic peptides. *Eur. J. Heart Fail.* **2017**, *19*, 710–717. [CrossRef]
20. Gremmler, B.; Kunert, M.; Schleiting, H.; Kisters, K.; Ulbricht, L.J. Relation between N-terminal pro-brain natriuretic peptide values and invasively measured left ventricular hemodynamic indices. *Exp. Clin. Cardiol.* **2003**, *8*, 91–94. [PubMed]
21. Linde, C.; Daubert, C.; Abraham, W.T.; Sutton, M.S.J.; Ghio, S.; Hassager, C.; Herre, J.M.; Bergemann, T.; Gold, M.R. Impact of Ejection Fraction on the Clinical Response to Cardiac Resynchronization Therapy in Mild Heart Failure. *Circ. Heart Fail.* **2013**, *6*, 1180–1189. [CrossRef] [PubMed]
22. Balmforth, C.; Simpson, J.; Shen, L.; Jhund, P.S.; Lefkowitz, M.; Rizkala, A.R.; Rouleau, J.L.; Shi, V.; Solomon, S.D.; Swedberg, K.; et al. Outcomes and Effect of Treatment According to Etiology in HFrEF. *JACC Heart Fail.* **2019**, *7*, 457–465. [CrossRef] [PubMed]
23. Cicoira, M.; Zanolla, L.; Rossi, A.; Golia, G.; Franceschini, L.; Brighetti, G.; Marino, P.; Zardini, P. Long-term, dose-dependent effects of spironolactone on left ventricular function and exercise tolerance in patients with chronic heart failure. *J. Am. Coll. Cardiol.* **2002**, *40*, 304–310. [CrossRef]

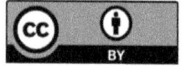

© 2020 by the authors. Licensee MDPI, Basel, Switzerland. This article is an open access article distributed under the terms and conditions of the Creative Commons Attribution (CC BY) license (http://creativecommons.org/licenses/by/4.0/).

MDPI
St. Alban-Anlage 66
4052 Basel
Switzerland
Tel. +41 61 683 77 34
Fax +41 61 302 89 18
www.mdpi.com

Diagnostics Editorial Office
E-mail: diagnostics@mdpi.com
www.mdpi.com/journal/diagnostics

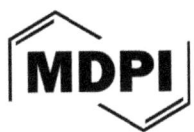

www.ingramcontent.com/pod-product-compliance
Lightning Source LLC
LaVergne TN
LVHW070725100526
838202LV00013B/1170